American Society of PeriAnesthesia Nurses

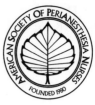

CERTIFICATION REVIEW FOR
PERIANESTHESIA NURSING

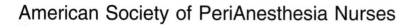

Second Edition

Barbara Putrycus, RN, MSN, CCRN

Surgical Services
QA/Regulatory Compliance/Infection Control
Oakwood Hospital & Medical Center
Dearborn, Michigan

Jacqueline Ross, RN, MSN, CPAN

Perianesthesia Nursing Consultant
Patient Safety Analyst
OHIC Insurance/The Doctors Company
Columbus, Ohio

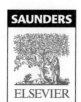

SAUNDERS

ELSEVIER

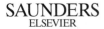

SAUNDERS
ELSEVIER

11830 Westline Industrial Drive
St. Louis, Missouri 63146

CERTIFICATION REVIEW FOR PERIANESTHESIA NURSING, 2/e   ISBN: 978-1-4160-3124-6

Notice

Knowledge and best practice in this field are constantly changing. As new research and experience broaden our knowledge, changes in practice, treatment and drug therapy may become necessary or appropriate. Readers are advised to check the most current information provided (i) on procedures featured or (ii) by the manufacturer of each product to be administered, to verify the recommended dose or formula, the method and duration of administration, and contraindications. It is the responsibility of the practitioner, relying on their own experience and knowledge of the patient, to make diagnoses, to determine dosages and the best treatment for each individual patient, and to take all appropriate safety precautions. To the fullest extent of the law, neither the Publisher nor the Editors assumes any liability for any injury and/or damage to persons or property arising out of or related to any use of the material contained in this book.

The Publisher

Library of Congress Control Number: 2007940826

Executive Publisher: Darlene Como
Acquisitions Editor: Tamara Myers
Associate Developmental Editor: Tina Kaemmerer
Publishing Services Manager: Jeff Patterson
Project Manager: Jeanne Genz
Designer: Elaine Rickles

Working together to grow
libraries in developing countries

www.elsevier.com | www.bookaid.org | www.sabre.org

ELSEVIER   BOOK AID International   Sabre Foundation

Printed in the United States of America

Last digit is the print number: 9 8 7 6 5 4 3 2 1

To my parents Arnold and Shirley
for the many years of love and encouragement
you provided me during my nursing career.

To my sisters, Diane and Susan
for your ongoing support and continued
encouragement for me to pursue my goals.

I am especially grateful to the many professional mentors and friends
I have had in my career.
Your support and guidance have provided me the ability to work
through challenges and fulfill dreams.

Barbara

To my husband, Brad,
who provided me support
and encouragement during this process.

To my daughter, Savannah,
whose humor assisted me during the tedious periods.

I also extend my sincere gratitude to my mentors,
both professional and personal—without your guidance and vision my professional
career would not be as fulfilling and challenging as it is today.

Jackie

Contributors

Joni M. Brady, RN, MSN, CAPA
Breathline Editor
American Society of PeriAnesthesia Nurses
Stuttgart, Germany

Matthew D. Byrne, RN, MS, CPAN
Adjunct Instructor
College of St. Benedict
Saint John's University
Saint Joseph, Minnesota

Theresa Clifford, RN, MSN, CPAN
Perianesthesia Staff Nurse and Educator
Mercy Hospital
Portland, Maine

Vallire D. Hooper, RN, MSN, CPAN, FAAN
Co-editor, Journal of PeriAnesthesia Nursing
Assistant Professor
School of Nursing
Medical College of Georgia
Augusta, Georgia

Dolly Ireland, RN, MSN, CAPA, CPN
Clinical Nursing Educator
Perianesthesia Surgical Services and Ambulatory Services
Mount Clemens Regional Medical Center;
Nursing Faculty
University of Phoenix—Macomb Michigan Campus
Mount Clemens, Michigan

Stephanie Kassulke, RN, CPAN
Staff Nurse
Aurora Sinai Medical Center
Milwaukee, Wisconsin

Bonnie S. Niebuhr, RN, MS, CAE
Chief Executive Officer
ABPANC
New York, New York

Denise O'Brien, MSN, APRN, BC, CPAN, CAPA, FAAN
Clinical Nurse Specialist, UH PACU
Department of Operating Rooms/PACU
University of Michigan Health System
Ann Arbor, Michigan

Jan Odom-Forren, RN, BSN, MS, CPAN, FAAN
Perianesthesia Nursing Consultant
Co-editor, Journal of PeriAnesthesia Nursing
Louisville, Kentucky

Lois Schick, MN, MBA, CPAN, CAPA
Per Diem Staff Nurse and Entrepreneur
Lutheran Medical Center
Wheatridge, Colorado;
Littleton Adventist Hospital
Littleton, Colorado;
Ambulatory Surgery Center at Lutheran Medical Center
Wheatridge, Colorado

Mary Seitenbach, RN, BSN, CPAN
Exempla Lutheran Medical Center
Wheat Ridge, Colorado

Barbara A. Struthers, RN, BSN, CPAN, CAPA
Manager Ambulatory Services
Mercy Hospital—Cadillac
Cadillac, Michigan

Nancy M. Strzyzewski, RN, BSN, CPAN, CAPA
Nurse Clinician
William Beaumont Hospital
Royal Oak, Michigan

Candace Taylor, RN, BSN, CPAN
PACU Supervisor, Patient Safety Officer
Cedar Oaks Surgery Center
Warrensburg, Missouri

Sara N. Waldron, RN, BSN, CPAN
PACU Staff Nurse and Clinical Educator
Carondelet St. Joseph's Hospital
Tucson, Arizona

Reviewers

Sandra Barnes, RN, MS, CPAN
Nurse Manager
Greenwich Hospital
Ambulatory Surgery and Post Anesthesia Care
  Unit
Greenwich, Connecticut

Marcia Bixby, RN, MS, CS, CCRN
Critical Care Clinical Nurse Specialist
Consultant for Critical Care Education
Beth Israel Deaconess Medical Center
Boston, Massachusetts

Linda Boyum, RN, BSN, CPAN, LHRM
Administrator
Lake Mary's Surgery Center
Lake Mary, Florida

Susan L. Carter, RN, BSN, CPAN, CAPA
Staff Nurse
University of California—San Diego
La Jolla, California

Marjorie A. Geisz-Everson, MS, CRNA
Certified Registered Nurse Anesthetist
Louisiana State University Health Sciences Center
Medical Center of Louisiana at New Orleans
New Orleans, Louisiana

Judy Graham-Garcia, MN, CRNA, FNA, ACNP
Staff Nurse Anesthetist
Anaesthesia Associates of Massachusetts
Boston, Massachusetts;
Clinical Site Manager
Northshore Medical Center
Salem and Lynn, Massachusetts;
Part-Time Faculty
Boston College
Chestnut Hill, Massachusetts

Debby Niehaus, RN, BS, CPAN
Clinical Nurse III
Bethesda North Ambulatory Surgery Center
PeriOperative Services
Cincinnati, Ohio

Twilla M. Shrout, RN, BSN, MBA, CAPA
Staff Nurse V
Boone Hospital Center
Columbia, Missouri

Annette S. Williams, RN, BSN, CPAN
Post Anesthesia Care Unit
Memorial Hospital at Gulfport
Gulfport, Mississippi

Preface

Taking the step towards certification marks an important milestone in your professional career. The purpose of the *Certification Review for Perianesthesia Nursing* in this, its second edition, remains as it was in its inception—to articulate the knowledge base that underlies perianesthesia nursing practice. Each edition of this book attempts to redefine that knowledge base for nurses who practice in this ever-expanding specialty area.

The specialty of perianesthesia nursing extends into many different settings. The book is designed to assist those nurses sitting for either the CPAN or the CAPA exams. Both of these credentials signify that the registered nurse possesses skill and knowledge related to either inpatient (the CPAN designation) or ambulatory (the CAPA designation) settings. Many perianesthesia nurses' practice extends into both areas, and these nurses can possess both credentials. Regardless of the credential you are aspiring to attain, this text is designed to assist in the preparation for the exam.

All of the authors that contributed to this text are experts in perianesthesia nursing. The rationales from their questions should fuel your critical-thinking skills. Take the time to reflect on the rationales. Like the prior edition, this book is designed to refresh and strengthen you, rather than start from the beginning, in areas that you already have some knowledge. In-depth information can be found in the books and articles listed in the references. You are encouraged to read these articles and immerse yourself in the literature. Expand your knowledge.

Remember, to pass the CPAN or CAPA examination, you need to begin preparing in advance. This is best accomplished if you study and use the information in clinical practice. This reinforces the material far better than if you just read the content in this book. We have included tips to help you take the test at the beginning of this review book.

Good luck in preparing for the exam and in using this book to guide your clinical practice. Your clinical expertise enables you to sit for this exam. Understand that you have the experience, knowledge, and confidence to pass this exam. It is a mark of a professional to want to expand your knowledge. You will find passing the CPAN or CAPA exam to be one of the most satisfying moments of your professional career. You can be proud of this accomplishment!

Acknowledgments

This text has been an adventure in extending the knowledge base for perianesthesia nurses around the world. Each chapter presented an array of challenges to assure that the content was timely and concise. The questions and their rationale will provide perianesthesia nurses a wealth of understanding that will extend far beyond the certification exam. Patients can be assured that they will be receiving the most evidence-based care from perianesthesia nurses.

We recognize, however, that we are not alone in this project. We would like to acknowledge the following individuals:

- First, we would like to thank ASPAN for giving us the opportunity to co-edit this endeavor.
- Kathy Carlson, who as the first editor for the *Certification Review for Perianesthesia Nursing*, had the vision to improve the education for perianesthesia nurses through the first edition of this text. Thank you for your time and effort!
- Each contributor for this text provided countless hours of research and writing questions and well-thought out rationales.
- Bonnie Niebuhr and ABPANC for their reviews of content. The questions were reviewed to ensure that the format was similar to the certification exams.
- Perianesthesia nurses can be assured that this text represents the formatting of the certification exam.
- For each respected perianesthesia reviewer of this text—each of them took time from their busy schedules to read over the content, seek clarification, and promote a well-developed text.
- To our perianesthesia colleagues who offered suggestions and support for revisions and updates to this edition.
- Tamara Myers, Tina Kaemmerer, and Jeanne Genz for their support and understanding over this publication process. We have both learned a lot about the publication process, and we could not have been successful without their dedication to this project.
- To the numerous other members of the Elsevier team who helped us throughout the many stages of this edition, we extend our sincere gratitude.
- And certainly not last, every perianesthesia nurse who strives to learn and apply more within their daily practice—their quests are what inspired us to continue with the text.

Contents

Chapter 1

Certification of Perianesthesia Nurses

The CPAN® and CAPA® Certification Programs

For the most up-to-date information about the Certified Post Anesthesia Nurse (CPAN) and Certified Ambulatory Perianesthesia Nurse (CAPA) certification programs, contact the American Board of Perianesthesia Nursing Certification, Inc. (ABPANC) directly at 800-6ABPANC or e-mail abpanc@proexam.org or visit the website at www.cpancapa.org.

AMERICAN BOARD OF PERIANESTHESIA NURSING CERTIFICATION

ABPANC is a not-for-profit corporation established in 1985 for the purpose of sponsoring specialty nursing certification programs for registered nurses caring for perianesthesia patients. Its mission "to assure a certification process for perianesthesia nurses that validates the achievement of knowledge gained through professional education and experience, ultimately promoting quality patient care"[1] is driven by its commitment to:

- Professional practice
- Advocating the value of certification to health care decision-makers and the public
- The administration of valid, reliable, and fair certification programs
- Ongoing collaboration with the American Society of PeriAnesthesia Nurses (ASPAN), other specialty organizations, and key stakeholder groups
- Evolving psychometric and technologic advances in testing

ABPANC's mission and related activities are aimed at achieving its compelling vision,

"Recognizing and respecting the unequaled excellence in the mark of the CPAN and CAPA credentials, perianesthesia nurses will seek it, managers will require it, employers will support it and the public will demand it"![1]

Definition of Certification

ABPANC has adopted the following definition of certification as defined by the American Board of Nursing Specialties (ABNS): "Certification is the formal recognition of the specialized knowledge, skills, and experience demonstrated by the achievement of standards identified by a nursing specialty to promote optimal health outcomes."[2] State licensure, on the other hand, provides the legal authority for an individual to practice professional nursing.[3] Private, voluntary certification, as sponsored by ABPANC, reflects achievement of a standard beyond licensure for specialty nursing practice.

CPAN and CAPA Credentials

The CPAN and CAPA credentials, granted to qualified registered nurses by ABPANC, are federally registered service marks and are protected by law. Registered nurses who have not achieved CPAN and/or CAPA certification status or whose certification status has lapsed are not authorized to use these credentials.

HISTORICAL PERSPECTIVE

ABPANC offered the CPAN certification examination for the first time in 1986. Given the changing health care environment and the emerging trend of outpatient surgery, ABPANC began to investigate the need for a separate certification examination related to ambulatory nursing in 1991. The first CAPA certification examination related to this emerging specialty area was given in 1994. Two subsequent role delineation studies or studies of perianesthesia nursing practice, conducted by ABPANC, have validated the need for two separate certification examinations.

ABOUT THE CPAN AND CAPA CERTIFICATION PROGRAMS

ABNS Accreditation

Both the CPAN and CAPA certification programs are accredited by the American Board of Nursing Specialties (ABNS). Accreditation status must be renewed every 5 years.

ABNS is the standard-setting body for specialty nursing certification programs and offers a stringent and comprehensive accreditation process. ABPANC provided extensive documentation demonstrating that it has met the 18 ABNS standards of quality. ABNS accreditation signifies that a nationally recognized accrediting body has determined that the CPAN and CAPA credentials are based on a valid and reliable examination process and that the structures in place to administer the examinations meet and even exceed the standards of the certification industry from a legal, regulatory, and association management perspective.

For further information about ABNS and the accreditation process and standards, visit their website at www.nursingcertification.org.

Basis for CPAN and CAPA Examinations—A Role Delineation Study

The CPAN and CAPA examinations are each based on the results of a Role Delineation Study (RDS), also called a *Study of Practice*. This type of study is conducted every 5 years to ensure that examination content remains relevant and current to the practice specialty. A variety of methods may be employed to gather data, the findings of which are reflected in the newly designed or revised examination blueprints.

Based on the findings of the 1999-2000 RDS, the CPAN and CAPA examination blueprints were reconceptualized to focus on four domains of perianesthesia patient needs: physiologic, behavioral and cognitive, safety, and advocacy

needs.[4] These needs, as well as the knowledge base required of perianesthesia nurses to meet these needs, were defined.[3]

An RDS was repeated in 2005-2006 and resulted in minor updates to the listing of patient needs and nursing knowledge, as well as a revision to the percentage of examination questions asked in each of the four domains of patient needs.

Examination Blueprints

The CPAN and CAPA examination blueprints are based on data from the RDS. Although it was determined that patient needs and the knowledge base of the nurse to meet those needs are the same, the percentage of questions asked in each domain or category of patient need varies, depending on whether the candidate is taking the CPAN or CAPA examination. A complete listing of the most current patient needs and related nursing knowledge that make up the examination blueprints can be found on the ABPANC website (www.cpan-capa.org).

Examination Questions

Examination questions are written by practicing CPAN and CAPA certified nurses. Item Writer/Reviewer Committees (IWRC) and Examination Review Committees (ERC) for both the CPAN and CAPA programs are made up of individuals who currently practice in a variety of settings in various roles throughout the country. This ensures that the examination reflects the diversity of practice around the country. Each question is reviewed a minimum of three times before use on an examination. Each question is judged against the criteria of relevance, currency, and criticality to the care of perianesthesia patients. Each question must also have a current, related reference no older than 5 years. In addition, editors at ABPANC's testing company review each question for proper format as a multiple-choice question and ensure that item bias is not present. This very complex process ensures that the CPAN and CAPA examinations are current and relevant to perianesthesia nursing and are reflective of the content identified in the most recent RDS. Questions in this text are comparable to questions on the examinations.

In addition, examination questions are written at various cognitive levels based on a condensed version of Bloom's Taxonomy. The three cognitive levels used by ABPANC are:

- **Level 1**—Knowledge and Comprehensive: questions examine one's ability to recall a fact or understand a principle.
- **Level II**—Application and Analysis: questions examine one's ability to relate two or more facts to a situation or analyze a group of facts.
- **Level III**—Synthesis and Evaluation: questions examine one's ability to evaluate a situation using facts or make recommendations based on analysis and evaluation of facts.

The majority of CPAN and CAPA questions are focused at levels II and III.

Each CPAN and CAPA examination is a 3-hour examination consisting of 165 questions. In addition to the 150 questions that are scored, 15 questions are being pre-tested (piloted) and these will not count toward the candidate's final score. These 15 piloted questions are randomly distributed through the examination and will not be specifically identified. Each scored question is carefully written, referenced, and validated to ensure accuracy and correctness.

ELIGIBILITY REQUIREMENTS

To sit for either the CPAN or CAPA certification examination, the applicant must:

- Possess a current, unrestricted registered nurse license in the United States or any of its territories that use the NCLEX as the basis for determining RN licensure
- Meet a clinical experience requirement
- Submit a complete application and fee

A complete description of eligibility requirements is found in the *Candidate Handbook and Application.*

The policy of ABPANC is that no individual shall be excluded from the opportunity to participate in the CPAN and/or CAPA certification programs on the basis of ethnic origin, national origin, religion, sex, age, disability, marital status, or sexual orientation.

DETERMINING WHICH EXAMINATION TO TAKE

Determining which examination is most relevant to an examination candidate's practice is based on patient needs and the amount of time patients spend in the specific phases described by the Perianesthesia Continuum of Care (as defined in ASPAN's Scope of Practice, Perianesthesia Nursing).[4] Regardless of the setting in which the examination candidate practices, if most of the examination candidate's time is spent caring for patients in Phase I, the CPAN examination is most relevant. If most of his or her time is spent caring for patients in the Preanesthesia phases, Phase II, and/or Extended Observations, the CAPA examination is most relevant.

CERTIFICATION PERIOD

To ensure that certified perianesthesia nurses possess the most up-to-date knowledge and current experience, CPAN and CAPA certification status is granted for a period of 3 years and must be renewed. To renew credentials, CPAN and CAPA certified nurses must meet certain RN licensure and clinical experience eligibility requirements and either successfully complete the examination OR earn contact hours related to continual learning. Acceptable activities for obtaining contact hours are:

- Attendance at formal continuing education offerings
- Attendance at hospital and unit in-services
- Participation in home study or self-study programs that grant contact hours via computer or in professional journals

A complete description of acceptable activities is found in the recertification handbook.

STUDYING FOR THE CPAN AND CAPA CERTIFICATION EXAMINATIONS

Perianesthesia nurses considering seeking CPAN and/or CAPA certification should be congratulated! They are taking the next step in their professional careers. The following study tips have been identified by those candidates who have successfully gone before them.[5]

Rally Support

Form a study group, or identify a study buddy (coach or mentor). Study groups of three to six people have been shown to be the most effective. A clear benefit of forming a study group is the psychologic support that members receive from each other throughout the study process. If no one from their unit is interested, perianesthesia nurses at other local institutions can be contacted. Members of an ASPAN component near them may have plans to form a study group, or they may know of people who would be interested. If forming a study group is not possible, a study group of "one" will work.

Once the study group is formed, begin by setting some ground rules regarding meeting times, study timelines, and responsibilities of group members. Carefully read the *Candidate Handbook and Application*—noting all application postmark deadlines. For any questions about information in the *Handbook*, contact the ABPANC national office.

Identifying a study buddy may be the approach that best fits one's needs. In addition, seeking an already certified CPAN or CAPA certified nurse to serve as a coach or mentor is also useful.

Develop a Study Plan

This is the first step to beginning a study plan, whether studying alone or with others. Begin by carefully reading the ABPANC *Candidate Handbook and Application*. Using the examination blueprint published in it, develop an outline of study topics, focusing on areas of weakness first. Identify a schedule for studying those topics, and assign one individual to coordinate that study topic.

Determining a study schedule depends on whether studying each topic in depth or taking a review approach is preferred. A study schedule may take 6 to 12 weeks or longer, depending on individual needs.

Identify Study Resources

Once study topics are determined, identify references for each subject. Refer to the list of references noted in the *Candidate Handbook and Application*. Journal articles published in the past 2 to 3 years are very helpful. The study group can prepare a list of relevant articles and then divide the list among the members to write or present a short synopsis of the articles to the group. Do not forget to use a variety of resources, including:

- CPAN/CAPA colleagues
- Staff development educators
- Clinical nurse specialists
- Journals in related fields
- Local conferences or review courses
- ASPAN videos or other electronic media
- Internet continuing education courses

Do not limit study references to only one or two. Individuals or study groups cannot possibly study all the references listed and should pick those references found to be most relevant to their study needs and weaknesses.

General Study Tips

Whether studying alone or in a group, consider the following tips:

- Start with a positive attitude—be proud of what you know.
- Study some every day. A little each day is much better than a lot all at once.
- Avoid cramming.
- Spend more time on subjects that are your greatest weakness.
- Pick a time to study when you are most alert. Research indicates that morning and early evening are the most productive times to study.
- Stick to your study schedule!
- Your study place should be conveniently located, quiet, well lit, cool, undisturbed, and comfortable.
- Take breaks, but rest for only about 3 to 5 minutes.
- Each day, briefly review what you have learned. At the end of a week, conduct a weekly review.
- When taking notes, mapping may be helpful. Use brief outlines.
- Write out 10 questions from your notes and then answer them.
- Read aloud.
- Avoid studying two related subjects in the same study period. Take a rest in between.
- Tape record important key items from references and listen to tapes to and from work or other travels.
- Make flash cards and use with a study buddy.
- Make index cards with important facts highlighted—carry in your pocket at work to review.
- Post a drug of the week or topic of the week by the work phone.
- Do dress rehearsals—make up a self-examination.

- Purchase the Practice Examinations from ABPANC.
- Allow time for family and fun!

Dealing with Test-taking Anxiety

Many adults suffer from test-taking anxiety and may wish to consider taking a course at a local college designed to teach test-taking strategies. The Internet is a great place to find strategies— enter *examination taking* or *studying* as key words.

As the examination date nears, study preparations should come to a close. Spend the last week before the examination reviewing materials rather than trying to learn new information.

If taking an examination review course, decide if the purpose of doing so is to learn new material or to review material. Learning new material should take place earlier in the study program, whereas reviewing material can occur later in the process.

In the days before the examination, concentrate on healthy living! Eat sensibly, and get plenty of rest. To reduce anxiety on the day of the examination, locate the examination site before the need to travel to it.

Do not study the night before the examination. Get a good night's rest.

Dress in layers for the examination. Wear bright, upbeat colored clothing to the examination!

Upon arrival at the examination, do not panic. Sit quietly and practice relaxation techniques. Have confidence—you have studied and prepared well.

Read all examination directions before beginning. Pace yourself. Divide the time given to take the examination according to the number of questions and the time allotted. Read each question carefully. Usually one's first response is the correct one. Avoid changing answers.

As of this writing, the CPAN and CAPA examinations are given via paper/pencil but will be administered via computer in the future. Regarding taking an examination using paper/pencil, if leaving an answer blank, upon going back, be certain to fill in the correct response on the answer sheet. However, avoid skipping around on the answer sheet. After finishing the examination, review the answer sheet to be certain that every circle is filled in.

Upon leaving the examination, do not discuss the questions with colleagues—this only heightens one's anxiety.

Celebrate!

Plan a celebration after taking the examination! Congratulations are in order for taking the next step in one's professional career. The study process, in and of itself, is a wonderful opportunity. You are a better perianesthesia nurse for having taken the journey!

REFERENCES

1. ABPANC: *About Us*. Website: www.cpanca-pa.org/about/index.htm. Accessed June 18, 2007.
2. ABNS: *Definition of Certification*. Website: www.nursingcertification.org. Accessed June 18, 2007.
3. Niebuhr B, Muenzen P: A study of perianesthesia nursing practice: the foundation for newly revised CPAN and CAPA certification examinations. *J PeriAnesth Nurs* 16(3): 163–173, 2001
4. ASPAN: *2006-2008 Standards of perianesthesia nursing practice*, Cherry Hill, NJ, 2006, ASPAN.
5. ABPANC: *Study tips for nurses seeking perianesthesia certification*, New York, 2001, ABPANC.

Professional Issues Applied to Perianesthesia Nursing Practice

LEGAL CONCEPTS

Question Sets 1, 2

Scenarios and items in this section reflect the legal dimensions of professional nursing practice in the perianesthesia environment. These issues represent only a small portion of the diverse situations encountered by the nurse in clinical practice and are important because:

- Each nurse is responsible for practicing in accordance with recognized standards of professional nursing practice and professional performance.
- Professional practice reflects the application of knowledge of current practice standards, guidelines, statutes, rules, and regulations.
- Professional growth and delivery of high-quality patient care preserve and protect patient autonomy, dignity, rights, and confidentiality within legal and regulatory parameters.

ESSENTIAL CORE CONCEPTS	AFFILIATED CORE CURRICULUM CHAPTERS
Legal Concepts	**Chapter 6**
Liability Issues	
The Legal Process	
Issues of Consent	
Ethical Standards	**Chapter 2**
Ethical Principles	
Ethical Decision Making	
Competency-based Practice	

ETHICAL DILEMMAS IN CLINICAL PRACTICE

Question Set 3

Scenarios and items in this section reflect the ethical dilemmas encountered in professional nursing practice in the perianesthesia environment. This is only a small sampling of the many ethical situations and dilemmas that the perianesthesia nurse may encounter in daily practice. The perianesthesia nurse practices by providing nursing care to preanesthesia and postanesthesia patients. The perianesthesia nurse accepts the responsibility bestowed upon him or her by the state, the profession, and society. Standards for ethical practice demonstrate accountability to the public and to the profession and are important because:

- They assist the perianesthesia nurse to relate the American Nurses Association (ANA) Code of Ethics to his or her own practice.
- They identify the use of appropriate mechanisms to resolve ethical dilemmas.
- They provide a specific context for applying the Code of Ethics to perianesthesia practice and serve as a resource to develop ethically sound practices.

SET 1

ITEMS 2.1–2.31

2.1. The type of law associated with medical malpractice is:
a. criminal law.
b. common law.
c. procedural law.
d. civil law.

2.2. To proceed with a claim of medical malpractice, it is necessary to have which of the following four key elements?
a. Policy, breach of duty, complaint, and filing
b. Breach of duty, damages, causation, and duty
c. Competency, failure of competency, damages, and incident report
d. Damages, incident report, duty, and loss of work

2.3. An 86-year-old man was admitted to an outpatient facility for a minor urology procedure. After signing his hospital consent form, he proceeded to the preoperative holding area. After his procedure and initial recovery, the patient was moved to the post anesthesia care unit (PACU) Phase II. While moving from the stretcher to the chair, he fell and suffered a fractured right hip. The patient's family is considering a malpractice claim. The patient established a relationship (duty) with the outpatient facility by:
a. agreeing to the procedure with his doctor.
b. choosing a specific outpatient facility.
c. arriving and signing his hospital consent form.
d. arriving on time for his scheduled procedure.

2.4. Standards of care are:
a. the highest degree of professional behavior.
b. the minimum requirement of acceptable level of care.
c. established professional requirements by the state.

d. policies required by the hospital.

2.5. Professional standards of care are established to provide:
a. an example of provided care for legal purposes.
b. a basis or framework for quality nursing care.
c. a comparison between intended care and established policy.
d. an orientation guide for new nurses.

NOTE: Consider the scenario and items 2.6-2.7 together.

The American Society of PeriAnesthesia Nurses (ASPAN) *2006-2008 Standards of Perianesthesia Nursing Practice* states that two licensed nurses, one of whom is a RN competent in Phase II postanesthesia nursing, are *present* whenever a patient is receiving Phase II level of care. A registered nurse (RN) must be present at all times during Phase II.

2.6. ASPAN defines "present" as meaning:
a. available within 5 minutes of the PACU.
b. present in the physical surgical suite area.
c. present in the place where the patient is receiving care.
d. present in the operating room (OR) as part of the surgical team.

2.7. Examples of patients who may be cared for in this phase include all of the following *except:*
a. patient awaiting discharge instructions and transportation home with family.
b. patient requiring extended observation/interventions but is stable hemodynamically.
c. patient who is extremely sleepy, has a 92% SaO_2, and must be encouraged to take deep breaths.
d. patient without a companion present who no longer needs airway management.

2.8. In addition to caring for an adult male patient, the Phase II PACU nurse was also caring for a very sleepy 10-year-old whose mother was at his side and an adult who had just been transferred from Phase I. The nurse was just asked to admit and care for an endoscopy patient. After reviewing ASPAN's recommended patient classification staffing guidelines, it is determined that the nurse's assignment was:
a. appropriate if the unlicensed assistive personnel assigned to Phase II admits the new patient.
b. inappropriate because there is a one-nurse-to-three-patient ratio in Phase II at all times.
c. inappropriate because the 10-year-old patient requires a one-to-one patient ratio at all times.
d. appropriate for the condition of the patients described and necessary level of care.

2.9. Two clinical RNs working in the Phase I PACU already have the following assignments: Nurse One has an adult, conscious, stable, and free of complications; nurse Two has a 9-year-old conscious patient who is stable, and free of complications. The operating room (OR) wants to send a 7-year-old tonsillectomy patient who still has an oral airway in place. Which nurse should receive this assignment?
a. Neither one; the child should remain in the OR until the oral airway is removed and then proceed to Phase II.
b. Nurse One; the patient he or she has is an adult and can be watched easily while caring for an additional patient, making the assignment a one-nurse-to-two-patient ratio.
c. Nurse Two; the 10-year-old patient is already awake and a parent should be called in to sit at the bedside so that the nurse can care for the unconscious child.
d. The two patients already admitted should be combined into one assignment, freeing one nurse to take the new patient, which is a one-to-one patient ratio.

2.10. Privacy, informed consent, confidentiality of communications, and continuity of care are expectations mandated by:
a. The Joint Commission.
b. the Patient Self-Determination Act.
c. the Patient's Bill of Rights.
d. Health Insurance Portability and Accountability Act (HIPAA).

2.11. To maintain confidentiality in a busy Phase I PACU with two patients next to each other, the nurse should:
a. move one patient to the end of the room when discussing specific information.
b. ask the patient not being spoken to to please not listen to the adjacent conversation.
c. pull the curtain around the patient being spoken to and lower your voice.
d. write everything down and do not speak aloud.

2.12. A hospital is located in an area with diverse multicultural populations. The staff demonstrates competency in:
a. an additional language besides English.
b. communicating by using a sign board.
c. transcultural nursing issues.
d. gender differences.

2.13. As patients are discharged from the Phase I area, monitors are cleared of memory, strips are discarded, and cubicles are cleaned. With regard to patient information, which important regulations went into effect in 2004 that increased sensitivity to all patient information?
a. The Joint Commission sentinel alert
b. HIPAA regulations
c. Hospital department policies
d. Occupational Safety and Health Administration (OSHA) standards

2.14. The staffing and personnel management standard of ASPAN's *2006-2008 Standards of Perianesthesia Nursing Practice* indicates that the professional perianesthesia nurse providing Phase I level of care will maintain certain competencies concerning Advanced Cardiac

Life Support (ACLS) and Pediatric Advanced Life Support (PALS), and the expectation is:

a. an equivalent course of ACLS/PALS is provided and maintained by each individual facility.
b. current ACLS and/or PALS provider status is maintained appropriate to the patient population served.
c. current ACLS provider status is maintained and PALS offered when pediatric population exceeds 10 pediatric cases/day.
d. current Basic Life Support (BLS) provider status and be encouraged to seek ACLS/PALS.

2.15. A normally busy Phase II PACU is starting to discharge patients for the day. At 3 PM only two patients are remaining in the Phase II area. The normal staffing at this time if patient census is three or fewer is one licensed practical nurse/licensed vocational nurse (LPN/LVN) and one certified nursing assistant. After reviewing Standard III, the staff determines that this staffing assignment is:

a. appropriate only for one or two patients.
b. inappropriate; one more nursing assistant should be available.
c. appropriate as suggested.
d. inappropriate because one of the personnel must always be an RN.

2.16. It is an extremely busy day in the preanesthesia unit. There have been three staffing call-ins and four emergency cases added to the surgical schedule. Eight patients are already admitted to the unit, you have two RNs, one LPN, one certified nursing assistant, and one transporter. A new patient needs to be admitted, and you assign the LPN to this patient. This staffing assignment is:

a. inappropriate because the LPN is already watching two other patients.
b. appropriate because the RN is needed to administer medication.
c. inappropriate because the preanesthesia assessment is performed by an RN competent in preanesthesia nursing.

d. appropriate because the unit is short-staffed.

NOTE: Consider the scenario and items 2.17-2.21 together.

A 19-year-old patient is scheduled for a laminectomy. The doctor explained the procedure to the patient, explained alternatives to the proposed surgery, and then said "That's it." The patient had the surgery and suffered paralysis, a devastating complication.

2.17. Using the information given in the scenario just described, identify an important aspect that is missing when referring to "informed consent."

a. Length of time of proposed surgery
b. Rehabilitation time after surgery
c. Risks and benefits of proposed surgery
d. Choice of anesthesia for proposed surgery

2.18. In a medical malpractice case, the court imposes the liability and responsibility for informed consent on:

a. the hospital and the physician.
b. solely the physician.
c. the preadmission nurse admitting the patient.
d. solely the patient.

2.19. Informed consent consists of:

a. the written document, signed by the patient explaining the proposed procedure.
b. explanation by preadmission nurse about procedure and what to expect.
c. explanation by physician about diagnosis, significant complications, benefits, and alternatives of surgery.
d. a written document detailing the surgical procedure and the proposed anesthetic plan.

2.20. The young patient in this scenario became paralyzed as a result of the laminectomy. There was considerable dispute in the resulting medical malpractice testimony as to what the patient was told. The patient stated he was not told about any possible complications or specifically about the risk of paralysis. The court held the:

a. nurses in the preadmission holding unit liable for not explaining possible postoperative complications.

b. physician liable for lack of an informed consent based on what a reasonable person would want to know.

c. hospital liable for failure to obtain an informed consent.

d. hospital and the physician liable for failure to obtain a written consent form detailing possible complications.

2.21. A patient must consent to being touched; otherwise a patient can claim:

a. breach of confidentiality.

b. battery.

c. assault and battery.

d. invasion of privacy.

NOTE: Consider the scenario and items 2.22-2.25 together.

A group of PACU nurses are eating together in the cafeteria. They begin talking about several of the young teenage girls they took care of that morning and accidentally interchange names and diagnoses. One of the nurses incorrectly identified the wrong girl as having been pregnant.

2.22. This discussion involves a quasi-intentional tort called:

a. invasion of privacy.

b. defamation of character.

c. disclosure of confidential information.

d. misrepresentation and fraud.

2.23. The nurses continue discussing these young patients they have been caring for, commenting on information the girls relayed to them during the admission process. Discussing this information in the cafeteria involves a quasi-intentional tort called:

a. breach of confidentiality.

b. disclosure of confidential information.

c. defamation of character.

d. invasion of privacy.

2.24. One of the visitors sitting in the cafeteria overheard the conversation. He was a school teacher at the incorrectly identified teenager's school. He shared the information he had heard with the school principal. This resulting tort is called:

a. a HIPAA violation.

b. fraud.

c. invasion of privacy.

d. misrepresentation.

2.25. The majority of lawsuits brought against nurses are based on negligence; a significant number involve an area of law known as *intentional* and *quasi-intentional torts*. Intentional torts most often seen in health care are:

a. breach of duty, unprofessional conduct, and defamation of character.

b. assault and battery, false imprisonment, and conversion of property.

c. breach of confidentiality, professional incompetence, and invasion of privacy.

d. misrepresentation, fraud, slander, and libel.

NOTE: Consider the scenario and items 2.26-2.28 together.

Three clinical RNs working in the Phase I PACU anticipate five patient admissions during the next 90 minutes and collaboratively plan nursing care assignments. Patients already in the PACU include a sedated 13-year-old boy whose oral airway was just removed and now has an SpO_2 of 98% and respiratory rate of 15 breaths per minute and an awake 9-year-old girl who is accompanied by her mother. The staff intends to provide safe nursing care that aligns with staffing recommendations in ASPAN's *2006-2008 Standards of Perianesthesia Nursing Practice*. One suggested assignment option is to have one nurse care for both children and to admit one adult woman after her cardioversion ends in 5 minutes.

2.26. After reviewing ASPAN's recommended patient classification guidelines, the staff determines that this assignment option is:

a. appropriate if a medical aide admits the new woman.

b. inappropriate; only two patients per nurse in Phase I.

c. inappropriate; the 13-year-old boy requires one-to-one care.

d. appropriate as suggested; and meets staffing recommendations.

2.27. The nurse to patient ratio changes to a one-on-one ratio with children when the child is:
   a. 9 years old, awake, but without a parent to sit with him or her.
   b. 13 years old without an artificial airway.
   c. younger than 8 years and unconscious.
   d. 8 years old and conscious with a parent at the bedside.

2.28. ASPAN's patient classification guidelines give specific criteria for nurse to patient ratios in the Phase I PACU. Ratios include:
   a. one nurse to one patient, one nurse to two patients, and two nurses to one patient.
   b. one nurse to one patient, two nurses to one patient, and one nurse to three patients.
   c. two nurses to one patient, one nurse to two patients, and one nurse to three patients.
   d. one nurse to three patients with a second nurse available to assist as necessary.

2.29. Conditions most associated with increased risk of nosocomial infection include all of the following *except:*
   a. broad-spectrum antibiotics.
   b. applied asepsis principles.
   c. multiple invasive catheters.
   d. concurrent multisystem illnesses.

2.30. The nurse obtains the most appropriate supplies, as recommended by the Malignant Hyperthermia Association of the United States, including dantrolene sodium and:
   a. bag-valve-mask unit with oxygen, iced crystalloid, and sodium bicarbonate.
   b. succinylcholine, ventilator, and renal-dose dopamine.
   c. chilled gastric lavage, lidocaine, and pressure monitoring equipment.
   d. phenylephrine, cooling blanket, and midazolam.

2.31. To reconstitute dantrolene, you will need:
   a. sterile water.
   b. normal saline.
   c. normal saline without additives.
   d. sterile water without preservatives.

SET 2

NOTE: Consider the scenario and items 2.32-2.33 together.

During a postoperative transfusion of banked packed red blood cells through an electrically operated blood warmer, the patient's temperature increases to 39° C (102.2° F). The nurse observes the color of blood entering the patient is bright red; the blood tubing feels hot. The transfusion is immediately discontinued and returned to the blood bank, where the blood temperature registers 42° C (107.6° F). An "overtemperature" alarm failed to signal increasing blood temperature before cell hemolysis.

2.32. The clinical nurse's responsibility includes:
   a. determining whether long-term patient harm occurred.
   b. reporting the incident directly to the manufacturer.
   c. informing facility managers of the malfunction.
   d. returning the equipment for quick biomedical repair.

2.33. In addition to the reporting process concerning equipment failure, what additional piece of documentation should be completed concerning the patient's problem?
   a. A root cause analysis form
   b. A hospital incident report
   c. A medical equipment log
   d. A biomedical safety alert form

NOTE: Consider the scenario and items 2.34-2.38 together.

The orthopedist orders 5 mg midazolam and 25 mg meperidine intravenously for an adult male patient's moderate sedation. The orthopedist then gives the nurse a list of supplies, sterile gloves, antibiotics, and additional medications, which are needed from the pre-anesthesia holding unit.

2.34. In this situation, the PACU nurse's primary responsibility is to:
   a. administer medications as ordered and then obtain the necessary supplies.
   b. locate an anesthesia-certified colleague to administer medications as ordered.
   c. collaborate with the surgeon to adjust and individualize the medication doses as monitoring of the patient indicates.
   d. obtain the supplies while the orthopedist medicates the patient and begins the procedure.

2.35. The PACU nurse reminds the orthopedist that the patient takes phenelzine (Nardil) each day for depression. His last dose was 9 PM last evening. One medication to avoid is:
   a. streptomycin.
   b. midazolam.
   c. ketorolac.
   d. meperidine.

2.36. Physiologic measurements should include but not be limited to:
   a. level of consciousness, temperature, pain assessment, and ability to talk.
   b. respiratory rate, oxygen saturation, blood pressure, cardiac rate/rhythm, and level of consciousness.
   c. respiratory rate, oxygen saturation, blood pressure and pulse, and temperature.
   d. blood pressure, pulse, respirations, and oxygen saturation.

2.37. Which of the following emergency equipment must be immediately available during the administration of and recovery from sedation?
   a. Oxygen, airways, suction, bag-valve-mask devices, and an emergency cart with defibrillator and resuscitative medications, including reversal agents

b. Oxygen, appropriate airways, reversal agents, and code button to summon emergency cart

c. Emergency cart with defibrillator, respiratory equipment, and all medications

d. Bag-valve-mask devices, oxygen, and emergency plan to transfer patient if needed

NOTE: The scenario continues.

2.38. The nurse assesses that the patient is wincing and is not relaxed; the orthopedist now asks the nurse to administer methohexital 50 mg. When the orthopedist asks the nurse to administer methohexital 50 mg, a legally appropriate response for the PACU nurse to ask the physician is to delay further manipulation and:

a. observe the patient while the nurse obtains methohexital.

b. ask an anesthesia provider to administer methohexital.

c. quickly review the state's nurse practice act.

d. attach a pulse oximeter and cardiac and blood pressure monitors.

NOTE: Consider the scenario and items 2.39-2.40 together.

A PACU nurse is named in a malpractice lawsuit 6 months after a patient alleges she developed a back wound infection on the day of her L3-L4 hemilaminectomy and microdiskectomy surgery. The complaint states that the PACU was busy and that her nurse care provider improperly changed her bleeding back wound dressing after caring for another patient with hepatitis and then failed to inform the neurosurgeon of bleeding.

2.39. To demonstrate negligence, this patient must prove:

a. legal duty.

b. harmful intent.

c. undesirable outcome.

d. damaging conduct.

2.40. Criteria used to measure this nurse's clinical performance may include

showing that her nursing care aligned with accepted community practice and demonstrating:

a. that a nurse is accountable only to the unit manager.

b. compliance with *2006-2008 Standards of Perianesthesia Nursing Practice.*

c. a lack of proximate cause during wound assessment.

d. that her skills equal the performance of a certified colleague.

2.41. A 6-year-old patient is undergoing a tonsillectomy, adenoidectomy, and bilateral myringotomy. At the end of the surgical procedure, the child is still unresponsive, placed on the stretcher, and transferred by the anesthesiologist alone to the PACU. The operating room suite is the last room in a long hallway. The child begins to wake up while en route to the PACU, starts thrashing, and before the anesthesiologist can intercede, has struck his arm on the stretcher rail, resulting in a fracture. Because of this injury, the hospital may have placed itself in jeopardy of a medical malpractice claim. What part of the scenario would be the probable cause based on understanding of the *2006-2008 Standards of Perianesthesia Nursing Practice?*

a. Children should not be transported unresponsive.

b. Children should not be transported alone by one person.

c. Appropriate safety features should be used, especially when transporting children.

d. Children should be transferred by carrying them to the PACU.

2.42. When describing something that you observe with a patient, it is very important that you chart:

a. immediately.

b. objectively.

c. sequentially.

d. subjectively.

2.43. A particularly troubling problem in writing orders and in taking both verbal and telephone orders prompted The Joint Commission to put out a list of:

a. grammar mistakes.
b. frequently misspelled medications.
c. abbreviations not to use.
d. incorrect dosages.

2.44. When documenting patient assessments, it is important to:

a. leave several blank lines so that you can be sure to have enough space to finish your narrative charting.
b. date and time each entry and sign your name at the end of the documentation.
c. include every single comment made by the patient.
d. document an assessment every 10 minutes, even if nothing has changed.

2.45. The nurse working 7 AM-3:30 PM has left for the day. She calls on her cell phone at 4:15 PM and asks you to chart a medication that was given to a patient who was transferred to Phase II just before she left. What should you do?

a. Take down the exact information (drug, dose, and time given) and chart it on the patient's chart.
b. File an incident report and ask her to come back to work immediately and chart this information.
c. Report the information to the nurse caring for the patient and save the chart for a late entry to be made.
d. Refer the call to the manager and let him or her decide what to do.

2.46. The purpose of taking a deposition is to:

a. let everyone involved in the care know what to say in case there is a trial.
b. get testimony from anyone thought to have information pertaining to the case.
c. practice the testimony you will actually give in court.
d. allow you to meet the patient's attorney and learn why they are claiming medical malpractice.

2.47. A deposition is:

a. a friendly gathering to discuss the details of the case.
b. testimony given under oath, recorded by a court reporter.
c. an informal hearing to establish who needs to testify.
d. a formal hearing with judge and witnesses.

2.48. All of the information given during the deposition is:

a. inadmissible during a real medical malpractice trial.
b. can be used in future examination and testimony.
c. used, but only with consent of those at the deposition.
d. admitted into the trial with the judge's approval.

2.49. A critical element of the perianesthesia nurse's educational growth is willingness to:

a. work alone to provide care and education for four patients in a Phase II PACU.
b. demonstrate selected PACU competencies each year.
c. delegate mandibular support to the medical aide.
d. attend one educational seminar and adapt content to orient a colleague.

2.50. The PACU nurse reviews literature describing visitation by family members in the PACU for the unit's monthly journal club meeting. After critiquing several studies that report anxiety reduction among visited patients, the perianesthesia nurse supports incorporating study recommendations into unit practice. When preparing his journal club presentation, this nurse carefully phrases research conclusions as:

a. proof that visited patients have shorter PACU stays.
b. decisive evidence that refutes skepticism of peers.
c. a technique to encourage family bonding.
d. information to support PACU policy for visitation.

2.51. ASPAN's *2006-2008 Standards of Perianesthesia Nursing Practice* recommends current ACLS provider certification for perianesthesia nurses. The American Heart Association (AHA) recommends that ACLS provider status occur:

a. annually.
b. every 2 years.
c. every 3 years.
d. before The Joint Commission visitation.

SET 3

2.52. A 95-year-old resident of a long-term care facility with a "do not resuscitate or intubate" (DNR/DNI) advance directive fell and broke her hip. The physician orders a "no cardiopulmonary resuscitation (CPR)" status for the duration of the hospitalization. Her family signs consent for surgical repair. With regard to the advance directive in the PACU, ethical guidelines as interpreted by recent literature recommend:
   a. perioperative continuation of the DNR/DNI directive.
   b. automatic revocation until return to long-term care.
   c. focused review of intent for perianesthesia period.
   d. suspension of the DNI directive and retention of the DNR portion.

2.53. The nurse's advocacy role to promote patient well-being is predicated on the ethical principle of:
   a. beneficence.
   b. autonomy.
   c. fidelity.
   d. justice.

2.54. The word "ethical" is used to refer to:
   a. moral principles.
   b. reasons for decisions about how one ought to act.
   c. nonnegotiable care.
   d. explicit primary obligations.

2.55. The next patient admitted to the PACU, Phase I, is a 32-year-old woman who had a breast biopsy. She was extremely anxious in the preoperative holding area. The anesthesiologist tells you that the physician believes the biopsy is definitely positive but wants you to tell the patient that "everything is fine" until he sees her in the office. Which ethical principle does this challenge?
   a. Justice
   b. Fidelity
   c. Double-effect
   d. Veracity

2.56. A 17-year-old patient is scheduled for an abortion. Three staff nurses are on duty during the afternoon shift. Two nurses have assignments, and nurse C is free to accept a patient. Nurse C objects to this assignment. Ethical responsibility to patients includes ensuring that all patients are cared for by a professional nurse. This responsibility can be challenged when:
   a. there are too many patients and not enough staff, causing an inequity in patient ratios.
   b. the perianesthesia nurse's personal convictions prohibit participation.
   c. the patient is aborting with a large amount of blood loss and is in emergent danger.
   d. the nurse disapproves of the physician's choice of procedures.

2.57. Perianesthesia nurse A observes nurse B consistently having discrepancies with the narcotic documentation record. Nurse B is then seen dropping a suspicious vial into her lab coat while signing the same out to a patient. To follow policies, procedures, and laws to protect patients from incompetent, unethical, or illegal practice, nurse A must:
   a. approach her colleague, tell her she saw her take drugs, and tell her to put it back and stop this practice immediately.
   b. call the police, and tell them to come immediately because drugs have been stolen.
   c. appropriately report the nurse exhibiting questionable practice to her manager.
   d. do nothing.

2.58. A perianesthesia nurse is caring for a precocious 3-year-old who whispers

"my throat hurts" after a tonsillectomy procedure. She is also caring for a 17-year-old male who was involved in a motor vehicle accident while driving impaired. He also has a previous history of drug abuse. The nurse's ethical role in medicating both of these patients in the same manner is based on the ethical principle of:
a. nonmaleficence.
b. double indemnity.
c. respect.
d. justice.

2.59. The word "moral" refers to:
a. the proper respect given to an individual.
b. personal beliefs and cultural values.
c. following the "right" laws in the "right" way.
d. being a nice person and following the "golden rule."

2.60. A prominent businessman in the community has entered the hospital to have surgery and is very concerned about keeping his information private. His surgery is completed, and he has been admitted into the PACU. The chief of staff, who also happens to be a neighbor of the patient, enters the PACU and asks the nurse caring for him about his condition. The nurse:
a. answers all his questions because he is the chief of staff.
b. asks if he has the family's permission to be in the PACU checking on the patient.
c. gives the chief of staff the patient's chart to read.
d. refers the chief of staff to the family, maintaining confidentiality of patient information.

2.61. The complexity of health care collaboration requires:
a. good communication, budgetary responsibility, and competence.
b. mutual trust, recognition, and respect among the health care team.
c. personal goals, compliance with regulations, and shared decision making.

d. open dialogue, incentive systems, and conflict resolution.

2.62. In determining the appropriate delegation of tasks consistent with the nurse's obligation to provide optimum patient care, two ethical attributes are necessary for the nurse to exhibit. What are they?
a. Respect and accountability
b. Perseverance and benevolence
c. Accountability and responsibility
d. Integrity and responsibility

2.63. Initial assessment of a newly admitted patient to the Phase I PACU is delegated to a:
a. graduate nurse with no other assignment or patients.
b. registered nurse with one patient who is awake and stable.
c. student nurse observing care in the PACU.
d. registered nurse with a child who has an artificial airway.

2.64. Maintenance of competence and ongoing professional growth describes a nurse's:
a. duty to self.
b. evidence-based competence.
c. professional integrity.
d. lifelong learning goals.

2.65. Nurse educators must ensure that students possess:
a. optimal standards of nursing education.
b. essential knowledge, skills, and competencies.
c. accepted standards of professional nursing practice.
d. professional autonomy and self-regulation.

2.66. When an ethical dilemma arises:
a. the legal interpretation takes precedence over all moral decisions.
b. the consequences of right or wrong are determined by ethics.
c. law influences ethical decisions, and ethics influences legal decisions.
d. the deontology system interprets correct ethical decision making.

2.67. Utilitarianism is a theory that promotes:
a. dignity for everyone.
b. resolving conflicts.
c. fairness to all people.
d. the greatest good for the greatest number of people.

2.68. The patient is given a full, informed explanation concerning a proposed surgical procedure while being admitted in the preoperative holding area. All the risks and benefits are explained by the surgeon, as well as possible alternatives to the surgery. The patient, in refusing to consent to the surgery, is exercising what ethical principle?
a. Justice
b. Autonomy
c. Equality
d. Nonmaleficence

NOTE: Consider items 2.69-2.72.

Never before have end-of-life decision-making issues been more significant for health care professionals, particularly nurses. Rapid advances in biotechnology and medical science and their life-prolonging capabilities bring nurses into daily contact with potential ethical dilemmas.

2.69. The shared decision-making framework is based on everything *except:*
a. respect.
b. truth-telling.
c. doing good for patients.
d. deontology.

2.70. Using a moral framework for ethical decision-making enables nurses to:
a. identify sources of ethical conflict.
b. determine whether the patient has a living will.
c. advise the uses of all possible technologies.
d. decide upon the best patient surrogate.

2.71. Life-sustaining therapy is:
a. always given to dying patients.
b. used to maintain bodily function of dying patients.
c. always appropriate for dying patients.
d. restricted to medically provided nutrition and hydration.

2.72. Intentionally ending the life of a terminally ill, competent person with his or her consent is:
a. assisted suicide.
b. nonvoluntary euthanasia.
c. euthanasia.
d. voluntary euthanasia.

2.73. The professional code of ethics obligates all nurses to address pain management. This is accomplished by all of the following *except:*
a. subjective assessment of pain using recognized pain scales.
b. provision of effective pain control for dying patients.
c. continuing education/competence in pain management.
d. relief of patient suffering at end of life even if it hastens death.

2.74. The PACU's competency-based continuing education program reviews the Malignant Hyperthermia Association of the United States (MHAUS) recommendations for necessary equipment and supplies to respond to malignant hyperthermia (MH) crisis. Evaluation and successful completion of the competency include gathering initial supplies for a mock MH situation in the PACU. The nurse obtains the most appropriate supplies including dantrolene sodium and:
a. bag-valve-mask unit with oxygen, cold saline/sterile water solution, and blood tubes for electrolyte blood draw.
b. succinylcholine, ventilator, and renal-dose dopamine.
c. chilled gastric lavage, lidocaine, and pressure monitoring equipment.
d. phenylephrine, cooling blanket, and sodium bicarbonate.

2.75. When presenting the structure and function of the PACU to a nurse who is being oriented, the preceptor describes available equipment as recommended in ASPAN's *2006-2008 Standards of*

20

Perianesthesia Nursing Practice. In addition to a pulse oximeter, necessary equipment for each patient in Phase I includes a/an:

a. portable end-tidal CO_2 monitor.
b. active rewarming system.
c. ECG monitor.
d. pulmonary artery pressure transducers.

2.76. A student nurse is assigned to work with an expert PACU nurse. During delivery of care, the PACU nurse "thinks aloud." This process demonstrates a teaching strategy that primarily:

a. decreases student anxiety in clinical settings.
b. improves a student's decision making skills.
c. confuses the student with multiple options.
d. increases the student's technical skill.

2.77. In an inservice conducted for nurses who will assist in data collection for a research project, a graduate nursing student explains the study's procedures and tools. This inservice is necessary to improve the study's:

a. interrater reliability.

b. construct validity.
c. internal consistency.
d. content analysis.

2.78. The surgical services business manager chooses to orient interested medical-surgical nurses for weekend and on-call positions in the Phase I PACU. The professional practice arm of the PACU collaborative governance structure crafts a proposal that recommends only nurses with critical care experience be placed in these positions. The proposal cites ASPAN's *2006-2008 Standards of Perianesthesia Nursing Practice*, which recommends that a Phase I nurse demonstrate competence in:

a. identifying heart block and stating indications for beta blockers.
b. adjusting pacemaker parameters and administering intracardiac epinephrine.
c. interpreting electroencephalogram patterns and managing phenytoin protocols.
d. cardioversion techniques, intubation skill, and central venous cannulation.

SET 1

ANSWER KEY

2.1.	d		2.17.	c
2.2.	b		2.18.	b
2.3.	c		2.19.	c
2.4.	b		2.20.	b
2.5.	b		2.21.	b
2.6.	c		2.22.	b
2.7.	c		2.23.	a
2.8.	b		2.24.	c
2.9.	d		2.25.	b
2.10.	c		2.26.	b
2.11.	c		2.27.	c
2.12.	c		2.28.	a
2.13.	b		2.29.	b
2.14.	b		2.30.	a
2.15.	d		2.31	d
2.16.	c			

SET 1

RATIONALES AND REFERENCES

2.1. Correct Answer: **d**
In this situation, medical malpractice is associated with civil law. Civil law is based on rules and regulations and includes tort law. Tort law includes negligence and professional negligence. The word tort comes from the Latin word "tortus." In the French language, a tort is a civil wrong, other than breach of contract, for which the law will provide an injured person to seek damages. (Quinn D, Schick L, editors: *PeriAnesthesia nursing core curriculum: preoperative, Phase I and Phase II PACU nursing*, Philadelphia, 2004, Saunders; Brent NJ: *Nurses and the law*, ed 2, Philadelphia, 2001, Saunders.)

2.2. Correct Answer: **b**
In every negligence action, four essential elements must be proven for a cause of action in tort to be successful: a duty must exist between the injured party and the person who allegedly caused the injury; a breach of duty must occur; the breach of duty must be the proximate cause of the injury; and damages or injuries or both, which are recognizable and compensable by law, must be experienced by the injured party. (Quinn D, Schick L, editors: *PeriAnesthesia nursing core curriculum: preoperative, Phase I and Phase II PACU nursing*, Philadelphia, 2004, Saunders; Brent NJ: *Nurses and the law*, ed 2, Philadelphia, 2001, Saunders.)

2.3. Correct Answer: **c**
Duty is the particular relationship that has arisen between the plaintiff and defendant. Historically, hospitals were free to determine who would receive treatment, including emergency cases. Currently, hospitals that maintain emergency facilities are obligated to care for those in need of emergency treatment. Thus the hospital's duty has been expanded. Courts and legislatures have determined that a legal relationship arises when an injured patient in need of emergency care visits an emergency room. Likewise, when a patient enters the hospital for surgery and signs the general consent for treatment or surgery, a "duty" is established. The criterion of duty is usually easy to satisfy in terms of the nurse-patient relationship and is rarely challenged in legal decisions, since the nurse is an employee of the institution providing care for the patient. (Quinn D, Schick L, editors: *PeriAnesthesia nursing core curriculum: preoperative, Phase I and Phase II PACU nursing*, Philadelphia, 2004, Saunders; Fiesta J: *The law and liability: a guide for nurses*, New York, 1983, A Wiley Medical Publication; Brent NJ: *Nurses and the law*, ed 2, Philadelphia, 2001, Saunders.)

2.4. Correct Answer: **b**
There are many definitions of standards of care. Professional negligence involves the conduct of professionals that falls below a professional standard of due care. The law requires that professional caregivers conform to the applicable standard of care for that professional group. The applicable standard includes a "standard minimum of special knowledge and ability." Conduct should be compared with that of other ordinary, reasonable, and prudent professionals in the same or similar circumstances, and in the same or

similar locality. (Brent NJ: *Nurses and the law*, ed 2, Philadelphia, 2001, Saunders.)

2.5. Correct Answer: **b**
Professions have a responsibility to identify and define their practice to protect consumers by ensuring the delivery of quality service. Standards of practice are a means to fulfill this professional charge. The purpose of professional standards of care is to provide a basis or framework for quality nursing care. (ASPAN: *2006-2008 Standards of perianesthesia nursing practice*, Cherry Hill, NJ, 2006, ASPAN.)

2.6. Correct Answer: **c**
In ASPAN's *2004 Standards of Perianesthesia Nursing Practice*, "present" was defined as being in the particular place where the patient is receiving care. It was necessary to define 'present' because the statement for Phase I and Phase II read: "Two licensed nurses, one of whom is a RN competent in Phase I or II Post Anesthesia Nursing, are present whenever a patient is receiving Phase I or II level of care." The Phase II statement continued by stating: "A RN must be present at all times during Phase II." Many facilities were defining very loosely what the term 'present' meant. To more clearly define this requirement in *Standards of perianesthesia nursing practice* the term 'present' was replaced with the phrase "in the same room where the patient is receiving Phase I level of care" to reduce any interpretation of this intent. (ASPAN: *2006-2008 Standards of perianesthesia nursing practice*, Cherry Hill, NJ, 2006, ASPAN.)

2.7. Correct Answer: **c**
As the patient progresses and no longer requires the intensive nursing care provided in a PACU, a second phase of recovery is appropriate. Phase II is used to describe this area. The professional perianesthesia nursing role during Phase II focuses on preparing the patient/family/significant other for care in the home, for care in a Phase III setting, or for care in an extended care environment. For patients to be in the Phase II setting they must have met the discharge criteria from Phase I, which would require them to have an adequate airway, vital signs, and oxygen saturation. (ASPAN: *2006-2008 Standards of perianesthesia nursing practice*, Cherry Hill, NJ, 2006, ASPAN; Burden N: *Ambulatory surgical nursing*, ed 2, Philadelphia, 2000, Saunders.)

2.8. Correct Answer: **b**
In this scenario, a staffing assignment is described in which the Phase II nurse is already caring for three patients. It is not appropriate to take report or accept care for another patient because this would exceed the recommended nurse to patient ratio according to ASPAN's *Standards of Perianesthesia Nursing Practice*, supported in Resource 3. (ASPAN: *2006-2008 Standards of perianesthesia nursing practice*, Cherry Hill, NJ, 2006, ASPAN.)

2.9. Correct Answer: **d**
In this scenario, each nurse present already has one patient; neither nurse can accept the new patient according to the description presented in the scenario. However, the two patients already admitted can be safely combined into one assignment, allowing a nurse to admit and accept the new assignment. (ASPAN: *2006-2008 Standards of perianesthesia nursing practice*, Cherry Hill, NJ, 2006, ASPAN.)

2.10. Correct Answer: **c**
In ASPAN's *2006-2008 Standards of Perianesthesia Nursing Practice*,

the rationale for Patient Rights states that consideration of social and economic status, culture, personal attributes, and the nature of the health care problem must be given when working with patients, families, and the community. In 1992 The American Hospital Association revised the document "A Patient's Bill of Rights," which guarantees certain rights and privileges to every patient. (ASPAN: Resource 3 in *2006-2008 Standards of perianesthesia nursing practice*, Cherry Hill, NJ, 2006, ASPAN; O'Keefe ME: *Nursing practice and the law*, Philadelphia, 2001, FA Davis.)

2.11. Correct Answer: **c**
In 2004 the Health Insurance Portability and Accountability Act (HIPAA) went into effect. A covered entity must have in place appropriate administrative, technical, and physical safeguards that protect against uses and disclosures not permitted by the privacy rule and that limit incidental uses or disclosures. *Reasonable and appropriate measures to protect the patient's privacy* is the key phrase to remember. (OCR HIPAA Privacy. Incidental Uses and Disclosures [45 CFR 164.502 (a) (1) (iii)], December 3, 2002.)

2.12. Correct Answer: **c**
As communities become more multicultural, it is important for health care workers to become competent in transcultural nursing care. Age-specific competencies were required some time ago by both The Joint Commission and individual hospital standards. Many programs are available to inservice staff on multicultural issues that will prepare the nurse to care for diverse populations. The goal is to provide respectful, meaningful, and competent care to people of diverse cultures that leads to health and

well-being or to face death or disabilities of individuals or groups. Cultural caring rituals of patients are powerful forces to know, understand, assess, and respectfully use. (ASPAN: Resource 3 in *2006-2008 Standards of perianesthesia nursing practice*, Cherry Hill, NJ, 2006, ASPAN; Leininger M, McFarland MR: *Transcultural nursing: concepts, theories, research, & practice*, ed 3, New York, 2002, McGraw-Hill.)

2.13. Correct Answer: **b**
Patient information cannot be left in the open for anyone to view or find. Therefore if the monitors that are being used have a patient name and/or hospital number built in that reads out on the printed strips, those monitors must be cleared from memory when that patient is discharged. Likewise, any remaining strips not being mounted into the patient chart should be discarded into the shredder so that vital patient information is not accidentally retrieved by someone else. (Joint Commission on Accreditation of Healthcare Organizations: *Standards*, JCAHO, 2005.)

2.14. Correct Answer: **b**
ASPAN's Standard III, Staffing and Personnel Management, states that staffing patterns will reflect ASPAN's Patient Classification/Recommended Staffing Guidelines (Resource 3). Under this section, it specifies that "the professional perianesthesia nurse providing Phase I level of care will maintain a current advanced cardiac life support (ACLS) and/or pediatric advanced life support (PALS) provider status, as appropriate to the patient population served." (ASPAN: Resource 3 Patient Classification/Recommended Staffing Guidelines in *2006-2008 Standards of*

perianesthesia nursing practice, Cherry Hill, NJ, 2006, ASPAN; Burden N: *Ambulatory surgical nursing,* ed 2, Philadelphia, 2000, Saunders.)

2.15. Correct Answer: **d**
In this scenario, the staffing criteria and designation are applied according to ASPAN's *2006-2008 Standards of Perianesthesia Nursing Practice,* Resource 3. In Phase II, it specifies that "a RN must be in the Phase II PACU at all times while a patient is present." (ASPAN: Resource 3 in *2006-2008 Standards of perianesthesia nursing practice,* Cherry Hill, NJ, 2006, ASPAN.)

2.16. Correct Answer: **c**
This scenario deals with the staffing assignment in a preanesthesia area. The scope of perianesthesia nursing practice involves the assessment for, diagnosis of, intervention for, and evaluation of physical or psychosocial problems or risks for problems that may result from the administration of sedation/analgesia or anesthetic agents and techniques. This specialty of perianesthesia nursing encompasses the care of the patient and family/significant other along the perianesthesia continuum of care—preanesthesia, postanesthesia Phase I, Phase II, and Phase III. Characteristics unique to the preanesthesia phase are a focus on preparing the patient/family/significant other physically, psychologically, socioculturally, and spiritually for his or her experience. Interviewing and assessment techniques are used to identify potential or actual problems that may result. Education and interventions are initiated to optimize positive outcomes. ASPAN's *Standards of Perianesthesia Nursing Practice* identifies that the preanesthesia assessment is performed by an RN competent in preanesthesia

nursing; this is supported by Resources 3, 4, and 15. (ASPAN: Standard III and Resources 3, 4, and 15 in *2006-2008 Standards of perianesthesia nursing practice,* Cherry Hill, NJ, 2006, ASPAN.)

2.17. Correct Answer: **c**
The law concerning consent in health care situations is based on informed consent. This doctrine of informed consent has developed from negligence law as the courts began to realize that, although consent may have been given, not enough information was imparted from the foundation of an informed decision. Informed consent mandates to the physician or independent health care practitioner the separate legal duty to disclose necessary facts in language that the patient can reasonably understand so that the patient can make an informed choice. There should be a description of the procedure, available alternatives, possible risks and expected benefits, as well as the side effects of the treatment or procedure. Because all the possible risks and/or benefits of the proposed surgery were not disclosed, this 19-year-old patient was unable to make an informed choice about the proposed procedure. (Brent NJ: *Nurses and the law,* ed 2, Philadelphia, 2001, Saunders; Burden N: *Ambulatory surgical nursing,* ed 2, Philadelphia, 2000, Saunders; O'Keefe ME: *Nursing practice and the law,* Philadelphia, 2001, FA Davis.)

2.18. Correct Answer: **b**
Nurses should understand that the responsibility for informed consent rests with the physician who is going to perform the procedure. This is a principle that is misunderstood by many health care practitioners. However, courts have consistently held the physician rather than the

CHAPTER 2 • **Professional Issues Applied to Perianesthesia Nursing Practice**

nurses or hospital liable for failure to obtain an informed consent. In some medical malpractice cases, courts have imposed joint liability on the hospital and the physician. However, current case law is clear that in the area of informed consent, courts recognize clearly that it is the responsibility of the physician to obtain an informed consent. (Fiesta J: *The law and liability: a guide for nurses*, New York, 1983, A Wiley Medical Publication; Brent NJ: *Nurses and the law*, ed 2, Philadelphia, 2001, Saunders; Burden N: *Ambulatory surgical nursing*, ed 2, Philadelphia, 2000, Saunders; O'Keefe ME: *Nursing practice and the law*, Philadelphia, 2001, FA Davis.)

2.19. Correct Answer: **c**
This scenario poses another interesting concept of the *informed consent*. The documentation of the consent process through the use of a printed form should not be confused with the actual explanation given to the patient and the informed consent itself. The nurse's role in obtaining an informed consent is being clearly delineated by the courts. The physician bears the direct responsibility of explaining the diagnosis, the significant complications, benefits, risks, possible alternatives, and anything else having to do with the proposed procedure. (Fiesta J: *The law and liability: a guide for nurses*, New York, 1983, A Wiley Medical Publication; Brent NJ: *Nurses and the law*, ed 2, Philadelphia, 2001, Saunders; Burden N: *Ambulatory surgical nursing*, ed 2, Philadelphia, 2000, Saunders; O'Keefe ME: *Nursing practice and the law*, Philadelphia, 2001, FA Davis.)

2.20. Correct Answer: **b**
This scenario examines the informed consent process even more deeply, looking at exactly what the physician said to the

patient and what the patient reasonably would want to know about the procedure. The physician could be held liable for lack of an informed consent based on what the *reasonable* patient would want to know. Many states have a reasonable person standard or prudent patient standard when applying the law to informed consent. This means that the situation in question is analyzed depending on what a reasonable person or a prudent patient would have done if placed in the same situation. Or, in addition, what information should a reasonable person or a prudent patient have received to make an informed decision about the treatment being offered by the health care provider. (Fiesta J: *The law and liability: a guide for nurses*, New York, 1983, A Wiley Medical Publication; Burden N: *Ambulatory surgical nursing*, ed 2, Philadelphia, 2000, Saunders; O'Keefe ME: *Nursing practice and the law*, Philadelphia, 2001, FA Davis.)

2.21. Correct Answer: **b**
Consent becomes an important issue from a legal perspective in that the patient may sue for a battery (unconsented touching) if he or she does not consent to the procedure or treatment and the health care provider goes ahead with the procedure or treatment. The theory contends that an adult of sound mind has the right to decide when treatment is necessary and advisable. This is the basic principle of all consents—the patient's right to consent to being touched. Obtaining informed consent is also important for the health care provider, for without it, he or she may be subject to a lawsuit alleging assault, battery, negligence, or a combination of these causes of action. (Fiesta J: *The law and liability: a guide for nurses*, New York, 1983, A Wiley Medical Publication;

Brent NJ: *Nurses and the law*, ed 2, Philadelphia, 2001, Saunders; Burden N: *Ambulatory surgical nursing*, ed 2, Philadelphia, 2000, Saunders.)

2.22. Correct Answer: **b**

Quasi-intentional torts are those torts in which the intent of the actor may not be as clear as with the intentional torts but a voluntary act on the defendant's part takes place. Common quasi-intentional torts seen in health care are defamation, breach of confidentiality, invasion of privacy, and malicious prosecution. Defamation includes the "twin torts" of libel (written word) and slander (spoken word). It involves wrongful injury to an individual's reputation (i.e., his or her good name, respect, or esteem) through either oral or written communication to persons other than the person defamed. Nurses are advised to avoid any type of subjective language when charting and to avoid derogatory comments about patients or their family members. *Defamation* is a communication that "tends to hold the plaintiff up to hatred, contempt, or ridicule, or to cause him or her to be shunned or avoided (Brent, 2001)." (Brent NJ: *Nurses and the law*, ed 2, Philadelphia, 2001, Saunders; Burden N: *Ambulatory surgical nursing*, ed 2, Philadelphia, 2000, Saunders; O'Keefe ME: *Nursing practice and the law*, Philadelphia, 2001, FA Davis; Keeton, Dobbs, Keeton, & Owen, 1984, Ï 111 citing *Kimmerle v. New York Evening Journal, 1933*.)

2.23. Correct Answer: **a**

Breach of confidentiality is another one of the quasi-intentional torts. The law of breach of confidentiality protects a patient's sharing of information with a health care provider without fear that the information will be released to those not involved in his or her care. In today's electronic and information age, the tort of breach of confidentiality, like the tort of invasion of privacy, takes on new legal concerns in health care. Information about the patient is confidential and may not be disclosed without authorization. The patient's right to privacy and *confidentiality* is a key concept in both the American Nurses Association Code for Nurses and the Canadian Nurses Association Code of Ethics for Nursing, as well as the nurse practice acts for each state. Nurses need to be familiar with what information their agency considers confidential and in what manner and by whom it may be revealed. (Brent NJ: *Nurses and the law*, ed 2, Philadelphia, 2001, Saunders; Burden N: *Ambulatory surgical nursing*, ed 2, Philadelphia, 2000, Saunders; O'Keefe ME: *Nursing practice and the law*, Philadelphia, 2001, FA Davis; American Nurses Association, 1985; Canadian Nurses Association, 1991.)

2.24. Correct Answer: **c**

The quasi-intentional tort of invasion of privacy is quite different from breach of confidentiality. With invasion of privacy, the interest protected is the individual's right to be free from unreasonable intrusions into his or her private affairs. It involves four separate possible invasions of this overall interest, which have greatly expanded the interest the tort originally protected.

Use of likeness or name without consent for commercial advantage: Occurs when name, photograph, or other likeness is used as a symbol of his or her identity to further the product or service of another. An example in health care would be showing photographs of a patient who has had successful cosmetic surgery to advertise.

Unreasonable intrusion into private affairs and seclusions:

This category takes place when conduct pries or intrudes upon a person's private affairs or seclusions and is objectionable to a reasonable person. The conduct can be physical intrusion, peering into a private area, or eavesdropping. A good example of this point took place in a PACU when a former employee who was now a patient had her sheet lifted by a supervisor to look at her abdominal incision. The patient had not given consent for this supervisor to be present, much less invade her privacy in the manner in which she did.

Public disclosure of private facts:

To satisfy the elements of this invasion of privacy action, (1) there must be public disclosure of private facts; (2) the disclosure must be objectionable to someone of ordinary sensibilities; and (3) the information disclosed must be the type that the public has no legitimate interest in knowing. This type of invasion takes place when the discussion of an identified patient's treatment or information takes place during a public gathering. A nurse shares medical information with other employees and with the public, and there is a special relationship with the public and the person (dissemination to that special group).

Placing a person in a false light in the public eye:

This occurs when an individual publishes false facts about another—attributing views not held or actions not taken—that would be objectionable to a person of ordinary sensibilities. A picture of a patient is used in the advertising of the new infectious disease unit, but the patient has never been a recipient of those services.

In this particular scenario, discussing this private information in the cafeteria was a public disclosure to everyone within hearing distance. As it turned out, one of those people overhearing the conversation had "special interest" in the patient and passed this information on to another party, causing additional invasion of privacy. (Brent NJ: *Nurses and the law*, ed 2, Philadelphia, 2001, Saunders; O'Keefe ME: *Nursing practice and the law*, Philadelphia, 2001, FA Davis.)

2.25. Correct Answer: **b**
Although most personal injury lawsuits are based primarily on claims of negligence, a person may also sue someone for intentionally injuring him or her. Unlike the concept of failure to use ordinary care, as in a claim of negligence, intentional conduct is designed to bring about a particular result. The law, therefore, calls these acts *intentional torts*. The intentional torts most often seen in health care are assault, battery, false imprisonment, and conversion of property. (Brent NJ: *Nurses and the law*, ed 2, Philadelphia, 2001, Saunders; O'Keefe ME: *Nursing practice and the law*, Philadelphia, 2001, FA Davis.)

2.26. Correct Answer: **b**
In this scenario, one must assess the patients already admitted and the expected admissions about to arrive. One nurse would be able to combine the two children already in the room and provide care based on their current stage of recovery. However, unless discharge of one of these patients is anticipated, the proposed staffing option is inappropriate. According to ASPAN's *2006-2008 Standards of Perianesthesia Nursing Practice,* Resource 3, the highest level of nurse:patient ratio is one nurse to two patients. (ASPAN: *2006-2008 Standards of perianesthesia*

nursing practice, Cherry Hill, NJ, 2006, ASPAN.)

2.27. Correct Answer: **c**
As stated in the rationale for 2.26, the recommended classification guidelines for Phase I PACU are very important for the perianesthesia nurse to be familiar with, especially when determining admission status. With this scenario the answer is **c** because any unconscious patient 8 years of age and under requires a one-nurse-to-one-patient ratio. A 9-year-old awake patient is appropriate for a two-patient-to-one-nurse assignment. The 13-year-old patient is also an appropriate choice for a two patient to one nurse assignment; however if this patient had an artificial airway then this patient would become a one nurse to one patient assignment. Any patient requiring mechanical life support and/or artificial airway requires a one nurse to one patient assignment. An awake 8 year old or under who has family or competent support staff present is also an appropriate choice for a two patient to one nurse assignment. (ASPAN: Resource 3 in *2006-2008 Standards of perianesthesia nursing practice,* Cherry Hill, NJ, 2006, ASPAN.)

2.28. Correct Answer: **a**
It is recommended that nurses working in the perianesthesia practice setting be aware of the *2006-2008 Standards of Perianesthesia Nursing Practice,* specifically Resource 3, Patient Classification/Recommended Staffing Guidelines. These guidelines give nurse-to-patient ratios, which detail nurse:patient ratios defined as Class 1:2, Class 1:1 and Class 2:1. Each specific class delineates exact patient criteria.
Class 1:2 indicates one nurse to two patients who are: One unconscious, stable without artificial airway, and older than 8 years; and one conscious, stable, and free of

complications. Two conscious, stable, and free of complications. Two conscious, stable, 8 years of age and younger, with family or competent support staff person.
Class 1:1 indicates one nurse to one patient: At the time of admission, until the critical elements are met. Requiring mechanical life support and/or artificial airway. Any unconscious patient 8 years of age and younger. A second nurse must be available to assist as necessary.
Class 2:1 indicates two nurses to one patient: One critically ill, unstable, complicated patient.
When aware of these guidelines, it is much easier to triage patients arriving in the PACU and thus any child younger than 8 years and unconscious would require a one-to-one nurse-to-patient ratio. (ASPAN: Resource 3 in *2006-2008 Standards of perianesthesia nursing practice,* Cherry Hill, NJ, 2006, ASPAN.)

2.29. Correct Answer: **b**
Health care providers who follow principles of asepsis and standard precautions reduce the spread of nosocomial, or hospital-acquired, infections. Handwashing and attention to cleanliness limit microorganism numbers. Coexisting illnesses, many care providers, prolonged hospitalization, and multiple invasive procedures are conditions most associated with increased risk of nosocomial infection. Indwelling catheters, including monitoring lines and urinary catheters, introduce exogenous infection. Broad-spectrum antibiotics alter the patient's normal body flora, creating imbalance and allowing microorganisms, including antibiotic-resistant strains, to colonize and rapidly proliferate. (Burden N: *Ambulatory surgical nursing*, ed 2, Philadelphia, 2000, Saunders; Black JM, Hawks JH, Keene AM: *Medical-surgical nursing*, vol 1,

Philadelphia, 2001, Saunders; Potter PA, Perry AG: *Fundamentals of nursing*, ed 5, St. Louis, 2001, Mosby.)

2.30. Correct Answer: **a**
Initial treatment of malignant hyperthermia (MH) crisis requires many vials of dantrolene sodium, cold IV saline for infusion, cooling blankets, sodium bicarbonate, mannitol, and 100% oxygen for possible delivery with positive pressure. The patient may or may not be intubated. IV lidocaine and succinylcholine are considered possible triggers of MH and are not given to any patient with suspected MH. (ASPAN: Resource 5 in *2006-2008*

Standards of perianesthesia nursing practice, Cherry Hill, NJ, 2006, ASPAN; www.MHAUS.org; 1-800-MHHYPER.)

2.31. Correct Answer: **d**
Reconstitution of dantrolene is time-consuming and requires several people for its rapid preparation. The powdered drug dissolves slowly and requires 60 mL of diluent added to each vial. Because of the large volume of diluent used to reconstitute a full course of the drug, diluents should not contain bacteriostatic agents. (Burden N: *Ambulatory surgical nursing*, ed 2, Philadelphia, 2000, Saunders; www.MHAUS.org.)

SET 2

ANSWER KEY

2.32.	c		**2.42.**	b
2.33.	b		**2.43.**	c
2.34.	c		**2.44.**	b
2.35.	d		**2.45.**	c
2.36.	b		**2.46.**	b
2.37.	a		**2.47.**	b
2.38.	b		**2.48.**	b
2.39.	d		**2.49.**	b
2.40.	b		**2.50.**	d
2.41.	c		**2.51.**	b

SET 2

RATIONALES AND REFERENCES

2.32. Correct Answer: **c**

Any patient complication related to medical device use must be reported to the Food and Drug Administration (FDA) and the manufacturer. The staff nurse need not directly inform these agencies but must set the facility protocol in motion so mandatory reporting is completed within 10 days of an incident. In 1990 a federal law, the Safe Medical Devices Act (SMDA), was established to protect consumers from product-related illness, injury, or death. The law requires the health care worker in hospitals, ambulatory facilities, and nursing homes to report device malfunctions. (Allen A: Medical device reporting: a new challenge for perioperative nurses, *J Post Anesth Nurs* 7(5):352-353, 1992. News notes: *J Post Anesth Nurs* 7(5):135, 1992.)

2.33. Correct Answer: **b**

A second form of documentation is an unusual occurrence report, sometimes called an *incident report* or a *variance report*. These reports are created and designed to be part of the risk management process by allowing written documentation of issues that concern patient care in the aggregate. Documentation that is pertinent to the follow-up care after patient incidents or injuries, documentation that is needed to ensure the smooth functioning of all departments, and documentation that is required to report occurrences not directly concerning patients may be found on incident reports. Nurses are cautioned to remember that the purpose of incident reports is confidential and that no reference to the report should be included in the patient care record.

(ASPAN: Standard IV in *2006-2008 Standards of perianesthesia nursing practice,* Cherry Hill, NJ, 2004, ASPAN; Burden N: *Ambulatory surgical nursing,* ed 2, Philadelphia, 2000, Saunders.)

2.34. Correct Answer: **c**

The nurse must recognize the need for dose reduction in an elderly, small, or debilitated patient and then collaborate with the physician to adjust the patient's dose. In addition, the nurse assigned to the patient's care must *establish priorities:* continuously monitoring his response during moderate sedation and emergency intervention are the nurse's *only* responsibilities. Obtaining supplies, not patient observation, must be delegated. Even though he is a healthy man, a 5-mg dose of midazolam likely will over-sedate an elderly man like the patient; his ability to independently maintain his airway, a requirement of moderate sedation, could also be eliminated. Meperidine augments these effects. (ASPAN: *2006-2008 Standards of perianesthesia nursing practice,* Cherry Hill, NJ, 2006, ASPAN.)

2.35. Correct Answer: **d**

Meperidine and antidepressant monoamine oxidase inhibitors (MAOIs) like phenelzine (Nardil) do not mix well together. The combination could produce profound hypertension. MAOIs promote storage of epinephrine, which meperidine releases. In some patients, this catecholamine surge can produce wildly fluctuating blood pressures with agitation and headache. Appreciating the potential consequences of combining meperidine with an MAOI medication and then questioning the physician's order are nursing responsibilities related to drug administration. (Burden N: *Ambulatory surgical nursing*, ed 2, Philadelphia, 2000, Saunders.)

2.36. Correct Answer: **b**
The RN managing the care of the patient receiving sedation shall have no other responsibilities that would leave the patient unattended or compromise continuous monitoring. Physiologic measurements should include but are not limited to respiratory rate, oxygen saturation, blood pressure, cardiac rate and rhythm, and patient's level of consciousness. (ASPAN: Resource 9 in *2006-2008 Standards of perianesthesia nursing practice*, Cherry Hill, NJ, 2006, ASPAN.)

2.37. Correct Answer: **a**
Resource 9 is intended to provide a guideline for care and monitoring of patients receiving sedative medications in any setting, for any purpose, and by any route. The following emergency equipment must be immediately available during the administration of and recovery from sedation: supplemental oxygen and delivery systems; appropriate airways; suction; bag-valve-mask device; and an emergency cart with a defibrillator and all resuscitative medications including reversal agents. (ASPAN: Resource 9 in *2006-2008 Standards of perianesthesia nursing practice*, Cherry Hill, NJ, 2006, ASPAN.)

2.38. Correct Answer: **b**
Methohexital is classified as an anesthetic medication for intravenous (IV) induction; therefore administration is usually beyond the scope of practice of the non-anesthetist RN. Any nurse who assists with moderate sedation should review and understand in advance which medications can be given with a physician's order. Institutional policy, standards of care, and that state's nurse practice act specify this information. The nurse managing care must then demonstrate competence in care of patients receiving IV moderate sedation, including monitoring of blood pressure, heart rate, and oxygen saturation. (ASPAN: Resource 9 in *2006-2008 Standards of perianesthesia nursing practice*, Cherry Hill, NJ, 2006, ASPAN; Burden N: *Ambulatory surgical nursing*, ed 2, Philadelphia, 2000, Saunders.)

2.39. Correct Answer: **d**
A charge of negligence means the patient (plaintiff) must *prove* that damage (the wound infection) actually occurred as a direct result of the accused nurse's actions (changing the dressing after caring for a patient with an infection). Even undesirable outcomes must be directly linked to a specific alleged action. Negligence commonly includes failure to monitor condition and failure to accurately document observed events and physician notification. The nurse has a legal responsibility (duty) to provide safe patient care without the intention to harm. (Brent, NJ: *Nurses and the law*, ed 2, Philadelphia, 2001, Saunders; Quinn D, Schick L, editors: *PeriAnesthesia nursing core curriculum: preoperative, Phase I and Phase II PACU nursing*, Philadelphia, 2004, Saunders; O'Keefe ME: *Nursing practice and the law*, Philadelphia, 2001, FA Davis.)

2.40. Correct Answer: **b**
Standards of care (whether established by state or federal law, nursing and specialty organization, or accrediting agencies) are legal measures to determine the acceptability of a nurse's professional actions. Nurses must meet the same

standard of acceptable care whether certified or not. Expert witnesses may attest to whether this nurse acted responsibly to provide nursing care as another "ordinary, prudent nurse would have performed in the same or similar manner" and in a similar circumstance. The plaintiff who brings the lawsuit, not the nurse-defendant, must prove both proximate cause and damage. (Brent, NJ: *Nurses and the law*, ed 2, Philadelphia, 2001, Saunders; Quinn D, Schick L, editors: *PeriAnesthesia nursing core curriculum: preoperative, Phase I and Phase II PACU nursing*, Philadelphia, 2004, Saunders.)

2.41. Correct Answer: **c**
This scenario depicts an anesthesiologist transporting a pediatric patient, alone, to the PACU. The OR is the last room in a long hallway, and pediatric patients can begin to wake up from anesthesia very quickly. Therefore this child should have had safety features in place. These safety features include the safety strap on the stretcher, rail pads to protect the side rails, and/or more personnel to assist if the child did start waking up while proceeding to the PACU. None of these factors were in place according to the scenario given. ASPAN's *Standards of Perianesthesia Nursing Practice* addresses environment of care issues. Standard II states that perianesthesia nursing practice promotes and maintains a safe, comfortable, and therapeutic environment for patients, staff, and visitors. It further delineates in the criteria that a policy will exist to ensure safe transportation of patients and refers the reader to Resource 10. Resource 10 is safe transfer of care and states that in accordance with Standards II and VIII and Resource 4, the perianesthesia nurse is responsible for the safe transfer of care of patients from

each phase of the perianesthesia continuum. (ASPAN: Standard II and Resource 10 in *2006-2008 Standards of perianesthesia nursing practice,* Cherry Hill, NJ, 2006, ASPAN.)

2.42. Correct Answer: **b**
Comprehensive documentation provides accurate information on which care can be based. Accurate charting of nursing actions and interventions has multiple purposes. It is necessary to chart care given objectively and accurately. Chart the facts and only the facts; do not embellish documentation. It is important to chart what is observed, what was done, and what the outcomes were. It is very difficult to prove legally that something was done if it is not charted. The medical record is used in litigation in which professional negligence is alleged; therefore it must be viewed as a viable way by which to defend against allegations of professional negligence. Factual, objective entries are essential. The medical record is no place for opinions, assumptions, or meaningless words or statements. The entry should be factual, complete, and accurate, containing observations, clinical signs and symptoms, patient quotes, interventions, and patient reactions. (ASPAN: Standard II and Resource 10 in *2006-2008 Standards of perianesthesia nursing practice,* Cherry Hill, NJ, 2006, ASPAN; Brent NJ: *Nurses and the law*, Philadelphia, 2001, Saunders; Burden N: *Ambulatory surgical nursing*, ed 2, Philadelphia, 2000, Saunders; Quinn D, Schick L, editors: *PeriAnesthesia nursing core curriculum: preoperative, Phase I and Phase II PACU nursing*, Philadelphia, 2004, Saunders.)

2.43. Correct Answer: **c**
All nursing documentation should support the policies and standards

of the facility and of the profession and regulating bodies. All the abbreviations nurses use must be appropriate, unambiguous, communicated to the entire staff, and incorporated into the standard policy of the facility. Abbreviations should be confined to those adopted by the health care delivery system only and used according to the meaning assigned to them. If there is no adopted policy concerning abbreviations, then the nurse should not use them. (Brent NJ: *Nurses and the law*, Philadelphia, 2001, Saunders; Burden N: *Ambulatory surgical nursing*, ed 2, Philadelphia, 2000, Saunders; The Joint Commission on Accreditation of Healthcare Organizations: 2005 National Patient Safety Goals, 2005, JCAHO.)

2.44. Correct answer: **b**
The medical record is an essential part of patient care. The medical record is to be a complete and accurate account of the patient's care while receiving treatment in the health care delivery system. In ASPAN's *2006-2008 Standards of Perianesthesia Nursing Practice*, Standard VI states that the professional perianesthesia nurse performs a systematic and continuous assessment of the patient and ensures that all data are collected, documented, and communicated. Every entry must be accounted for; the nurse must sign his or her name and list credentials and other required data for every entry reflecting patient care. (ASPAN: Standard VI in *2006-2008 Standards of perianesthesia nursing practice*, Cherry Hill, NJ, 2006, ASPAN; Brent NJ: *Nurses and the law*, Philadelphia, 2001, Saunders; Quinn D, Schick L, editors: *PeriAnesthesia nursing core curriculum: preoperative, Phase I and Phase II PACU nursing*, Philadelphia, 2004, Saunders.)

2.45. Correct Answer: **c**
Two documentation issues are discussed in this item. The first issue is that something needs to be added to the patient chart that occurred at an earlier time. The second issue is that a nurse is asking another nurse to make that entry. When it is necessary to add omitted information to an already existing entry, policies and procedures should be consulted and followed. Usually, the addition of information is coded on the next available line or space as a "late entry" or "addition to nursing note of _____," the date and time of the information that is being added is documented, and the additional information is then placed in the record. Some facilities also call this an "addendum." No nurse should document in the medical record for another person unless that practice is "standard" practice, as in an emergency code. Even so, when documenting for another in an emergency, the nurse "scribe" must accurately reflect who is providing care and who is documenting. Under **NO** circumstances, however, should the nurse sign another nurse's name in any portion of the record. (Brent NJ: *Nurses and the law*, Philadelphia, 2001, Saunders.)

2.46. Correct Answer: **b**
The depositions of the parties are usually taken in their attorney's offices, but depositions of fact witnesses and experts may be taken anywhere and at any time that is reasonable. Oral testimony is given under oath by any person thought to have information pertaining to the case. The format in a deposition is a question-and-answer format. Depositions are used by attorneys in several ways. They help the parties develop the evidence needed to prosecute or defend their case. At the time of trial, should the

witness testify in a manner that is inconsistent with his or her prior deposition testimony, an attorney may **impeach** his or her credibility by confronting the witness with that inconsistency. (Brent NJ: *Nurses and the law*, Philadelphia, 2001, Saunders; Quinn D, Schick L, editors: *PeriAnesthesia nursing core curriculum: preoperative, Phase I and Phase II PACU nursing*, Philadelphia, 2004, Saunders; O'Keefe ME: *Nursing practice and the law*, Philadelphia, 2001, FA Davis.)

2.47. Correct Answer: **b**
A *deposition* is a procedure whereby a party in the case or a witness gives his or her statement concerning the case under oath with all parties and their attorneys present. To request the deposition of a party to the case, one serves notice to the party's attorney. The witness is sworn in by a court reporter who takes transcription of all that is said during the course of the deposition. (Brent NJ: *Nurses and the law*, Philadelphia, 2001, Saunders; Quinn D, Schick L, editors: *PeriAnesthesia nursing core curriculum: preoperative, Phase I and Phase II PACU nursing*, Philadelphia, 2004, Saunders; O'Keefe ME: *Nursing practice and the law*, Philadelphia, 2001, FA Davis.)

2.48. Correct Answer: **b**
The format in a deposition is a question-and-answer format. Depositions are used by attorneys in several ways. They help the parties develop the evidence needed to prosecute or defend their case. At the time of trial, should the witness testify in a manner that is inconsistent with his or her prior deposition testimony, an attorney may impeach his or her credibility by confronting the witness with that inconsistency. (Brent NJ: *Nurses and the law*,

Philadelphia, 2001, Saunders; Quinn D, Schick L, editors: *PeriAnesthesia nursing core curriculum: preoperative, Phase I and Phase II PACU nursing*, Philadelphia, 2004, Saunders; O'Keefe ME: *Nursing practice and the law*, Philadelphia, 2001, FA Davis.)

2.49. Correct Answer: **b**
Staff members participate in annual perianesthesia nursing competency validation and continuing educational opportunities. Working alone with any perianesthesia patient or delegating a nursing function like jaw support does not comply with the established standards. (ASPAN: Standard III and Resource 13 in *2006-2008 Standards of perianesthesia nursing practice*, Cherry Hill, NJ, 2006, ASPAN.)

2.50. Correct Answer: **d**
Using evidence to support a policy change is appropriate, though this critic should describe a variety of studies to present balanced and well-supported positions. Researchers' (or research consumers') bias or judgments might mean a study's conclusions are interpreted in ways that stretch beyond information provided in the study. For example, permitting visitation does not cause shorter PACU stays but may be one supportive factor in anxiety reduction, so the end result is earlier discharge. (Smykowski L, Rodriguez W: The post anesthesia care unit experience: a family-centered approach, *J Nurs Care Qual* 18(1): 5-15, 2003; Poole EL: The effects of postanesthesia care unit visits on anxiety in surgical patients, *J Post Anesth Nurse* 8(6):386-394, 1993.)

2.51. Correct Answer: **b**
Renewal of ACLS provider status is every 2 years. These renewal requirements are established by the American Heart Association.

(American Heart Association: www.americanheart.org; ASPAN: Standard III and Resource 13 in

 2006-2008 Standards of perianesthesia nursing practice, Cherry Hill, NJ, 2006, ASPAN.)

Set 3

Answer Key

2.52.	c		**2.66.**	c
2.53.	a		**2.67.**	d
2.54.	b		**2.68.**	b
2.55.	d		**2.69.**	d
2.56.	b		**2.70.**	a
2.57.	c		**2.71.**	b
2.58.	d		**2.72.**	d
2.59.	b		**2.73.**	a
2.60.	d		**2.74.**	a
2.61.	b		**2.75.**	c
2.62.	c		**2.76.**	b
2.63.	b		**2.77.**	a
2.64.	a		**2.78.**	a
2.65.	b			

SET 3

2.52. Correct Answer: **c**

A specific "no-CPR" request is only one portion of an advance directive. The American Heart Association recommends that "no CPR" or "DNR/DNI" orders be reviewed with the surgical patient and family by the attending physician and anesthesiologist. Discussion focuses on the desired response by the health care team for specific perioperative potential events. Based on this discussion, the orders may be continued or suspended. Individual health care facilities often establish specific protocols to consider DNR/DNI orders for the perianesthesia period; situational concerns can be directed to a facility's ethics committee. (Schneiderman LJ, Jecker NS, Jonsen AR: Medical futility: response to critiques, *Ann Intern Med* 125(8):669-674, 1996; Drain CB: *Perianesthesia nursing: a critical care approach*, ed 4, Philadelphia, 2003, Saunders.)

2.53. Correct Answer: **a**

The ethical principle of beneficence obligates a health care provider to act in ways to provide more benefit than harm or burden. Whether positive benefit occurs is established from the patient's perspective. (ASPAN: *2006-2008 Standards of perianesthesia nursing practice*, Part II, Cherry Hill, NJ, 2006, ASPAN; American Nurses Association: *Code for nurses with interpretive statements*, Washington, DC, 2001, The Association.)

2.54. Correct Answer: **b**

There are numerous approaches for addressing ethics; these include adopting or subscribing to ethical theories including humanist, feminist, and social ethics; adhering to ethical principles; and cultivating virtues. The Code of Ethics for Nurses reflects all these approaches. The words "ethical" and "moral" are used throughout the Code of Ethics. "Ethical" is used to refer to reasons for decisions about how one ought to act, using the approaches just mentioned. (American Nurses Association: *Code for nurses with interpretive statements*, Washington, DC, 2001, The Association.)

2.55. Correct Answer: **d**

Veracity is an ethical and legal principle, simply defined as truthfulness. Most of the literature identifies truth as an important component of nursing practice. Not telling the truth may show lack of respect for others and non-trustworthiness of the person telling the lies. Under therapeutic privilege, patients may not be given information about health care if the information would cause further harm to the patient. (O'Keefe ME: *Nursing practice and the law*, Philadelphia, 2001, FA Davis.)

2.56. Correct Answer: **b**

The "Responsibility to Patients" section of ASPAN's *Perianesthesia Standards for Ethical Practice* states that the perianesthesia nurse ensures that all patients are cared for by a professional nurse. (∗) The asterisk signifies this statement. Where the perianesthesia nurse's personal convictions prohibit participation, that nurse may remove himself or herself from a patient care situation as long as such removal does not harm the patient or constitute a breach of duty. The professional nurse should provide his or her manager with information about the specific situations that would be difficult to participate in so that the manager is better able to plan for patient needs. However, if an unplanned situation arises in which no other professional nurse is available to care for the patient, then the objecting nurse must ensure that the care needs of the patient are met. (ASPAN: *2006-2008 Standards of perianesthesia nursing practice,* Part II, Cherry Hill, NJ, 2006, ASPAN.)

2.57. Correct Answer: **c**
Nurses must be vigilant to protect the patient, the public, and the profession from potential harm when a colleague's practice, in any setting, appears to be impaired. In a situation in which a nurse suspects another's practice may be impaired, the nurse's duty is to take action designed both to protect patients and to ensure that the impaired individual receives assistance in regaining optimal function. Action begins with consulting supervisory personnel and may also include confronting the individual in a supportive manner. If impaired practice poses a threat or danger to self or others, regardless of whether the individual has sought help, the nurse must take action to report the individual to persons authorized to address the problem. (American Nurses Association: *Code for nurses with interpretive statements,* Washington, DC, 2001, The Association; ASPAN: *2006-2008 Standards of perianesthesia nursing practice,* Part II, Cherry Hill, NJ, 2006, ASPAN.)

2.58. Correct Answer: **d**
Justice is one of the key ethical principles described in the perianesthesia core curriculum. It describes justice as a duty to be fair to all people. Justice can be further defined as the nurse's duty to be fair and equitable and to provide access and appropriate care to all patients. Two types of justice are described within ethics. **Distributive justice** contemplates the fair and equitable distribution of health care goods and nursing services; **procedural justice** is described as a known, fair process within which distributive justice occurs. (Quinn D, Schick L, editors: *PeriAnesthesia nursing core curriculum: preoperative, Phase I and Phase II PACU nursing,* Philadelphia, 2004, Saunders; O'Keefe ME: *Nursing practice and the law,* Philadelphia, 2001, FA Davis.)

2.59. Correct Answer: **b**
The words "ethical" and "moral" are used throughout the Code of Ethics. In general, the word "moral" overlaps with ethical but it is more aligned with personal beliefs and cultural values. Morals are one's sense of good and bad, right and wrong. Moral reasoning is the psychologic interpretive process that helps connect one's moral values with one's ethical choices. Through moral reasoning, one examines the salient features in an ethical situation and makes a judgment or chooses a course of action that is, presumably, congruent with one's moral beliefs and values. Moral values are not static; they change as persons mature. Theorists such as Piaget, Kohlberg, Gilligan, and Rest are attempting to look at the developmental patterns of moral values. (American Nurses Association: *Code for nurses with interpretive statements,* Washington, DC, 2001, The Association; Brent NJ: *Nurses and the law,* Philadelphia, 2001, Saunders; O'Keefe ME: *Nursing practice and*

the law, Philadelphia, 2001, FA Davis.)

Washington, DC, 2001, The Association.)

2.60. Correct Answer: **d**
Associated with the right to privacy, the nurse has a duty to maintain confidentiality of all patient information. The rights, well-being, and safety of the individual patient should be the primary factors in arriving at any professional judgment concerning the disposition of confidential information received from or about the patient, whether oral, written, or electronic. The standard of nursing practice and the nurse's responsibility to provide quality care require that data be shared with those members of the health care team who have an explicit need to know. Only information pertinent to a patient's treatment and welfare is disclosed. (American Nurses Association: *Code for nurses with interpretive statements*, Washington, DC, 2001, The Association.)

2.61. Correct Answer: **b**
In health care, the goal is to address the health needs of the patient and the public. The complexity of health care delivery systems requires a multidisciplinary approach to the delivery of services that has the strong support and active participation of all the health professions. Nursing's contribution, scope of practice, and relationship with other health professions needs to be clearly articulated, represented, and preserved. Collaboration requires mutual trust, recognition, and respect among the health care team, shared decision making about patient care, and open dialogue among all parties who have an interest in and a concern for health outcomes. (American Nurses Association: *Code for nurses with interpretive statements*,

2.62. Correct Answer: **c**
The *Code of Ethics for Nurses with Interpretive Statements* explains in interpretive statement 4 that the nurse is responsible and accountable for individual nursing practice and determines the appropriate delegation of tasks consistent with the nurse's obligation to provide optimum patient care. Nursing practice includes direct care activities, acts of delegation, and other responsibilities such as teaching, research, and administration. Nurses are faced with decisions in the context of the increased complexity and changing patterns in the delivery of health care. As the scope of nursing changes, the nurse must exercise judgment in accepting responsibilities, seeking consultation, and assigning activities for others who carry out nursing care. *Accountability* means to be answerable to oneself and others for one's own actions. *Responsibility* refers to the specific accountability or liability associated with the performance of duties of a particular role. Individual nurses are responsible for assessing their own competence. When the needs of a patient are beyond the nurse's qualifications and competencies, consultation and collaboration must be sought from a qualified nurse, other heath professionals, or other appropriate sources. (American Nurses Association: *Code for nurses with interpretive statements*, Washington, DC, 2001, The Association.)

2.63. Correct Answer: **b**
ASPAN's *2006-2008 Standards of Perianesthesia Nursing Practice* provides sound rationale for this scenario. Standard VI states that the professional perianesthesia nurse

42

performs a systematic and continuous assessment of the patient and ensures that all data are collected, documented, and communicated. Assessment and data collection provide a clinical basis for nursing interventions. In Resource 3, the staffing classification and recommended staffing guidelines show the appropriate nurse to patient ratios for Phase I. By looking at Standard VI and Resource 3 together, the proper delegation in this scenario is evident. A graduate nurse and/or a student nurse cannot admit and perform the initial assessment on a new patient. The nurse who is caring for a child is not able to accept another patient because the child is still unconscious. The RN with one awake and stable patient is able to accept another patient and can perform the admission assessment to the PACU. (ASPAN: Standard VI and Resource 3 in *2006-2008 Standards of perianesthesia nursing practice*, Cherry Hill, NJ, 2006, ASPAN.)

2.64. Correct Answer: **a**
The Code of Ethics interpretive statement 5 indicates that the nurse owes the same duties to self as to others, including the responsibility to preserve integrity and safety, to maintain competence, and to continue personal and professional growth. Respect extends to oneself as well; the same duties that nurses owe to others they owe to themselves. *Self-regarding duties* refer to a realm of duties that primarily concern oneself and include professional growth and maintenance of competence, preservation of wholeness of character, and personal integrity. Although competence, integrity, and learning goals are seemingly correct answers, duty to self describes this scenario in whole. (American Nurses Association: *Code for*

nurses with interpretive statements, Washington, DC, 2001, The Association.)

2.65. Correct Answer: **b**
Nurse educators act in collaboration with their students to assess the learning needs of the student, the effectiveness of the teaching program, the identification and utilization of appropriate resources, and the support needed for the learning process. Nurse educators must ensure that only those students who possess the knowledge, skills, and competencies that are essential to the nursing graduate from their respective nursing programs. (American Nurses Association: *Code for nurses with interpretive Washington, DC, 2001, The Association.*)

2.66. Correct Answer: **c**
In ethical decision making, the goal is to determine right from wrong in certain situations. There are legal parameters to consider that look at the rules and regulations, and there are values to look at that are subject to philosophic, moral, and individual interpretation. When ethical dilemmas arise, the law influences the ethical decision and ethics influences the legal decision. They are interwoven and overlapping. (Quinn D, Schick L, editors: *PeriAnesthesia nursing core curriculum: preoperative, Phase I and Phase II PACU nursing*, Philadelphia 2004, Saunders.)

2.67. Correct Answer: **d**
There are three fundamental theories or systems within which the nurse makes bioethical decisions: utilitarianism, deontology, and virtue ethics. Utilitarianism is a moral theory or system in which nursing action is judged on the outcomes or consequences. Specifically, the nurse chooses the action that has the greatest usefulness for

the greatest number of people. Under deontology, the action of the nurse is right or wrong based on ethical principles, not the consequences. It is a system of ethics in which ethical decisions are made based on the duty of the nurse specified within ethical principles. Virtue ethics is synonymous with character ethics and is based on the assumption that nursing actions are determined by innate moral virtues. Utilitarianism allows for decisions to be based on the "greatest good for the greatest number." (Quinn D, Schick L, editors: *PeriAnesthesia nursing core curriculum: preoperative, Phase I and Phase II PACU nursing*, Philadelphia, 2004, Saunders; O'Keefe ME: *Nursing practice and the law*, Philadelphia, 2001, FA Davis.)

2.68. Correct Answer: **b**
Freedom of action as chosen by an individual is the definition of the ethical principle of autonomy. In this scenario, even after a thorough explanation of the proposed surgery with benefits, risks, and alternatives explained, the patient has decided to refuse consent for the surgery. He is exercising his autonomy by freely choosing an action and making that decision. Autonomy is the freedom to be self-regulating. According to E.K. Dvorak, the principle of autonomy has two distinct features that allow: (1) the patient the right to be left alone or untreated and/or (2) the patient to be considered the best judge of the best treatment for his or her needs. This ethical concept is perhaps the first and the most important consideration in patient care. (Quinn D, Schick L, editors: *PeriAnesthesia nursing core curriculum: preoperative, Phase I and Phase II PACU nursing*, Philadelphia, 2004, Saunders; O'Keefe ME: *Nursing practice and the law*, Philadelphia, 2001, FA Davis; Personal

communication with E.K. Dvorak, noted in O'Keefe ME, November 22, 1998.)

2.69. Correct Answer: **d**
The most common forms of ethical analysis and ethical decision making in nursing practice are conducted through the following models: (1) principled ethics, (2) clinical ethics, (3) feminist ethics, and (4) casuistry. Casuistry refers to a variety of forms of case-based reasoning. All these decision-making models are based on respect, truth-telling, and doing well for the patient. Deontology is an ethical system or theory of ethics within which the nurse makes bioethical decisions. (Drain CB: *Perianesthesia nursing: a critical care approach*, ed 4, Philadelphia, 2003, Saunders; O'Keefe ME: *Nursing practice and the law*, Philadelphia, 2001, FA Davis.)

2.70. Correct Answer: **a**
Morals are one's sense of good and bad, right and wrong. The evolution of the nursing code of ethics, or professional values and standards of nursing practice, has been of historical significance to the development of health care and thus nursing practice. It is believed that the spiritual beliefs and religious practices and the evolution of the role of women have specifically influenced the moral foundation of nursing practice. The use of a moral framework allows nurses to identify sources of ethical conflict. (O'Keefe ME: *Nursing practice and the law*, Philadelphia, 2001, FA Davis; Drain CB: *Perianesthesia nursing: a critical care approach*, ed 4, Philadelphia, 2003, Saunders.)

2.71. Correct Answer: **b**
Life-sustaining medical treatment is health care used to maintain the patient's life, which may be categorized as ordinary or extraordinary.

Ordinary medical treatment offers the patient a good prognosis, without excessive pain or expense. Extraordinary medical treatment, synonymous with the term *heroic measures*, offers the patient little to no hope, with the prospect of a prolonged, expensive, and/or painful life. If the prognosis is dire and a fatal outcome is likely, discussion of treatment options should include realistic options that will promote the medical treatment goals agreed on by both physician and patient. If patients are offered marginally effective or futile medical treatment that will not change the outcome, they may be very disappointed. (O'Keefe ME: *Nursing practice and the law*, Philadelphia, 2001, FA Davis; Drain CB: *Perianesthesia nursing: a critical care approach*, ed 4, Philadelphia, 2003, Saunders.)

2.72. Correct Answer: **d**
Euthanasia means an action or inaction designed to result in an easy, painless, or good death. There are three subcategories of euthanasia. The first subcategory, voluntary euthanasia, occurs when the patient, after informed consent, refuses treatment. The second subcategory, involuntary euthanasia, results when treatment is withheld or withdrawn without informed consent. The third subcategory, nonvoluntary euthanasia, results when treatment is withheld or withdrawn without knowledge of what the patient would have wanted. Intentionally ending the life of a terminally ill, competent patient occurs when the patient, after being informed of all of the outcomes, refuses treatment of any kind and prefers to die. (O'Keefe ME: *Nursing practice and the law*, Philadelphia, 2001, FA Davis.)

2.73. Correct Answer: **a**
Nurses are obligated by their professional code of ethics with certain responsibilities to patients. ASPAN's *Perianesthesia Standards for Ethical Practice* indicates in the "Responsibility to Patients" section that the perianesthesia nurse "aggressively provides pain control and other comfort measures." The measures nurses take to care for the patient enable the patient to live with as much physical, emotional, social, and spiritual well-being as possible. Nursing care aims to maximize the values that the patient has treasured in life and extends supportive care to the family and significant others. Nursing care is directed toward meeting the comprehensive needs of patients and their families across the continuum of care. This is particularly vital in the care of patients and their families at the end of life to prevent and relieve the cascade of symptoms and suffering that are commonly associated with dying. The nurse should provide interventions to relieve pain and other symptoms in the dying patient even when those interventions entail risks of hastening death. (American Nurses Association: *Code for nurses with interpretive statements*, Washington, DC, 2001, The Association; ASPAN: *2006-2008 Standards of perianesthesia nursing practice*, Part II, Cherry Hill, NJ, 2006, ASPAN; Scanlon C: *End-of-life care: ethical dimensions*, 2002, Glaxo Wellcome, Inc.)

2.74. Correct Answer: **a**
Initial treatment of malignant hyperthermia (MH) crisis requires many vials of dantrolene sodium, sterile water for injection to mix the dantrolene, cold IV saline for infusion, cooling blankets, and hyperventilation of 100% oxygen via bag-valve-mask. The patient may or may not be intubated. Electrolytes are checked initially, especially potassium. Succinylcholine and all volatile inhalation anesthetics are

considered triggering agents of MH and are not given to any patient with suspected MH. Sodium bicarbonate is considered a secondary step. (ASPAN: Resource 5 in *2006-2008 Standards of perianesthesia nursing practice,* Cherry Hill, NJ, 2006, ASPAN; Malignant Hyperthermia Association of the United States. Website: www.mhaus. org/index.cfm/fuseaction/Content. Display/PagePK/Home.cfm. Accessed February 2007.)

2.75. Correct Answer: **c**
Resource 5 states that each patient bedside will be equipped with eight types of equipment or supplies. These include various types and sizes of artificial airways, constant and intermittent suction; various means of oxygen delivery; means to monitor blood pressure; adjustable lighting; capacity to ensure patient privacy; ECG monitor; and pulse oximeter. (ASPAN: Resource 5 in *2006-2008 Standards of perianesthesia nursing practice,* Cherry Hill, NJ, 2006, ASPAN.)

2.76. Correct Answer: **b**
When an expert nurse "thinks aloud," the student hears the rationale behind specific nursing actions. Narratives reveal a nurse's judgment and reflect the skills embedded in patient assessment and nurse decision making. Sharing these will assist the student's learning process and help nurses highlight essential elements of practice. (Corcoran S, Narayan S, Moreland H: "Thinking aloud" as a strategy to improve clinical decision making, *Heart Lung* 17(5):465-568, 1988; Feldman ME: Uncovering clinical knowledge and caring practices, *J Post Anesth Nurs* 8(3):159-162, 1993; Benner P: *From novice to expert: excellence and*

power in clinical nurse practice, Menlo Park, Calif, 1984, Addison-Wesley.)

2.77. Correct Answer: **a**
Research consistency requires each data collector (rater) to consider each subject with identical tools and criteria. Observational research methods are vulnerable to human error. Researchers educate observers to maximize accuracy and reliability of data and to minimize bias and then evaluate the observers in a practice session and compare their answers for agreement. (Polit DF, Hungler BP: *Nursing research: principles and methods,* ed 5, Philadelphia, 1995, Lippincott; Litwack K, editor: *ASPAN's core curriculum for post anesthesia nursing practice,* ed 3, Philadelphia, 1994, Saunders.)

2.78. Correct answer: **a**
The PACU is considered a critical care area. ASPAN's *2006-2008 Standards of Perianesthesia Nursing Practice* recommends that the RN practicing in a perianesthesia area achieve competencies related to airway management, circulatory support, comfort, and thermoregulation. In addition, ASPAN standards recommend ACLS certification. Content in a recommended competency-based education program includes critical care concepts for dysrhythmia identification, pharmacologic interventions, and defibrillation or cardioversion techniques. Appropriate documentation includes written tests, algorithm knowledge, and return demonstration. (ASPAN: Standard III and Resource 13 in *2006-2008 Standards of perianesthesia nursing practice,* Cherry Hill, NJ, 2006, ASPAN.)

Chapter 3

Perianesthesia Considerations Across the Life Span

Caring for pediatric, adolescent, obstetric, and older adult patients in the perianesthesia setting can be challenging. Pregnancy and age—either young or old—challenge the perianesthesia nurse to look closely at the specific needs of these populations. The anatomic and physiologic changes in these populations profoundly influence the way patients recover from the stress of surgery and anesthesia. As you prepare for the certification examinations, much valuable information about the anesthesia and perianesthesia care these patient populations require can be found close to home. The Core Curriculum has several excellent chapters about these specialty populations. The *Journal of PeriAnesthesia Nursing* has provided some outstanding articles addressing the needs of these patients.

ESSENTIAL CORE CONCEPTS	AFFILIATED CORE CURRICULUM CHAPTERS
Nursing Process	**Chapters 3, 13, 14, 15, 16, 26**
Assessment	
Planning and Implementation	
Evaluation	
The Pediatric/Adolescent Patient	**Chapters 13, 14**
Anatomy: Child vs. Adult	
Developmental Concepts	
Education	
Family Dynamics	
Psychosocial	
Perianesthesia Issues	
Airway Compromises	
Anesthetic Specifics for Children	
Operative Specifics for Children	
Specific Patient Care Concerns	
Awakening, Restlessness, and Emesis	
Pain Management: Drugs and Alternatives	
Thermal Balance	
Parent Education	

The Obstetric Patient

Chapter 46

Physiology of Pregnancy
Expected Organ Systemic Changes
Managing Organ Pathophysiology
Pregnancy-associated Disorders
Assessing Preterm Labor
Hemorrhagic Emergencies
Hypertension: Eclampsia and Seizures
Postpartum/Postcesarean Observation
Perianesthesia Specifics
Anesthetic Options
Pharmacologic Interventions
Observation of Mother and Fetus After
  Surgery

The Geriatric Patient

Chapter 16

Physiology of Aging
Age-related Organ Dysfunction
Pharmacologic Responses
Anesthetic Options
Prescribed Medications
Perianesthesia Specifics
Barriers: Special Needs
Education Considerations
Risk Factors and Disease
Ventilation, Temperature, Fluids, and Comfort

SET 1

ITEMS 3.1-3.30

3.1. A 4-year-old boy is admitted to the PACU after a biopsy of a mass of the tibia under general anesthesia. He is incoherent, crying, thrashing, and kicking. His behavior is non-purposeful. The nurse should immediately assess the patient for signs and symptoms of:
a. hypoxemia and hypercarbia.
b. hemodynamic instability.
c. inadequate reversal.
d. fever and sepsis.

NOTE: Consider the scenario and items 3.2-3.3 together.

A 3 year-old girl is admitted to the preoperative unit for an elective tonsillectomy and adenoidectomy. She has a history of recurrent upper respiratory infections (URI) and currently has a runny nose with a slight, nonproductive cough.

3.2. A thorough preanesthesia assessment for this child will include assessing for these signs and symptoms.
a. Sore throat and tachycardia
b. Fever and congestion
c. Sneezing and clear secretions
d. Anxiety and history of asthma

3.3. Careful preoperative assessment of the pediatric airway is essential because postanesthesia pediatric patients are at great risk for:
a. emergence delirium.
b. airway hyperreactivity.
c. prolonged recovery.
d. pulmonary emboli.

3.4. The anesthesiologist has ordered midazolam to be given by mouth (PO) to a 15-kilogram 3-year-old child for preoperative sedation. What dosage of midazolam should the nurse administer?
a. 2.5 mg
b. 3 mg
c. 5 mg

d. 7.5 mg

3.5. A 9-month-old infant is admitted to the PACU after a Nissen fundoplication. His heart rate is 175 beats per minute (bpm), blood pressure is 50/38, and axillary temperature is 36.6° C (97.9° F). Admission assessment also reveals periorbital edema, grunting respirations, and adventitious lung sounds. The PACU nurse is most concerned about:
a. hyperthermia.
b. pain.
c. respiratory distress.
d. hypervolemia.

NOTE: Consider the scenario and items 3.6-3.8 together.

A 22-year-old woman who is 7 months pregnant is admitted to the PACU after a cholecystectomy under general anesthesia. The patient is placed on supplemental oxygen.

3.6. This patient has an increased potential for pulmonary aspiration because:
a. general anesthesia increases lower esophageal sphincter tone.
b. gastric acidity increases and varies widely during pregnancy.
c. gastric motility and emptying time are decreased in pregnancy.
d. uterine contractions stimulate the chemoreceptor zone.

3.7. A priority of care for the pregnant patient in the PACU is:
a. providing emotional support.
b. assessing and treating pain.
c. monitoring vital signs.
d. meeting oxygen demand.

3.8. After 10 minutes in the PACU, this patient states "All of a sudden I feel nauseated and faint." The patient's blood pressure has dropped from 130/70 to

110/60. An initial nursing intervention would be:

a. turning the patient to a left lateral position.
b. increasing the oxygen liter flow.
c. medicating the patient for nausea.
d. administering an IV fluid bolus.

3.9. Hypothermia in a small child can lead to:

a. hypoxemia, hypoglycemia, and metabolic acidosis.
b. hypercarbia, hypoglycemia, and metabolic alkalosis.
c. hypoxemia, hyperglycemia, and metabolic acidosis.
d. hypercarbia, hyperglycemia, and metabolic acidosis.

NOTE: Consider the scenario and items 3.10-3.11 together.

A 16-year-old male patient under general anesthesia is admitted to the PACU after an anterior cruciate ligament (ACL) reconstruction. On admission to the PACU, he is alert and oriented. Blood pressure is 100/50, heart rate is 120, and respiratory rate is 28 breaths per minute. Oxygen saturation is 88% with oxygen in use at 4 liters per nasal cannula. When the patient speaks, he becomes dyspneic after three or four words and his oxygen saturation drops to 82%. Auscultation of breath sounds reveals scattered rales heard throughout all lung fields.

3.10. Understanding postanesthesia complications, what does the nurse suspect?

a. Anaphylactic reaction
b. Noncardiogenic pulmonary edema
c. Cardiogenic shock
d. Inadequate reversal

3.11. What mechanism of injury would cause this to occur?

a. Exposure to latex
b. Inadequate reversal
c. Breathing against a closed glottis
d. Mitral valve dysfunction

3.12. Vagal stimulation during anesthesia and surgery place pediatric patients at risk for:

a. tachycardia and normotension.
b. tachycardia and hypoxia.
c. bradycardia and hypotension.
d. bradycardia and hypoxia.

3.13. Postanesthesia shivering increases an older adult patient's risk of:

a. delayed awakening, acidosis, and decreased renal perfusion.
b. delayed awakening, alkalosis, and cardiopulmonary compromise.
c. hypoxia, alkalosis, and delayed drug metabolism.
d. hypoxia, acidosis, and cardiopulmonary compromise.

3.14. In the pediatric postanesthesia population, the majority of cardiac dysrhythmias and arrests are related to:

a. medication error.
b. respiratory failure.
c. cardiac anomaly.
d. hypothermia.

3.15. In completing a preanesthesia history of a 79-year-old patient, the nurse is well aware that one of the leading issues contributing to anesthesia-related mortality and morbidity in the older population is:

a. concurrent diseases.
b. sedentary lifestyle.
c. heredity.
d. physiologic changes.

3.16. Children are at increased risk for hypoxia secondary to:

a. decreased functional residual capacity and greater oxygen consumption.
b. increased functional residual capacity and slower glomerular filtration rate.
c. increased tidal volume and proportionally larger tongue than head.
d. smaller nares, narrower airways, and increased cardiac output.

3.17. The normal infant response to hypoxia is:

a. tachycardia.
b. cardiac arrest.
c. respiratory arrest.
d. bradycardia.

3.18. A 28-year-old woman has been admitted to the PACU after a cesarean section under spinal anesthesia. A magnesium sulfate infusion to treat preeclampsia was initiated 24 hours earlier. One indication for the use of magnesium sulfate in the preeclamptic patient is for:

a. preventing clotting alterations.
b. improving fetal oxygenation.
c. preventing seizure activity.
d. improving uterine contractions.

3.19. While assessing a 79-year-old patient in the PACU, the nurse is aware that elderly patients are at an increased risk for intraoperative myocardial infarction because general anesthesia:

a. impairs gas exchange.
b. depresses the myocardium.
c. alters drug metabolism.
d. affects cardiac reserve.

3.20. What age-group may believe postoperative pain is "punishment" for their thoughts or deeds?

a. Adolescent
b. School age
c. Pre-school
d. Toddler

3.21. Polypharmacy is common in many older adult patients because older patients:

a. need multiple medications to manage symptoms from many concurrent diseases.
b. often misunderstand medication administration directions and may not discontinue medications as ordered.
c. add over-the-counter medications, vitamins, minerals and supplements, and folk remedies.
d. seek treatment from a variety of health care providers and receive multiple prescriptions.

3.22. PACU assessment after cesarean section includes assessment for full bladder. A full bladder after delivery can cause:

a. boggy uterus and increased lochia.
b. boggy uterus and decreased lochia.
c. uterine displacement and atony.
d. uterine displacement and decreased lochia.

NOTE: Consider the scenario and items 3.23-3.26 together.

An 86-year-old female was found on the floor of her apartment by a neighbor. It is estimated that she fell 2 days earlier and fractured her hip. She was sent directly to the preoperative department from the emergency room.

3.23. The patient is oriented to person only and is alone. What is one of the initial interventions the preoperative nurse should consider as part of the pre-anesthesia assessment of an elderly patient?

a. Start an IV
b. Locate family
c. Assess pain
d. Check blood glucose

3.24. Considering physiologic changes associated with aging, what other diagnostic information will the preoperative nurse be certain to include in the preanesthesia assessment?

a. Electrocardiogram (ECG) and blood urea nitrogen (BUN)
b. Chest X-ray
c. Liver enzymes
d. Blood gases

3.25. After undergoing a hip pinning under spinal anesthesia, the patient is in the PACU. Her blood pressure is 130/86, heart rate is 48 bpm, and oxygen saturation is 96% on oxygen at 2 liters per nasal cannula. Estimated blood loss (EBL) was 900 mL. She remains oriented to person only and is not moving her lower extremities. Considering the physiologic changes that occur with aging, which of the following choices will the PACU nurse utilize to improve this patient's neurologic status?

a. Increase oxygen delivery
b. Administer a fluid bolus
c. Administer atropine
d. Assess patient's ability to hear

3.26. The patient's blood pressure is now 150/90. Her rhythm is normal sinus bradycardia with frequent premature ventricular contractions (PVCs) at a rate of 48 bpm. She is still not moving her lower extremities. What intervention, if any, is needed?

a. No intervention at all
b. Medicate for pain
c. Consider hypovolemia
d. Consider atropine

3.27. Oxytocin infused faster than 500 mL per hour can cause:

a. severe cramping and respiratory distress.
b. severe cramping and uterine atony.
c. hypertension and cardiac dysrhythmias.
d. hypotension and cardiac dysrhythmias.

3.28. When assessing a patient after delivery in the PACU, the PACU nurse understands that lochia is considered normal when:

a. two pads or more are saturated per hour.
b. it is brown in color with no clots.
c. it is red to dark red with no clots.
d. it is red to dark red with clots.

3.29. Nasal airways are generally not used in children younger than 6 years because at this age children have:

a. adenoidal hypertrophy.
b. smaller nares.
c. shorter necks.
d. wider tongues.

3.30. What is the IV fluid of choice when replacing volume in the geriatric patient?

a. 0.9% normal saline
b. D_5 0.45% normal saline
c. Lactated Ringer's
d. D_5 0.2% normal saline

SET 2

ITEMS 3.31–3.60

3.31. A 76-year-old man has been admitted to the PACU after a rotator cuff repair. His blood pressure is 160/90, and heart rate is 92 bpm with normal sinus rhythm. Oxygen saturation is 98% on oxygen at 2 liters per nasal cannula. He was given 2 mg of morphine sulfate approximately 5 minutes ago before leaving the OR. On a scale of 1 to 10, he now reports his pain as a "20." Which of the following interventions is now most appropriate?
a. Administer 1 mg of morphine sulfate
b. Administer a nonsteroidal antiinflammatory drug (NSAID)
c. Assess for another 5 minutes
d. Administer a different opioid

3.32. Uncuffed endotracheal tubes are generally used in children up to what age?
a. 3 years
b. 6 years
c. 9 years
d. 10 years

3.33. In the immediate postanesthesia period, what is the staffing guideline recommended by the ASPAN *2006-2008 Standards of Perianesthesia Nursing Practice* for a 6-year-old intubated and unconscious child?
a. One nurse to two patients
b. One nurse to one patient
c. Two nurses to one patient
d. One nurse and one aide/tech to one patient

3.34. A 34-year-old woman is admitted to the PACU after cesarean section under general anesthesia. A magnesium sulfate infusion, started 10 hours earlier during labor, continues. The PACU nurse will monitor this patient for the development of:
a. uterine atony.
b. coagulopathy.
c. hypertension.
d. respiratory depression.

3.35. An 18-month-old child is admitted to the PACU after a hernia repair. On admission to the PACU, his oxygen saturation is 100% on 4 liters of oxygen delivered by blow-by. As the pulse oximeter begins to indicate a decreasing saturation, the nurse:
a. continues to monitor the patient.
b. assesses the monitor for problems.
c. stimulates the child to breath.
d. assesses heart rate for bradycardia.

NOTE: Consider the scenario and items 3.36-3.37 together.

A 42-year-old woman is admitted to the PACU after delivery of a healthy baby boy. EBL for the delivery was 1500 mL. Admission assessment revealed blood pressure 130/90, normal sinus rhythm with heart rate of 89 bpm, oxygen saturation of 98% on oxygen at 2 liters per nasal cannula, and profuse bright-red lochia. One IV is patent and infusing well with 10 units of Pitocin added to the solution in the bag.

3.36. The immediate nursing intervention is to:
a. draw a complete blood count (CBC).
b. assess for pain.
c. change perineal (peri) pad.
d. assess for full bladder.

3.37. Which of the following next interventions is most appropriate?
a. Setting up patient-controlled analgesia (PCA) as per order
b. Starting a second large-bore IV
c. Assessing that Foley catheter is draining
d. Bringing the baby to his mother

3.38. Which of the following is most consistent with Standard II (Environment of Care) in ASPAN's *2006-2008 Standards of Perianesthesia Nursing Practice*?
a. Allowing parents into the PACU before the child arrives from the OR

b. Arranging for walls of pediatric areas to be painted in bright, friendly colors

c. Stocking "kid-friendly" snacks such as pizza and ice cream in Phase II

d. Creating a tackle box for transport with various sizes of pediatric masks

3.39. A 92-year-old woman is admitted to the PACU after a bowel resection under general anesthesia. Her blood pressure is 110/70, and heart rate is 62 bpm with normal sinus rhythm. Oxygen saturation is 97% on oxygen at 2 liters per nasal cannula. Her temperature on admission to the PACU was 34.6° C (94.3° F) orally. She has been in the PACU for one hour and remains very sleepy. Which of the following interventions could the nurse consider to help this patient awaken?

a. Administer low dose Narcan

b. Administer a fluid bolus

c. Apply warm blankets

d. Wipe her face with a cool cloth

3.40. A 4-year-old boy is admitted to the PACU after a hernia repair under general anesthesia. He is thrashing and yelling incoherently. His blood pressure is 78/45, and his heart rate is 138 bpm. The nurse's first intervention is to:

a. listen to breath sounds.

b. medicate for pain.

c. provide for safety.

d. bring the parents to his bedside.

3.41. Sevoflurane is known for causing:

a. airway irritation and spasm.

b. rapid induction and emergence.

c. hypotension and bradycardia.

d. respiratory depression and hypoxia.

3.42. The PACU nurse expects to see which of the following respiratory patterns in a sleeping geriatric patient?

a. More periods of irregularity and apnea

b. Prolonged expiratory phase

c. Decreased depth of respirations

d. Prolonged inspiratory phase

3.43. A 4-year-old has been given chloral hydrate for outpatient magnetic resonance imaging (MRI). In the immediate postanesthesia phase of his care, the nurse is most concerned about which of the following complications?

a. Respiratory depression

b. Nausea and vomiting

c. Delayed recovery

d. Loss of airway patency

3.44. Factors that increase the potential for post-extubation laryngeal edema in children includes all of the following *except:*

a. coughing while intubated.

b. Down syndrome.

c. preoperative asthma.

d. surgery in prone position.

3.45. Which of the following most common beliefs among older adults must the nurse consider when teaching older patients about the use of pain medications?

a. Pain medication should not be taken because pain is healthy and necessary.

b. Medication should be taken only when pain is severe because of possibility of addiction.

c. Pain should be tolerated, and only "weak" people take pain medication.

d. Pain is expected, and taking pain medication will lead to tolerance.

3.46. Older adults are at greater risk for post-anesthesia respiratory complications, because in the older adult, common changes to anatomy and physiology include:

a. decreased lung compliance.

b. increased chest wall compliance.

c. decreased total lung capacity.

d. decreased area for gas exchange.

3.47. The endotracheal tube size required to reintubate an average-sized 6-year-old male patient is:

a. 2.5 mm.

b. 4.0 mm.

c. 5.5 mm.

d. 7.0 mm.

3.48. A 24-year-old woman is admitted to the PACU after a laparotomy for an ectopic pregnancy. What critical piece of

information is the PACU nurse most interested in hearing from the anesthesia care provider in report?
a. Time of last opioid
b. Preoperative emotional state
c. Amount of fluids given
d. Estimated blood loss

NOTE: Consider items 3.49-3.50 together.

3.49. An infant born 2 months premature is now 4 months old and has had general anesthesia for an ophthalmic procedure. The PACU nurse expects to observe a respiratory pattern characterized by:
a. episodic apnea.
b. stridor with retraction.
c. bradypnea and tachypnea.
d. a barking cough.

3.50. The management of this infant's care will most likely include close nursing observation and:
a. intubation and mechanical ventilation for 5 hours.
b. pulse oximeter in PACU for 10 hours.
c. overnight hospitalization and apnea monitoring.
d. discharge home if no apnea occurs in 4 hours.

3.51. Disseminating intravascular coagulation (DIC) in obstetric patients is treated with:
a. fresh frozen plasma (FFP), platelets, and cryoprecipitate.
b. packed red blood cells (PRBCs), platelets, and cryoprecipitate.
c. FFP, PRBCs, and platelets.
d. PRBCs, FFP, and hetastarch.

NOTE: Consider the scenario and items 3.52-3.53 together.

A 32-year-old woman who is 7 months pregnant is now in the PACU after an appendectomy under spinal anesthesia.

3.52. When the nurse asks the patient how she is feeling, the patient replies, "I feel a little odd. I'm feeling a lot of pressure, kind of like I have a full bladder but only more intense. I think I feel a little

crampy but that just might be from this backache." The nurse suspects:
a. that the spinal is resolving.
b. positioning discomfort.
c. preterm labor.
d. postoperative pain.

3.53. The nurse expects which of the following primary interventions?
a. Check blood pressure
b. Increase fluids
c. Reposition patient
d. Medicate for pain

3.54. A commonly held attitude among adolescent patients about pain is:
a. "The nurse should know I'm in pain. I should not have to ask for pain medication."
b. "I can't wait to get high. How much pain medication can I have?"
c. "I don't want any pain medication. I don't want to get addicted."
d. "I don't want to ask for pain meds. I don't want anyone to think I'm weak."

3.55. A 4-year-old boy is admitted to the PACU after a surgical procedure done under general anesthesia. He had been intubated for 90 minutes. As the patient wakes up, the nurse notices a mild degree of inspiratory stridor. The patient's oxygen saturation is 100% on oxygen at 10 liters delivered via blowby. The nurse is most concerned about:
a. laryngospasm.
b. respiratory depression.
c. croup.
d. aspiration.

3.56. All the following are associated with croup *except:*
a. irritation from intubation.
b. inspiratory stridor.
c. a hoarse bark-like cough.
d. a mucous plug.

3.57. Hypotension in pediatric patients is usually *not* related to:
a. inhalation agents.
b. inadequate fluid replacement.
c. opioid administration.

d. emergence delirium.

3.58. When communicating with adolescent patients, the nurse understands:
a. that they are generally not interested in interacting with adults.
b. that explanations should be directed to parents.
c. that they are not interested in a lot of information.
d. to avoid teasing and use humor cautiously.

3.59. In infants, a sign of respiratory distress is respirations that are:
a. 18 breaths/minute.
b. 20 breaths/minute.
c. 45 breaths/minute.
d. 65 breaths/minute.

3.60. In Phase II recovery, the nurse witnesses a 3-year-old patient hitting his mother. The nurse recognizes this behavior as:
a. a sign of poor parenting.
b. normal regressive behavior.
c. abnormal "spoiled" behavior.
d. an abused child acting out.

SET 1

ANSWER KEY

3.1.	a		**3.16.**	a
3.2.	b		**3.17.**	d
3.3.	b		**3.18.**	c
3.4.	d		**3.19.**	b
3.5.	d		**3.20.**	c
3.6.	c		**3.21.**	a
3.7.	d		**3.22.**	c
3.8.	a		**3.23.**	d
3.9.	a		**3.24.**	a
3.10.	b		**3.25.**	a
3.11.	c		**3.26.**	c
3.12.	c		**3.27.**	d
3.13.	d		**3.28.**	d
3.14.	b		**3.29.**	a
3.15.	a		**3.30.**	c

SET 1

3.1. Correct Answer: **a**
Postanesthesia agitation in children is usually the result of pain or anxiety. However, current research identifies that agitation can also be a sign of hypoxia and hypercarbia. Although it is difficult to assess an agitated child, current literature suggests that before medicating an agitated child with an analgesic or anxiolytic, the nurse should perform a thorough respiratory assessment to rule out hypoxia and/or hypercarbia. (Voepel-Lewis T et al: Nurses' diagnoses and treatment decisions regarding care of the agitated child, *J PeriAnesth Nurs* 20[4]:239-248, 2005.)

3.2. Correct Answer: **b**
The challenge to the preoperative nurse is to assess the child with an active URI to identify the origin of the infection. Children with URI caused by a viral infection have shown an increased risk of an irritable airway while under anesthesia and an increased risk of oxygen desaturation postanesthesia. Careful evaluation of the child with a URI in the preanesthesia holding room may indicate the need to postpone the surgical procedure for the safety of the patient. (Tait A, Voepel-Lewis T, Malviya S: Perioperative considerations for the child with an upper respiratory tract infection, *J PeriAnesth Nurs* 15[6]:392-396, 2000.)

3.3. Correct Answer: **b**
Children recovering from anesthesia are at risk for airway spasm. "Bronchospasm can occur as children are emerging from anesthesia, especially children with a history of hyperactive airway disease and long-term treatment with

bronchodilators (i.e., asthmatic patients)." (Zaglaniczny K, Aker J, editors: *Clinical guide to pediatric anesthesia*, Philadelphia, 1999, Saunders.)

3.4. Correct Answer: **d**
The correct dosage of oral midazolam for the pediatric patient is 0.5 mg/kg. (Malviya S et al: Sedation/analgesia for diagnostic and therapeutic procedures in children, *J PeriAnesth Nurs* 15[6]:415-422, 2000; Gregory G, editor: *Pharmacology in pediatric anesthesia*, ed 4, Philadelphia, 2002, Churchill Livingstone.)

3.5. Correct Answer: **d**
Infants and toddlers are at risk for hypervolemia via two mechanisms. Excessive fluid administration is one cause of hypervolemia in pediatric patients. A physiologic response to the stress of surgery provides the second mechanism that places infants and toddlers at risk for hypervolemia. In response to the stress of surgery, an increase in antidiuretic hormone and aldosterone is produced. This response causes the infant and toddler body to conserve fluids. (Quinn D, Schick L, editors: *ASPAN's perianesthesia nursing core curriculum: preoperative, Phase I and Phase II PACU nursing*, Philadelphia, 2004, Saunders.)

3.6. Correct Answer: **c**
Physiologic changes that occur during pregnancy include decreased gastric motility and gastroesophageal sphincter tone caused by increased maternal progesterone. As the uterus becomes larger, the stomach and intestines are displaced upward, which delays gastric

emptying time. The physiologic changes of pregnancy increase the patient's risk for aspiration. Because of this increased risk, pregnant patients should be treated with the same precautions used for a patient with a full stomach. (Shaver M, Shaver D: Perioperative assessment of the obstetric patient undergoing abdominal surgery, *J PeriAnesth Nurs* 20[3]:160-166, 2005; Quinn D, Schick L, editors: *ASPAN's perianesthesia nursing core curriculum: preoperative, Phase I and Phase II PACU nursing*, Philadelphia, 2004, Saunders.)

3.7. Correct Answer: **d**
During pregnancy, maternal cardiac output increases by 30% to 50% to meet an increasing metabolic rate of 15% to 20%. Maternal heart rate increases by 10 to 15 bpm to meet the increased oxygen requirements of both mother and baby. Respiratory changes also occur to help meet this increased demand for oxygen. Tidal volume and the rate of ventilation also increase to meet the increased demand for oxygen by both mother and fetus and the need for increased elimination of carbon dioxide. Physiologic changes of pregnancy and the demands of the fetus create an increased demand for oxygen. Surgical factors and anesthesia may also increase the demand for oxygen in both mother and fetus and alter carbon dioxide elimination through hypoventilation. Therefore meeting oxygen demand is a priority for the care of the pregnant patient in the PACU. (Noble K: The critically ill obstetric patient, *J PeriAnesth Nurs* 20[3]: 211-214, 2005; Quinn D, Schick L, editors: *ASPAN's perianesthesia nursing core curriculum: preoperative, Phase I and Phase II PACU nursing*, Philadelphia, 2004, Saunders.)

3.8. Correct Answer: **a**
"At approximately 24 weeks' gestation, the uterus is large enough to compress the vena cava when the mother is supine. This compression causes a decrease in venous return to the heart, a decrease in cardiac output, and a drop in maternal blood pressure, known as *supine hypotension*. When this occurs, the mother may feel faint or nauseated. Assisting the mother to assume a left lateral position will decrease the compression and relieves the symptoms." (Shaver M, Shaver D: Perioperative assessment of the obstetric patient undergoing abdominal surgery, *J PeriAnesth Nurs* 20[3]:160-166, 2005.)

3.9. Correct Answer: **a**
Several anatomic and physiologic factors place the infant and small child at an increased risk for hypothermia. Risk for hypothermia is increased as a result of physiologic stress, increased body surface area, decreased mass, and lack of insulating subcutaneous fat. Perioperative factors that increase the risk for hypothermia in this population are vasodilation from anesthetic agents and cool environment, room temperature, and IV fluids. Hypothermia increases oxygen consumption, depletes metabolic energy stores, and causes fluid and electrolyte imbalance. The end result of these changes to the pediatric patient is hypoxemia, hypoglycemia, and metabolic acidosis. (Quinn D, Schick L, editors: *ASPAN's perianesthesia nursing core curriculum: preoperative, Phase I and Phase II PACU nursing*, Philadelphia, 2004, Saunders.)

3.10. Correct Answer: **b**
The patient's age, type of anesthesia, and clinical symptoms suggest

noncardiogenic pulmonary edema. Noncardiogenic pulmonary edema can occur when a strong patient takes a breath against a closed glottis. Classic symptoms of pulmonary edema include dyspnea, wheezing, rales, hypoxia, and pink, frothy sputum. As a young healthy person, this patient is capable of creating the intrathoracic negative pressure that is needed to result in noncardiogenic pulmonary edema. General anesthesia offers the opportunity for the patient to breathe against a closed glottis. (Quinn D, Schick L, editors: *ASPAN's perianesthesia nursing core curriculum: preoperative, Phase I and Phase II PACU nursing*, Philadelphia, 2004, Saunders.)

3.11. Correct Answer: **c**
When a strong, young patient attempts to breathe against a closed glottis, negative pressure increases within the chest cavity. The increased negative pressure causes a sharp increase in hydrostatic pressure that in turn pulls water into the alveoli. The result is noncardiogenic pulmonary edema. (Quinn D, Schick L, editors: *ASPAN's perianesthesia nursing core curriculum: preoperative, Phase I and Phase II PACU nursing*, Philadelphia, 2004, Saunders.)

3.12. Correct Answer: **c**
Multiple factors may cause bradycardia and hypotension in infants and children. "The brisk nature of their vagal reflexes on instrumentation of the airway, especially during light levels of anesthesia, may lead to serious bradycardia." Gastric tube insertion in the neonate may result in significant bradycardia. Anesthetic agents such as succinylcholine can also cause bradycardia in infants and children. Halothane produces decreased myocardial contractility, heart rate, and cardiac output. Infants also respond to a variety of physiologic stimuli that occur during surgery and anesthesia by becoming seriously bradycardic. Bradycardia occurs in infants because the autonomic innervation of the heart is predominantly parasympathetic. Because cardiac output reflects heart rate multiplied by stroke volume, bradycardia results in hypotension. (Gregory G, editor: *Preoperative evaluation and preparation for surgery in pediatric anesthesia*, ed 4, Philadelphia, 2002, Churchill Livingstone.)

3.13. Correct Answer: **d**
Physiologic changes that occur with aging result in decreased renal perfusion and hepatic changes that result in slower drug metabolism. These changes ultimately do place the older adult patient at risk for delayed awakening. However, shivering increases oxygen consumption up to 400% in the older adult. This extreme increase in oxygen consumption increases the risk of hypoxia and acidosis and compromises the cardiopulmonary system. (Monarch S, Wren K: Geriatric anesthesia implications, *J PeriAnesth Nurs* 19[6]:379-384, 2004.)

3.14. Correct Answer: **b**
The majority of cardiac dysrhythmias and arrests in pediatric patients during the postanesthesia period are related to respiratory failure. The anatomy and physiology of the pediatric airway and medical conditions, such as asthma and allergies increase the pediatric patient's risk for respiratory failure. The PACU nurse places high priority on assessing, preventing, and treating respiratory issues because they may result in cardiac dysrhythmia or arrest. (Quinn D, Schick L, editors: *ASPAN's perianesthesia nursing core curriculum: preoperative, Phase I and Phase II PACU nursing*, Philadelphia, 2004, Saunders.)

3.15. Correct Answer: **a**
Active or unstable concurrent diseases present one of the biggest increased risk factors to older adults undergoing anesthesia. Although there are many predictable changes in the anatomy and physiology associated with aging, it is very difficult to predict where each patient is on the continuum of aging. Adults do not all age to the same extent at the same time. As we all have seen, not all 70-year-olds are alike! (Stevenson J: When the trauma patient is elderly, *J PeriAnesth Nurs* 19[6]:392-400, 2004.)

3.16. Correct Answer: **a**
"Children are at greater risk for hypoxia secondary to decreased functional residual capacity, higher closing volumes, and greater oxygen consumption." Pediatric airway issues, such as larger tongue proportionate to head, smaller nares, and narrower airways do contribute to postanesthesia airway concerns. However, functional residual capacity in children is of primary concern in the bigger picture of hypoxia. "Functional residual capacity is not nearly as effective in improving the oxygen reserve or acting as a buffer between pulmonary circulation and inspired gases because of the greater metabolic rate, the increased oxygen consumption, and the high degree of alveolar ventilation that exist." (Zaglaniczny K, Aker J, editors: *Clinical guide to pediatric anesthesia*, Philadelphia, 1999, Saunders.)

3.17. Correct Answer: **d**
Bradycardia occurs in infants because the autonomic innervation of the heart is predominantly parasympathetic. Because cardiac output reflects heart rate multiplied by stroke volume, bradycardia results in hypotension. (Gregory

G, editor: *Preoperative evaluation and preparation for surgery in pediatric anesthesia*, ed 4, Philadelphia, 2002, Churchill Livingstone.)

3.18. Correct Answer: **c**
"Magnesium sulfate is used in the preeclamptic patient to decrease the release of acetylcholine at the neuromuscular synapse, decreasing neuromuscular excitability, decreasing cerebral irritation, and depressing cardiac and smooth muscle contraction. Magnesium sulfate is used to decrease blood pressure, induce diuresis, and prevent seizure activity." (Noble K: The critically ill obstetric patient, *J PeriAnesth Nurs* 20[3]: 211-214, 2005.)

3.19. Correct Answer: **b**
Many changes to the cardiovascular system occur with normal aging. Decreases in cardiac output, valvular compliance, diastolic ventricular filling, chronotropic ability, coronary artery flow, and maximum achievable heart rate are all common changes. Cardiovascular diseases common in older adults include dysrhythmias, hypertension, and coronary artery disease. Anesthesia acts as a myocardial depressant. Other intraoperative events such as hypoxia, hypovolemia, and hypothermia also stress the myocardium. (Stevenson J: When the trauma patient is elderly, *J PeriAnesth Nurs* 19[6]:392-400, 2004.)

3.20. Correct Answer: **c**
The preschool child engages in magical thinking and views the world from a child's perspective. (Quinn D, Schick L, editors: *ASPAN's perianesthesia nursing core curriculum: preoperative, Phase I and Phase II PACU nursing*, Philadelphia, 2004, Saunders.)

3.21. Correct Answer: **a**
Older adults may need to take more than one medication to manage

symptoms from several different concurrent diseases. Older adults have more concurrent disease states and conditions that require medications to manage. (Kuchta A, Golembiewski J: Medication use in the elderly patient: focus on the perioperative/perianesthesia setting, *J PeriAnesth Nurs* 19(6):415-427, 2004.)

3.22. Correct Answer: **c**
"A full bladder may lead to uterine atony and increased vaginal bleeding. Careful assessment of urinary drainage tubing and the volume of urinary output is needed." (Noble K: The critically ill obstetric patient, *J PeriAnesth Nurs* 20(3):211-214, 2005.)

3.23. Correct Answer: **d**
The patient's baseline neurologic status is unknown. Her history includes potentially lying on the floor in her apartment for 2 days before admission. A valuable piece of assessment information is a blood glucose level. "Hypoglycemia may precipitate the alteration in the level of consciousness because glucose intolerance, insulin resistance, and diabetes exist on a larger scale in the elderly population." (Stevenson J: When the trauma patient is elderly, *J PeriAnesth Nurs* 19[6]:392-400, 2004.)

3.24. Correct Answer: **a**
The most common cause of injury in the geriatric population is falls. Falls often occur as a result of syncope or physiologic changes such as cardiac dysrhythmia and orthostatic hypotension. Many cardiovascular changes occur with aging as well as concurrent diseases that affect the heart. Beta-blocker use, implantable pacemakers, and defibrillators are common in the elderly. The liver and kidneys also change considerably with aging. It is important to understand how well the

elderly patient's kidneys are functioning before anesthesia. Many anesthetic agents are eliminated via the kidneys. (Stevenson J: When the trauma patient is elderly, *J PeriAnesth Nurs* 19[6]:392-400, 2004; Kuchta A, Golembiewski J: Medication use in the elderly patient: focus on the perioperative/ perianesthesia setting, *J PeriAnesth Nurs* 19[6]:415-427, 2004.)

3.25. Correct Answer: **a**
Normal physiologic changes associated with aging include decreased cardiac output and decreased response to hypoxia or hypercarbia. Other pulmonary changes combine to make it difficult for the patient to meet baseline oxygen demand. In the presence of confusion in the elderly patient, both hypoglycemia and hypoxia should be evaluated and treated. (Stevenson J: When the trauma patient is elderly, *J PeriAnesth Nurs* 19[6]:392-400, 2004.)

3.26. Correct Answer: **c**
Hypertension in the elderly should be looked at with suspicion. Elderly patients may have hypertension with increased systemic vascular resistance. The patient has had a spinal anesthetic and is not yet able to move her legs. This would indicate that she may be affected by vasodilation secondary to autonomic blockade of the spinal. (Stevenson J: When the trauma patient is elderly, *J PeriAnesth Nurs* 19[6]:392-400, 2004.)

3.27. Correct Answer: **d**
Oxytocin, used to control bleeding by causing uterine contractions, is infused up *to 500* mL per hour. Faster infusion may cause hypotension or cardiac dysrhythmias. (Chichester M: When your patient is from the obstetric department:

postpartum hemorrhage and massive transfusion, *J PeriAnesth Nurs* 20[3]:167-176, 2005.

3.28. Correct Answer: **d**
In the immediate postdelivery patient, lochia is considered "rubra"—dark in color with clots. An absence of clots may indicate a diagnosis of early DIC. (Noble K: The critically ill obstetric patient, *J PeriAnesth Nurs* 20[3]:211-214, 2005; Quinn D, Schick L, editors: *ASPAN's perianesthesia nursing core curriculum: preoperative, Phase I and Phase II PACU nursing*, Philadelphia, 2004, Saunders.)

3.29. Correct Answer: **a**
Nasal airways are not frequently placed in pediatric patients because of adenoidal hypertrophy. Adenoidal hypertrophy peaks between 2 and 6 years of age. Nasal airways can cause bleeding in small patients with small nares. Because of the small internal diameter, pediatric nasal airways can actually increase the work of breathing. (Zaglaniczny K, Aker J, editors: *Clinical guide to pediatric anesthesia*, Philadelphia, 1999, Saunders.)

3.30. Correct Answer: **c**
Lactated Ringer's is the fluid of choice when giving fluid replacement in the geriatric population. Normal saline has the potential to cause hyperchloremic acidosis secondary to impaired renal functioning that occurs with aging. (Stevenson J: When the trauma patient is elderly, *J PeriAnesth Nurs* 19[6]:392-400, 2004.)

SET 2

ANSWER KEY

3.31.	c		**3.46.**	d
3.32.	c		**3.47.**	c
3.33.	b		**3.48.**	d
3.34.	d		**3.49.**	a
3.35.	c		**3.50.**	c
3.36.	a		**3.51.**	a
3.37.	b		**3.52.**	c
3.38.	d		**3.53.**	b
3.39.	c		**3.54.**	a
3.40.	a		**3.55.**	c
3.41.	b		**3.56.**	d
3.42.	a		**3.57.**	b
3.43.	d		**3.58.**	d
3.44.	c		**3.59.**	d
3.45.	b		**3.60.**	b

SET 2

RATIONALES AND REFERENCES

3.31. Correct Answer: **c**
The major sites of drug metabolism, the hepatic and renal systems, progressively decline throughout the process of aging. "The number of drug receptor sites also decreases along with albumin levels. This results in an increase of unbound drug available and an increased pharmacological effect. Slower circulation times delay onset of intravenously administered drugs." As drug metabolism slows as well as cardiac output in the geriatric patient, opioids should be used with caution. The onset of action of morphine sulfate is 5 minutes after IV administration. The most prudent course of action when using narcotics in the geriatric patient is to allow extra time between dosages to allow for physiologic alterations. (Monarch S, Wren K: Geriatric anesthesia implications, *J PeriAnesth Nurs* 19[6]: 379-384, 2004.)

3.32. Correct Answer: **c**
Cuffed endotracheal tubes (ET) are rarely used in children younger than 9 years. There is a normal narrowing of the trachea at the cricoid cartilage ring. This narrowing provides an "anatomic cuff" that eliminates the need for a cuff on the ET. (Quinn D, Schick L, editors: *ASPAN's perianesthesia nursing core curriculum: preoperative, Phase I and Phase II PACU nursing*, Philadelphia, 2004, Saunders.)

3.33. Correct Answer: **b**
The recommended standard is one nurse to one patient when the patient is unconscious and 8 years of age or younger. (ASPAN's *2006-2008 Standards of perianesthesia nursing practice*, Cherry Hill, NJ, 2006, ASPAN.)

3.34. Correct Answer: **d**
Common side effects from magnesium sulfate include decreased or absent deep tendon reflexes, respiratory depression, and cardiac arrest. Magnesium sulfate also places this patient at an increased risk for respiratory depression as she recovers from general anesthesia. (Shaver M, Shaver D: Perioperative assessment of the obstetric patient undergoing abdominal surgery, *J PeriAnesth Nurs* 20[3]:160-166, 2005.)

3.35. Correct Answer: **c**
Several physiologic reasons explain the pediatric patient's intolerance for hypoxia. In an infant or small child, the functional residual capacity is not effective in improving oxygen reserve or acting as a buffer between pulmonary circulation and inspired gases. These children have a greater metabolic rate, increased oxygen consumption, and a high degree of alveolar ventilation. Because the demand is greater and the reserve is less, when a small child's oxygen saturation begins to drop, action should be taken immediately. (Zaglaniczny K, Aker J, editors: *Clinical guide to pediatric anesthesia*, Philadelphia, 1999, Saunders.)

3.36. Correct Answer: **a**
Physiologic changes that occur during pregnancy cause the maternal body to become hyperdynamic. Cardiac output increases by 30% to 50%. Heart rate increases 10% to 20% because of blood volume overload and hormonal changes. It is because of these changes that

blood loss may reach 35% before hypovolemic shock occurs or before a change in blood pressure and heart rate can be seen. By the time the patient exhibits tachycardia and lowered blood pressure, EBL is already nearing 2000 mL. Unlike surgical blood loss, postpartum blood loss may be indicative of serious complications such as life-threatening hemorrhage and DIC. (Quinn D, Schick L, editors: *ASPAN's perianesthesia nursing core curriculum: preoperative, Phase I and Phase II PACU nursing*, Philadelphia, 2004, Saunders; Chichester M: When your patient is from the obstetric department: postpartum hemorrhage and massive transfusion, *J PeriAnesth Nurs* 20[3]:167-176, 2005.)

3.37. Correct Answer: **b**
Considering the physiology of pregnancy and the risk this patient has for postpartum hemorrhage, the nurse should anticipate the need for transfusion of blood products. Initiating a second IV before the patient decompensates further would be a prudent intervention. (Chichester M: When your patient is from the obstetric department: postpartum hemorrhage and massive transfusion, *J PeriAnesth Nurs* 20[3]:167-176, 2005.)

3.38. Correct Answer: **d**
Standard II states "PeriAnesthesia nursing practice promotes and maintains a safe, comfortable, and therapeutic environment for patients, staff and visitors." This standard also highlights the importance of patient safety including safe transport of patients. (ASPAN: *2006-2008 Standards of perianesthesia nursing practice*, Cherry Hill, NJ, 2004, ASPAN; Collett L, D'Errico C: Suggestions on meeting ASPAN standards in a pediatric setting, *J PeriAnesth Nurs* 15[6]:386-391, 2000.)

3.39. Correct Answer: **c**
In the geriatric patient, a decrease in temperature causes a decrease in metabolism. When metabolism slows, the elimination of the anesthetic agents also slows, which then delays awakening. Geriatric patients also have a decrease in muscle mass that places them at increased risk for hypothermia. (Asher M: Surgical considerations in the elderly, *J PeriAnesth Nurs* 19[6]:406-414, 2004.)

3.40. Correct Answer: **a**
Although pain and anxiety are the most common causes of post anesthesia agitation in the pediatric patient, other physiologic sources should also be explored. Hypoxemia and hypercarbia should be ruled out before medicating the patient for pain or anxiety. "Hypercarbia, even in the absence of hypoxia, can lead to central nervous system excitability and mild-to severe agitation." (Voepel-Lewis T et al: Nurses' diagnoses and treatment decisions regarding care of the agitated child, *J PeriAnesth Nurs* 20[4]: 239-248, 2005.)

3.41. Correct Answer: **b**
Sevoflurane is an inhalation agent with a low blood/gas solubility. This property allows for rapid induction and emergence. Sevoflurane is also known to cause "minimal airway irritation, decreasing the incidence of bronchospasm and laryngospasm." (Moos D: Sevoflurane and emergence behavioral changes in pediatrics, *J PeriAnesth Nurs* 20[1]:13-18, 2005.)

3.42. Correct Answer: **a**
Many changes in pulmonary function occur during the process of aging that put geriatric patients at great risk for postanesthesia respiratory complications. Among these many changes is the change in respiratory pattern. The respiratory

pattern of the older adult does include more periods of irregularity and apnea during sleep. (Monarch S, Wren K: Geriatric anesthesia implications, *J PeriAnesth Nurs* 19[6]:379-384, 2004.

3.43. Correct Answer: **d**
"Chloral hydrate has not been associated with respiratory depression. However, this drug does have the potential to cause loss of airway patency caused by relaxation of the geniohyoid and genioglossus muscles that support the tongue and upper airway." (Malviya S et al: Sedation/analgesia for diagnostic and therapeutic procedures in children, *J PeriAnesth Nurs* 15[6]:415-422, 2000.)

3.44. Correct Answer: **c**
Asthma is a reactive lower airway spasm that results in bronchospasm. Laryngeal edema occurs in the upper airway. Upper airway edema occurs in children for several reasons. The narrowest part of the pediatric airway in children younger than 5 years is the cricoid cartilage. Edema in this area is common as a result of irritation from endotracheal tubes. Potential for airway edema increases when the patient is in any position other than supine during the surgical procedure. Children with Down syndrome have a congenitally narrow larynx, which predisposes them to upper airway edema. (Carlson K, editor: *Certification review for perianesthesia nursing*, Philadelphia, 1996, Saunders; Gregory G, editor: *Pediatric anesthesia*, ed 4, Philadelphia, 2002, Churchill Livingstone.)

3.45. Correct Answer: **b**
When providing patient teaching to older adults about pain medication, the nurse should remember that the patients themselves may provide barriers to effective pain management. Older people often refuse

pain medication because they fear addiction to pain medication. Another very common belief among older adults is that pain medication should be taken only when pain is severe. Nurses caring for older adults in all areas of perianesthesia care should include teaching about the proper use of pain medication to older adults. Patients should be reminded that the incidence of addiction to postoperative opioids is very rare (<1%). Nurses should also remind patients to treat pain before it becomes severe and out of control. (Paynter D, Mamaril M: Anesthesia challenges in geriatric pain management, *J PeriAnesth Nurs* 19[6]: 385-391, 2004.)

3.46. Correct Answer: **d**
"The primary effect of aging on the pulmonary system is loss of elastic recoil, impairing the alveoli's ability to remain open." As a result of this loss of elastic recoil, the alveoli collapse. The exchange of oxygen coming into the alveoli and carbon dioxide leaving the alveoli cannot occur when the alveoli are collapsed. Therefore the older adult is at greater risk for hypoxia. With aging, lung compliance increases, chest wall compliance decreases, and total lung capacity stays fairly constant. (Monarch S, Wren K: Geriatric anesthesia implications, *J PeriAnesth Nurs* 19[6]:379-384, 2004.)

3.47. Correct Answer: **c**
The size of endotracheal tube (ET) required to intubate a child 2 years old or older is calculated by using this formula: 16 + age (y) divided by 4 = approximate size of ET. For this child, 16 + 6 = 22, 22 ÷ 4 = 5.5 mm. It is recommended that for children 9 to 18 months old, ET size is 4.0 mm. For children 3 to 9 months old, the recommended ET size is 3.5 mm. The recommended

ET size for neonates and infants to 3 months of age is 3.0 mm. Recommended ET size for premature infants is based on weight. For premature infants weighing <1000 g, the recommended ET size is 2.5 mm. For premature infants weighing >1000 g, the recommended ET size is 3.0 mm. (Zaglaniczny K, Aker J, editors: *Clinical guide to pediatric anesthesia*, Philadelphia, 1999, Saunders; Carlson K, editor: *Certification review for perianesthesia nursing*, Philadelphia, 1996, Saunders.)

3.48. Correct Answer: **d**
Pregnancy implanted outside the uterus is considered ectopic. A common complication of ectopic pregnancy is preoperative or intraoperative hemorrhage leading to shock. A priority of PACU care is to monitor the patient for signs/symptoms of blood loss because preoperative and intraoperative blood loss may be more than other diagnoses. (Quinn D, Schick L, editors: *ASPAN's perianesthesia nursing core curriculum: preoperative, Phase I and Phase II PACU nursing*, Philadelphia, 2004, Saunders.)

3.49. Correct Answer: **a**
"Periodic breathing occurs in 78% of full-term neonates, usually during quiet sleep." Apnea is considered to be central when periods of apnea last 15 seconds or longer. Central apnea refers to when a part of the brain, which controls breathing, does not maintain or start the breathing process. Central apnea is rare in full-term infants but very common in premature infants. "This apnea can be life-threatening and can occur up to 41 to 55 weeks after conceptual age in the preterm infant, particularly after surgical procedures and anesthesia." (Zaglaniczny K, Aker J, editors: *Clinical guide to pediatric*

anesthesia, Philadelphia, 1999, Saunders; Carlson K, editor: *Certification review for perianesthesia nursing*, Philadelphia, 1996, Saunders.)

3.50. Correct Answer: **c**
"In the premature infant, postoperative apnea can occur as long as 4 hours or more after surgery. Therefore all these patients probably should be monitored for 24 hours after surgery to detect apnea or periodic breathing. Infants who develop apnea postoperatively require mechanical ventilation for several hours to several days." (Gregory G, editor: *Pediatric anesthesia*, ed 4, Philadelphia, 2002, Churchill Livingstone; Carlson K, editor: *Certification review for perianesthesia nursing*, Philadelphia, 1996, Saunders.)

3.51. Correct Answer: **a**
During postpartum hemorrhage, there is an "intrinsic activation of the clotting cascade and the development of microclotting. This consumes clotting factors and platelets needed to control uterine bleeding." "Fresh frozen plasma provides coagulation factors to correct prothrombin time (PT) or partial thromboplastin time (PTT)." Platelets are given to replace either lost or dysfunctional platelets. Cryoprecipitate is needed to replace fibrinogen lost during hemorrhage. (Noble K: The critically ill obstetric patient, *J PeriAnesth Nurs* 20[3]:211-214, 2005; Chichester M: When your patient is from the obstetric department: postpartum hemorrhage and massive transfusion, *J PeriAnesth Nurs* 20[3]:167-176, 2005.)

3.52. Correct Answer: **c**
Preterm labor and delivery is a concern after abdominal surgery. Intraoperative uterine manipulation may

provide enough irritation to the uterus to stimulate contractions. "Preterm labor may present as restlessness or vague complaints of abdominal discomfort. The mother may complain of lower abdominal pressure or have increased vaginal discharge." (Shaver M, Shaver D: Perioperative assessment of the obstetric patient undergoing abdominal surgery, *J PeriAnesth Nurs* 20[3]:160-166, 2005.)

3.53. Correct Answer: **b**
Initial interventions used to treat preterm labor include bedrest, hydration, emptying the bladder, and position the patient in a lateral position. Dehydration can cause preterm labor, so increasing IV fluids for this patient is the best intervention of the options offered by the question. (Quinn D, Schick L, editors: *ASPAN's perianesthesia nursing core curriculum: preoperative, Phase I and Phase II PACU nursing*, Philadelphia, 2004, Saunders.)

3.54. Correct Answer: **a**
Adolescent patients may deal with the stress of surgery by using regressive behaviors. They may become more dependent on their parents. They may also expect the nurse to know when they are in pain and believe they should not have to ask for pain medication. As a result of these beliefs, adolescents may not ask for pain medication. (Quinn D, Schick L, editors: *ASPAN's perianesthesia nursing core curriculum: preoperative, Phase I and Phase II PACU nursing*, Philadelphia, 2004, Saunders.)

3.55. Correct Answer: **c**
Common causes of croup include irritation caused by intubation, traumatic or repeated attempts at intubation, coughing with an endotracheal tube in place, change of patient position while intubated, and surgical procedures longer than 1 hour in duration. Signs and symptoms of croup include stridor, thoracic retractions, hoarseness, and crouplike cough. This child was intubated for longer than 1 hour and has stridor. This assessment information and the fact that he was intubated for longer than 1 hour should make the nurse suspect croup. (Quinn D, Schick L, editors: *ASPAN's perianesthesia nursing core curriculum: preoperative, Phase I and Phase II PACU nursing*, Philadelphia, 2004, Saunders.)

3.56. Correct Answer: **d**
Croup is associated with upper airway irritation. It is characterized by inspiratory stridor, croupy cough, hoarseness, and upper airway irritation from intubation. Mucous plugs generally occur in the lower portions of the airway. (Quinn D, Schick L, editors: *ASPAN's perianesthesia nursing core curriculum: preoperative, Phase I and Phase II PACU nursing*, Philadelphia, 2004, Saunders.)

3.57. Correct Answer: **b**
The most common causes of postanesthesia hypotension in pediatric patients are inhalation agents, administration of opioids, and may be a late sign of shock. Emergence delirium would not be related to postanesthesia hypotension. Fluid management in pediatric patients is usually carefully calculated and administered throughout the surgical procedure so there is a small likelihood of hypotension related to hypovolemia, which would lead the nurse to most likely suspect inhalation agents and opioid use as the main causes. (Quinn D, Schick L, editors: *ASPAN's perianesthesia nursing core curriculum: preoperative, Phase I and Phase II PACU*

nursing, Philadelphia, 2004, Saunders.)

3.58. Correct Answer: **d**
Although teasing an adolescent may be tempting and may seem to be accepted, adolescents are easily embarrassed and may not appreciate the humor. (Quinn D, Schick L, editors: *ASPAN's perianesthesia nursing core curriculum: preoperative, Phase I and Phase II PACU nursing,* Philadelphia, 2004, Saunders.)

3.59. Correct Answer: **d**
The normal respiratory rate for an infant is 30 to 60 breaths/minute. Any rate greater than 60 breaths per minute signifies respiratory

distress. (Quinn D, Schick L, editors: *ASPAN's perianesthesia nursing core curriculum: preoperative, Phase I and Phase II PACU nursing,* Philadelphia, 2004, Saunders.)

3.60. Correct Answer: **b**
When the pre-school child becomes stressed, it is normal for him or her to display regressive behavior as a coping mechanism. This behavior may also indicate the child is in pain. (Quinn D, Schick L, editors: *ASPAN's perianesthesia nursing core curriculum: preoperative, Phase I and Phase II PACU nursing,* Philadelphia, 2004, Saunders.)

Chapter 4

Pharmacologic Considerations

Scenarios and items in this section focus on the *pharmacologic concerns* encountered in the practice of perianesthesia nursing. These concepts are considered together because:

- Anesthetic medications alter and usually depress the function of vital organ systems.
- Interactions among medications produce varied patient responses indicated by allergic reactions, potentiated effects, compatibility concerns, altered neuromuscular and cardiopulmonary function, and side effects or contraindications.
- Assessment, intervention, and evaluation of the pharmacologic effects specifically related to anesthetic medications and techniques are *primary* and essential nursing responsibilities.

ESSENTIAL CORE CONCEPTS	AFFILIATED CORE CURRICULUM CHAPTERS
Nursing Process	**Chapters 2, 3**
Assessment	
Planning and Implementation	
Evaluation	
Scope of Practice	
Standards of Care	
Pharmacologic Principles in Action	**Chapters 26, 27**
Anatomy and Physiology	
Agonists and Antagonists	
Dose, Onset and Duration of Action, Clearance	
Neurotransmitters, Reversal and Toxicity	
Receptors, Synapses, Vascular Tone, and Target Organs	
Responses: Same Medication, Different Sites	
Anesthetic Techniques	
Balanced	
Dissociative (Neuroleptic)	
Epidural	
General	
Intravenous (IV) Regional Block	
Local Infiltration	
Spinal	
Conscious Sedation	

Dermatome Assessment
Efficacy, Potency, and Tolerance
Enhancing and Inhibiting Pharmacologic
   Environment
Minimum Alveolar Concentration
Pharmacodynamics
Clinical Consequences
Pharmacokinetics
Absorption, Distribution, and Elimination
Unique Properties and Effects

Anesthetic Medications   **Chapter 26**

Actions and Consequences for:
   Inhalation Anesthetics
   Gaseous Inhalants
   Volatile Liquids
   IV Medications
   Barbiturates, Hypnotics, and Sedatives
   Dissociative and Induction Agents
   Narcotics and Antagonists
   Reversal of Effect
   Local Anesthetics
   Amides and Esters
   Assessing Blockade
   Regional Techniques
   Muscle Relaxants
   Assessing Neuromuscular Blockade
   Depolarizing Medications
   Nondepolarizing Medications
Reversal Medications and Influencing
   Factors

Perianesthetic Medication Potpourri

Anticholinergics

Antiemetics   **Chapters 35, 36**

Benzodiazepines   **Chapters 26, 27**

Bronchodilators

Cardioactive Drugs and Diuretics   **Chapter 32**

Corticosteroids
Nonsteroidal Antiinflammatory Drugs
   (NSAIDs)
Oxygen

ESSENTIAL CORE CONCEPTS	AFFILIATED CORE CURRICULUM CHAPTERS
Pharmacology of Cardiac Life Support	**Chapter 32**
"Tuning" Electrolyte and Acid-Base Balance	**Chapters 24, 25**
Managing Analgesia	**Chapter 29**

Managing Analgesia

Agonistic and Antagonistic
Management and Monitoring IV,
 Intramuscular (IM), Regional, PCA
Pain Receptors
Physiologic Stress Response

SET 1

4.1. The primary neurotransmitter of the parasympathetic nervous system is:
a. acetylcholine.
b. dopamine.
c. epinephrine.
d. norepinephrine.

4.2. A 56-year-old woman is scheduled for a laparoscopic cholecystectomy. She has a history of mitral valve prolapse, moderate obesity, and a childhood history of polio and rheumatic heart disease. Particularly for this patient, the pre-anesthesia nurse recognizes the importance of prophylactic:
a. heparin anticoagulation.
b. loop or osmotic diuretics.
c. cardiac digitalization.
d. broad-spectrum antibiotics.

4.3. Eliminating the systemic effects of a volatile anesthetic medication **most** varies with:
a. alveolar ventilation.
b. volume of distribution.
c. renal blood flow.
d. rate of hepatic clearance.

4.4. To alter blood pressure, hydralazine's **primary** physiologic effect is to:
a. release renin by constricting renal vasculature.
b. reduce cardiac contractile force.
c. dilate arterial smooth muscle.
d. increase myocardial rate.

4.5. All of the following medications tend to cause pain on injection **except:**
a. diazepam.
b. propofol.
c. ketamine.
d. methohexital.

4.6. By definition, minimum alveolar concentration (MAC) is the lowest concentration of an inhalation anesthetic that:

a. allows spontaneous breathing in half of patients.
b. sustains an effective half-life for stage IV anesthesia.
c. eliminates ventilation in 50% of patients at 0.5% anesthetic concentration.
d. eradicates movement to pain in 50% of patients.

4.7. A factor that **least** affects a patient's minimum alveolar concentration (MAC) requirement is the patient's:
a. age.
b. gender.
c. temperature.
d. circulation.

4.8. Pharmacokinetics involves the study of all of the following **except:**
a. biotransformation.
b. mechanism of action.
c. distribution.
d. absorption.

4.9. When compared with diazepam, an equivalent dose of midazolam is:
a. not comparable.
b. 2 to 4 times greater.
c. equivalent, milligram for milligram.
d. one-half to two-thirds less.

4.10. The "antidote" to treat anticholinesterase medication overdose is intravenous:
a. atropine sulphate.
b. edrophonium chloride.
c. dexamethasone.
d. azathioprine.

4.11. A patient with a documented penicillin allergy should **not** receive:
a. gentamicin.
b. imipenem.
c. cefazolin.
d. ciprofloxacin.

4.12. Which of the following drugs is associated with a higher incidence of nausea and vomiting?
   a. Propofol
   b. Midazolam
   c. Ketamine
   d. Etomidate

4.13. An infant's and child's initial response to induction of anesthesia with inhalation agents varies from the adult's response *primarily* because the infant's and child's:
   a. tissues are highly vascular.
   b. vital organs slowly absorb medications.
   c. sensitive airway tissues easily spasm.
   d. metabolic rate and oxygen demand are lower.

4.14. Effective 5-HT$_3$ receptor antagonists used for decreasing the rate of postoperative nausea and vomiting (PONV) include all of the following *except:*
   a. ondansetron.
   b. dolasetron.
   c. dexamethasone.
   d. granisetron.

4.15. Which of the following does *not* increase the block of nondepolarizing muscle relaxants?
   a. Calcium channel blockers
   b. Aminoglycosides
   c. Halothane
   d. Theophylline

4.16. A healthy 28-year-old woman is awake, alert, and oriented when admitted to the Phase I PACU at 9:50 AM after a 20-minute right carpal tunnel release. Vital signs are within 20% of preoperative measures. Anesthesia was by IV regional block with sedation and analgesia. At 9:55 AM, the PACU nurse notes that this patient is not responsive and observes generalized tonic-clonic motor activity. The *most likely* reason for this activity is:
   a. unidentified idiopathic convulsive disorder.

   b. extreme hyperventilation related to pain and anxiety.
   c. generalized central nervous system toxicity.
   d. hypoxemic seizure related to oversedation.

4.17. An IV regional technique involves:
   a. infiltrating the surgical site with a narcotic.
   b. injecting local anesthetic after obliterating blood flow.
   c. infusing nitroprusside to suppress local blood loss.
   d. instilling local anesthetic into intracellular fluid.

4.18. The most common mechanism of action of local anesthesia is:
   a. inhibition of sodium influx.
   b. inhibition of potassium efflux.
   c. prevention of potassium influx.
   d. decrease of threshold of sodium channels.

4.19. After carpal tunnel release with IV regional block, the *most* positive patient outcomes are achieved by:
   a. 100 mL fluid in a wound drain and SpO$_2$ measures of more than 91%.
   b. pain level rating of "1 to 2" and gradual release of one tourniquet in the Phase I PACU.
   c. immediate return of arm sensation and overhead suspension to limit edema.
   d. moderate motor control of extremity and minimal bleeding.

4.20. The inhalation anesthetic that is *most likely* to induce airway spasm is:
   a. desflurane.
   b. enflurane.
   c. halothane.
   d. isoflurane.

4.21. An inhalation anesthetic is eliminated *most slowly* from:
   a. renal medulla.
   b. cardiac tissue.
   c. blood-brain barrier.
   d. skeletal muscle.

4.22. Systemic toxicity of local anesthetics is ***not*** potentiated by:
a. pregnancy.
b. hypercarbia.
c. acidosis.
d. alkalosis.

4.23. Compared with intramuscular morphine, providing analgesia with a continuous epidural morphine infusion decreases all the following effects ***except:***
a. episodic somnolence and variable duration.
b. muscle activity and vomiting.
c. neuroendocrine stress responses.
d. incidence of pneumonia.

4.24. The epidural space contains the following anatomic structures ***except:***
a. blood vessels.
b. adipose tissue.
c. cerebrospinal fluid.
d. lymph capillaries.

4.25. Addition of epinephrine to local anesthesia solutions results in all the following ***except:***
a. prolongation of duration of anesthesia.
b. decrease in blockade intensity.
c. minimization of peak blood levels.
d. reduced surgical bleeding.

SET 2

ITEMS 4.26-4.53

4.26. Cocaine-induced hypertension and tachycardia occur through:
a. direct cholinergic stimulation.
b. lacing cocaine doses with epinephrine.
c. indirect glucocorticoid reflexes.
d. blocked norepinephrine reuptake.

4.27. Muscle relaxants metabolized by plasma cholinesterase include:
a. succinylcholine and atracurium.
b. succinylcholine and mivacurium.
c. rocuronium and mivacurium.
d. atracurium and rocuronium.

4.28. Which of the following statements regarding usage of beta blockers is **not** true?
a. Metoprolol is used to treat patients having an acute myocardial infarction.
b. Toxic effects of metoprolol are potentiated by volatile anesthetics.
c. Metoprolol is used to treat the patient with ventricular dysrhythmias.
d. Metoprolol is used to treat hypertension associated with methamphetamine abuse.

4.29. The drug of choice to treat renal and biliary colic is:
a. morphine sulfate.
b. codeine.
c. meperidine.
d. hydromorphone.

4.30. Side effects occurring with the administration of ketorolac include all the following **except:**
a. reversible inhibition of platelet aggregation.
b. bronchospasm in patients with an asthma history.
c. bronchospasm in patients with aspirin (ASA) sensitivity.
d. a decrease in liver transaminase plasma levels.

4.31. Safe administration of parenteral ketorolac includes all the following factors **except:**
a. providing effective narcotic analgesia before dosing.
b. reducing the dose for a 75-year-old, 48-kg woman.
c. limiting an IV loading dose to 15 to 30 mg.
d. determining any "breathing difficulty" when using aspirin.

4.32. Nalbuphine's specific opioid receptor actions include:
a. mu antagonist, kappa and sigma agonist.
b. mu and sigma agonist, kappa antagonist.
c. mu agonist, kappa and sigma antagonist.
d. pure mu, sigma and kappa antagonist.

4.33. What effect does magnesium have on the potency of muscle relaxants?
a. Increases potency of both depolarizing and nondepolarizing muscle relaxants
b. Decreases potency of both depolarizing and nondepolarizing muscle relaxants
c. Increases potency of nondepolarizing muscle relaxants and decreases potency of depolarizing muscle relaxants
d. Increases potency of depolarizing muscle relaxants and increases potency of depolarizing muscle relaxants

4.34. A male patient sustained a tibial-fibular fracture in a motor vehicle accident 48 hours ago. He is admitted to PACU after an open reduction and internal fixation (ORIF) with tetracaine spinal anesthetic. During his first 30 minutes after admission, the PACU nurse observes increasing restlessness, disorientation, and tremulousness. He is currently diaphoretic, temperature is 36° C (96.8° F), heart rate is 128 bpm, cardiac rhythm is sinus, and blood pressure is 188/95. These symptoms are most likely caused by:

a. tetracaine toxicity.
b. cocaine overstimulation.
c. alcohol withdrawal syndrome.
d. deferred traumatic intraspinal bleeding.

4.35. A wildly restless, crying, and confused 12-year-old boy attempts to climb off the stretcher in the PACU. While assuring the physical safety of staff and patient, the nurse explains possible causes for the child's behavior to his mother, who visits in the PACU. Causes could include any of the following *except:*

a. hypoxemia.
b. central cholinergic effect.
c. bladder distention.
d. pseudocholinesterase toxicity.

4.36. Physostigmine is occasionally used to:

a. augment the analgesic effect of narcotics at the dorsal horn.
b. increase acetylcholine at the neuromuscular junction.
c. reverse consciousness-depressing effects of narcotics at the hypothalamus.
d. inhibit norepinephrine penetration of the blood-brain barrier.

4.37. A retrobulbar block is administered to a patient. The patient's level of consciousness decreases, and apnea ensues. The most likely cause of the decreased consciousness and apnea is:

a. intrathecal injection.
b. inadvertent intraocular injection.
c. retrobulbar hemorrhage.
d. inadvertent intravascular injection.

4.38. Nursing observations after administering physostigmine salicylate include monitoring:

a. temperature for hyperpyrexia.
b. consciousness for atypical hyperactivity.
c. cardiac rhythm for bradycardia.
d. muscle function for fasciculation.

4.39. After a total of 0.6 mg of IV flumazenil, the PACU nurse evaluates the patient's response for evidence of flumazenil-induced:

a. muscular re-relaxation.
b. emerging incisional pain.
c. sinus bradycardia.
d. respiratory depression.

4.40. Succinylcholine is classified as a(an):

a. depolarizing muscle relaxant.
b. anticholinesterase blocker.
c. calcium channel inhibitor.
d. nondepolarizing muscle relaxant.

4.41. An absolute contraindication to spinal anesthesia includes all the following *except:*

a. localized infection at the site.
b. patient refusal.
c. uncorrected coagulation deficit.
d. multiple sclerosis.

4.42. Sixty minutes after bupivacaine (Marcaine) is added to an epidural infusion of morphine sulfate (Duramorph), the patient complains of vertigo and tinnitus. The nurse observes muscle tremors, hypotension, and premature ventricular contractions. These symptoms are *most likely* related to:

a. early hyperdynamic sepsis.
b. local anesthetic toxicity.
c. systemic allergic response.
d. morphine overdose.

4.43. A 4-year-old child has vomited twice since her strabismus surgery ended an hour ago. She received small amounts of sevoflurane, fentanyl, and atracurium intraoperatively. Drugs of choice in the PACU for treating postoperative nausea and vomiting include:

a. ondansetron with dexamethasone.
b. droperidol with dexamethasone.
c. propofol with droperidol.
d. propofol with dexamethasone.

4.44. A patient who is wheelchair-dependent because of cerebral palsy from hypoxia at birth and who has had a mitral valve replacement 3 years ago is given nitrous oxide, ofloxacin, alfentanil, and

rocuronium for multiple dental extractions. In the immediate postanesthetic period, this patient is **most likely** to develop:
a. reflexive hyperventilation from diffusion hypoxia.
b. prolonged vomiting from swallowed blood.
c. malignant hypertension from autonomic dysreflexia.
d. painful sensations from early narcotic metabolism.

4.45. Metoclopramide affects postoperative nausea and vomiting by:
a. stimulating H_2 receptors and neutralizing gastric fluid.
b. suppressing CTZ dopamine receptors and increasing gastric motility.
c. suppressing H_1 receptors and decreasing gastric volume.
d. stimulating CTZ dopamine receptors and decreasing gastric emptying.

4.46. The most critical times to assess a patient's respiratory quality after a bolus dose of epidural morphine given just before arrival in the PACU is:
a. every hour for 18 hours.
b. 2 hours after injection.
c. 6 to 8 hours later.
d. when the patient complains of itching.

4.47. Which of the following nondepolarizing muscle relaxants has the most rapid onset?
a. Atracurium
b. Vecuronium
c. Succinylcholine
d. Rocuronium

4.48. For a brief period after a patient is given electroconvulsive therapy, which of the following is **most likely** to develop?
a. Hypertension with electromechanical dissociation
b. Hypotension with bundle branch block
c. Hypertension and supraventricular tachycardia
d. Hypotension and sinus bradycardia

4.49. The anesthesia provider accompanies a 45-year-old woman into the PACU after emergency appendectomy. The patient's medical history includes recent depression, treated with a monoamine oxidase inhibitor (MAOI). She is agitated, cries "Help me," and states her pain is "8" on a verbal pain scale of 0 to 10. This patient's pain is best managed with any of the following medications *except:*
a. fentanyl.
b. alfentanil.
c. hydrocodone (Dilaudid).
d. meperidine.

4.50. By definition, a patient under conscious sedation and analgesia may be amnesic or drowsy yet:
a. demonstrates airway patency with jaw support.
b. rouses to a supraorbital stimulus.
c. maintains independent, continuous airway patency.
d. transfers to a stretcher with minimal aid.

4.51. Medications considered appropriate for conscious sedation and analgesia include:
a. thiopental and meperidine.
b. diazepam and morphine sulfate.
c. methohexital and ketamine.
d. propofol and midazolam.

4.52. Biochemically, a local anesthetic affects nerve conduction by blocking:
a. acetylcholine release at the neuromuscular junction.
b. sodium entry into nerve cells to stabilize the membrane.
c. calcium channels at specific osmotic junctures.
d. norepinephrine effect to reverse an action potential.

4.53. A definitive treatment of postdural puncture headache is:
a. caffeine.
b. supine position.
c. epidural blood patch.
d. fluids.

Set 1

Answer Key

4.1.	a		**4.14.**	c
4.2.	d		**4.15.**	d
4.3.	a		**4.16.**	c
4.4.	c		**4.17.**	b
4.5.	c		**4.18.**	a
4.6.	d		**4.19.**	d
4.7.	b		**4.20.**	a
4.8.	b		**4.21.**	d
4.9.	d		**4.22.**	d
4.10.	a		**4.23.**	b
4.11.	c		**4.24.**	c
4.12.	d		**4.25.**	b
4.13.	a			

SET 1

4.1. Correct Answer: **a**

Acetylcholine is the primary neurotransmitter of both preganglionic and postganglionic fibers in the parasympathetic nervous system. This chemical is stored and then released at the neuromuscular junction to facilitate transmission of neurologic impulses. (Cole DJ, Schlunt M: *Adult perioperative anesthesia: the requisites in anesthesiology*, St. Louis, 2004, Mosby; Drain C, editor: *Perianesthesia nursing: a critical care approach*, ed 4, Philadelphia, 2003, Saunders; Faust RJ, editor: *Anesthesiology review*, ed 3, London, 2002, Churchill Livingstone; Miller RD et al, editors: *Anesthesia* (2-vol set with CD-ROM for Windows & Macintosh), ed 5, London, 2000, Churchill Livingstone.)

4.2. Correct Answer: **d**

This woman should receive an antibiotic dose within 1 hour before surgery. Her mitral valve dysfunction is likely related to her history of rheumatic heart disease; her risk of developing bacterial endocarditis is 5 to 8 times greater than that of another patient who has no cardiac disease. Antibiotic prophylaxis is especially important when the planned surgical procedure invades the genitourinary, oral, or upper respiratory system. Patients with multiple dental caries or orthopedic hardware also may receive antibiotic pretreatment. (Burden N et al: *Ambulatory surgical nursing*, ed 2, Philadelphia, 2000, Saunders; Cole DJ, Schlunt M: *Adult perioperative anesthesia: the requisites in anesthesiology*, St. Louis, 2004, Mosby; Quinn D, Schick L, editors: *ASPAN's perianesthesia nursing core curriculum: preoperative, Phase I and Phase II*

PACU nursing, Philadelphia, 2004, Saunders.)

4.3. Correct Answer: **a**

Volatile (inhaled) anesthetic agents rely on respiratory quality for clearance from the brain, the target organ for effect. The solubility coefficient (minimum alveolar concentration [MAC]) of the individual anesthetic and the patient's ability to breathe influence removal. After the flow of gas (exposure) is terminated, the effects of a highly soluble drug like halothane abate rapidly. A gas anesthetic is quickly eliminated when minute ventilation (increased rate and depth to remove alveolar gas) and cardiac output (rapid circulation time to quickly lower tissue saturation) are high. Renal and liver functions have minimal influence on elimination of a volatile anesthetic. (Drain C, editor: *Perianesthesia nursing: a critical care approach*, ed 4, Philadelphia, 2003, Saunders; Quinn D, Schick L, editors: *ASPAN's perianesthesia nursing core curriculum: preoperative, Phase I and Phase II PACU nursing*, Philadelphia, 2004, Saunders.)

4.4. Correct Answer: **c**

Hydralazine is an antihypertensive that decreases peripheral resistance by acting directly on peripheral vessels to relax and dilate arterioles. As blood pressure drops, compensatory mechanisms respond to prevent dire changes in cardiac output. Heart rate, renin production, myocardial contractility, and contractile force may increase as a result. (Drain C, editor: *Perianesthesia nursing: a critical care approach*, ed 4, Philadelphia, 2003, Saunders; Quinn D, Schick L, editors:

ASPAN's perianesthesia nursing core curriculum: preoperative, Phase I and Phase II PACU nursing, Philadelphia, 2004, Saunders; Skidmore-Roth L: *Mosby's 2006 nursing drug reference*, St. Louis, 2006, Mosby.)

4.5. Correct Answer: **c**
Diazepam contains propylene glycol, which has been associated with venous irritation and pain. Propofol has been noted to have a high incidence of pain on IV injection, and lidocaine is often used in conjunction with administration of propofol to decrease this pain. Methohexital is an alkaline solution and therefore burns on administration. Ketamine is the only agent listed above in which there has not been documentation of pain on injection. (Cole DJ, Schlunt M: *Adult perioperative anesthesia: the requisites in anesthesiology*, St. Louis, 2004, Mosby; Faust RJ, editor: *Anesthesiology review*, ed 3, London, 2002, Churchill Livingstone; Quinn D, Schick L, editors: *ASPAN's perianesthesia nursing core curriculum: preoperative, Phase I and Phase II PACU nursing*, Philadelphia, 2004, Saunders.)

4.6. Correct Answer: **d**
Minimum alveolar concentration (MAC) is the lowest concentration (partial pressure) of a specific inhalant anesthetic that obliterates movement in 50% of patients when a painful stimulus (like a surgical incision) is applied. MAC expresses the comparative (relative) potency of various inhalation anesthetic gases. The relationship is inverse: a low MAC indicates a very potent anesthetic. (Cole DJ, Schlunt M: *Adult perioperative anesthesia: the requisites in anesthesiology*, St. Louis, 2004, Mosby; Drain C, editor: *Perianesthesia nursing: a critical care approach*, ed 4, Philadelphia,

2003, Saunders; Quinn D, Schick L, editors: *ASPAN's perianesthesia nursing core curriculum: preoperative, Phase I and Phase II PACU nursing*, Philadelphia, 2004, Saunders.)

4.7. Correct Answer: **b**
Minimum alveolar concentration (MAC) is unaffected by anesthesia duration, a patient's gender, and $PaCO_2$ levels. Age, hypothermia, central nervous system depressants, and antihypertensives decrease MAC; hyperthermia, chronic alcohol use, and elevated levels of monoamine oxidase inhibitors (MAOIs) increase MAC. Inhalation anesthetics depress cardiac function and circulation. (Cole DJ, Schlunt M: *Adult perioperative anesthesia: the requisites in anesthesiology*, St. Louis, 2004, Mosby; Drain C, editor: *Perianesthesia nursing: a critical care approach*, ed 4, Philadelphia, 2003, Saunders; Quinn D, Schick L, editors: *ASPAN's perianesthesia nursing core curriculum: preoperative, Phase I and Phase II PACU nursing*, Philadelphia, 2004, Saunders.)

4.8. Correct Answer: **b**
Pharmacokinetics is the relationship between drug dose and plasma or effect-site concentration. It is what the body does to the drugs administered. The process of absorption, distribution, and clearance govern the relationship. (Miller RD et al, editors: *Anesthesia* (2-vol set with CD-ROM for Windows & Macintosh), ed 5, London, 2000, Churchill Livingstone; Quinn D, Schick L, editors: *ASPAN's perianesthesia nursing core curriculum: preoperative, Phase I and Phase II PACU nursing*, Philadelphia, 2004, Saunders.)

4.9. Correct Answer: **d**
Midazolam (Versed) is 2 to 3 times as potent as diazepam (Valium);

therefore the effective dose is at least 50% less. Small doses of IV midazolam are administered at intervals according to effect. Midazolam is lipophilic and nearly totally bound to serum albumin. Peak effect occurs quickly, within 3 to 5 minutes, though *duration* is 1 to 4 hours and half-life is from 1.2 to 12 hours. Effects are further increased by narcotics and sedatives. (Drain C, editor: *Perianesthesia nursing: a critical care approach*, ed 4, Philadelphia, 2003, Saunders; Quinn D, Schick L, editors: *ASPAN's perianesthesia nursing core curriculum: preoperative, Phase I and Phase II PACU nursing*, Philadelphia, 2004, Saunders; Skidmore-Roth L: *Mosby's 2006 nursing drug reference*, St. Louis, 2006.)

4.10. Correct Answer: **a**
Atropine sulfate (an anticholinergic) minimizes the bradycardia, salivation, gastrointestinal irritability, and miosis produced when muscarinic receptors are stimulated by anticholinesterase medications. Cholinesterase-inhibiting medications include neostigmine (Prostigmin) and edrophonium (Tensilon). These medications reverse the effects of nondepolarizing muscle relaxants (NDMR) by inactivating acetylcholinesterase. As a result, concentrations of the neurotransmitter acetylcholine increase and normal neuromuscular function resumes. Dexamethasone is a corticosteroid used for decreasing inflammation. Azathioprine is an immunosuppressant used with renal transplants, rheumatoid arthritis, and bone marrow transplants. (Burden N et al: *Ambulatory surgical nursing*, ed 2, Philadelphia, 2000, Saunders; Drain C, editor: *Perianesthesia nursing: a critical care approach*, ed 4, Philadelphia, 2003, Saunders; Skidmore-Roth L: *Mosby's 2006*

nursing drug reference, St. Louis, 2006, Mosby.)

4.11. Correct Answer: **c**
Up to 10% of patients with penicillin allergy are also sensitive to cephalosporin antibiotics. Consult with the surgeon before administering cefazolin and other antibiotics in this classification. Particularly if the patient has anaphylactic-type symptoms to penicillin, cephalosporins are usually avoided. Gentamicin and vancomycin protect against bacterial endocarditis but are associated with ototoxicity and renal failure. (Skidmore-Roth L: *Mosby's 2006 nursing drug reference*, St. Louis, 2006, Mosby.)

4.12. Correct Answer: **d**
Etomidate is associated with a high incidence (30%-40%) of nausea and vomiting, which is further enhanced by the addition of fentanyl. Propofol has been used successfully as an antiemetic in subanesthetic doses. Ketamine-propofol has gained popularity in the attempt to reduce opioid use and the incidence of PONV. (Cole DJ, Schlunt M: *Adult perioperative anesthesia: the requisites in anesthesiology*, St. Louis, 2004, Mosby; Quinn D, Schick L, editors: *ASPAN's perianesthesia nursing core curriculum: preoperative, Phase I and Phase II PACU nursing*, Philadelphia, 2004, Saunders; Thiemann LJ et al: *Nurse anesthetist exam review*, New York, 2006, McGraw Hill.)

4.13. Correct Answer: **a**
Compared with the adult, a greater proportion (about twice) of an infant's body weight comprises "vessel-rich" vital tissues. High respiratory rate and cardiac index and rapid blood flow through vital organs like heart, kidney, and liver mean rapid uptake of inhalation anesthetic medication. The result

may be a quick and significant depression of cardiac function. (Drain C, editor: *Perianesthesia nursing: a critical care approach*, ed 4, Philadelphia, 2003, Saunders; Litman RS: *Pediatric anesthesia: the requisites in anesthesiology*, St. Louis, 2004, Mosby.)

4.14. Correct Answer: **c**
The 5-HT$_3$ receptor antagonists, including ondansetron, dolasetron and granisetron, decrease PONV without the unwanted adverse effects such as dry mouth, sedation, and extrapyramidal symptoms. The 5-HT$_3$ receptor antagonists are more effective for vomiting than for nausea. Dexamethasone is a corticosteroid often used in conjunction with the 5-HT$_3$ receptor antagonists. (Cole DJ, Schlunt M: *Adult perioperative anesthesia: the requisites in anesthesiology*, St. Louis, 2004, Mosby; Drain C, editor: *Perianesthesia nursing: a critical care approach*, ed 4, Philadelphia, 2003, Saunders; Golembiewski J, Tokumaru S: Pharmacological prophylaxis and management of adult postoperative/postdischarge nausea and vomiting, *J PeriAnesth Nurs* 21[6]:385-397, 2006.)

4.15. Correct Answer: **d**
Theophylline has been known to antagonize the nondepolarizing muscle relaxants. Calcium channel blockers, aminoglycoside antibiotics, and volatile anesthetics including halothane can enhance nondepolarizing muscle relaxants. (Quinn D, Schick L, editors: *ASPAN's perianesthesia nursing core curriculum: preoperative, Phase I and Phase II PACU nursing*, Philadelphia, 2004, Saunders.)

4.16. Correct Answer: **c**
Local anesthetic toxicity results in seizures (neurotoxicity), hypotension, and bradycardia (cardiotoxicity) after initial hypertension with tachycardia. IV regional block (Bier block) involves injection of large volumes of local anesthetic, usually lidocaine, into the operative extremity. Deflation of the tourniquet(s) used to obstruct blood flow and contain the local anesthetic during a Bier block can allow unmetabolized local anesthetic to suddenly enter the bloodstream. A bolus dose of local anesthetic is most likely when the tourniquet(s) is (are) deflated early (less than 30 minutes after medication injection) or too rapidly or when a tourniquet cuff has technical faults. (Burden N et al: *Ambulatory surgical nursing*, ed 2, Philadelphia, 2000, Saunders; Karlet MC: *Nurse anesthesia secrets*, St. Louis, 2005, Mosby; Quinn D, Schick L, editors: *ASPAN's perianesthesia nursing core curriculum: preoperative, Phase I and Phase II PACU nursing*, Philadelphia, 2004, Saunders.)

4.17. Correct Answer: **b**
To establish an intravenous regional block, alias Bier block, the anesthesia provider applies a double-cuffed tourniquet to the surgical extremity. Blood is forcefully drawn from the vessels; a large bolus of local anesthetic is then injected into the venous system. The tourniquet both obstructs the extremity's blood flow and prevents movement of the anesthetic beyond the tourniquet. Anesthetic, typically lidocaine without epinephrine, then diffuses from vessels to bathe and numb tissues for approximately 90 minutes. (Burden N et al: *Ambulatory surgical nursing*, ed 2, Philadelphia, 2000, Saunders; Karlet MC: *Nurse anesthesia secrets*, St. Louis, 2005, Mosby; Quinn D, Schick L, editors: *ASPAN's perianesthesia nursing core curriculum: preoperative, Phase I and Phase II PACU nursing*, Philadelphia, 2004, Saunders;

Rathmell JP, Neal JM, Viscomi CM: *Regional anesthesia: the requisites in anesthesiology*, St. Louis, 2004, Mosby.)

4.18. Correct Answer: **a**
Local anesthetics reversibly block the sodium ion channels at the neuronal membrane, which inhibits neuronal transmission. Local anesthetics prevent the opening of the sodium channels and prevent the membrane potential from increasing threshold to open the additional sodium channels. (Cole DJ, Schlunt M: *Adult perioperative anesthesia: the requisites in anesthesiology*, St. Louis, 2004, Mosby; Drain C, editor: *Perianesthesia nursing: a critical care approach*, ed 4, Philadelphia, 2003, Saunders; Robertson KM et al: *Anesthesiology board review*, ed 2, New York, 2006, McGraw-Hill.)

4.19. Correct Answer: **d**
Ideally, a patient will have minimal bleeding and prompt return of arm function after an IV regional (Bier) block. However, the ongoing effect of local anesthetic medications can numb sensation and limit motor control in the extremity. Without support, protection, and cautious movement, the extremity can flail about, increasing potential for injury to the extremity or body. The PACU nurse should expect this patient to be alert but possibly have significant pain. Tourniquets create a relatively bloodless surgical field. However, if hemostasis is not ensured before tourniquet release, significant and reportable postsurgical bleeding can occur. (Burden N et al: *Ambulatory surgical nursing*, ed 2, Philadelphia, 2000, Saunders; Karlet MC: *Nurse anesthesia secrets*, St. Louis, 2005, Mosby; Quinn D, Schick L, editors: *ASPAN's perianesthesia nursing core curriculum: preoperative, Phase I and Phase II*

PACU nursing, Philadelphia, 2004, Saunders.)

4.20. Correct Answer: **a**
Desflurane (Suprane) acts quickly and dissipates quickly but is very likely to stimulate coughing and airway spasm. Inhalation anesthetics are generally known for their bronchodilating properties and low potential to irritate the airway. Halothane is a particularly appropriate choice for children and asthmatic patients. Enflurane (Ethrane) and isoflurane (Forane) have the most significant respiratory depressant effects. (Cole DJ, Schlunt M: *Adult perioperative anesthesia: the requisites in anesthesiology*, St. Louis, 2004, Mosby; Drain C, editor: *Perianesthesia nursing: a critical care approach*, ed 4, Philadelphia, 2003, Saunders.)

4.21. Correct Answer: **d**
Only about 25% of cardiac output perfuses skeletal muscle and fat, so release of any stored medication is gradual. Elimination of an inhaled anesthetic depends in part on blood flow (circulation) and also on distribution into body tissues, including brain, muscle, and fat. Some inhaled anesthetic agents are quickly absorbed into fat, which has low blood flow. Body tissues that receive the greatest proportion of cardiac output (perfusion) both absorb and eliminate anesthetic gases quickly. Vital organs like the heart, brain, and kidneys receive the largest blood flow, approximately 75% of cardiac output, and so quickly show both medication effects and clearance. (Cole DJ, Schlunt M: *Adult perioperative anesthesia: the requisites in anesthesiology*, St. Louis, 2004, Mosby; Drain C, editor: *Perianesthesia nursing: a critical care approach*, ed 4, St. Louis, 2003, Saunders; Litman RS: *Pediatric anesthesia:*

the requisites in anesthesiology, St. Louis, 2004, Mosby.)

4.22. Correct Answer: **d**
Hypoxia, acidosis, hypercarbia, and pregnancy potentiate systemic toxicity of local anesthetics. (Cole DJ, Schlunt M: *Adult perioperative anesthesia: the requisites in anesthesiology*, St. Louis, 2004, Mosby; Faust RJ, editor: *Anesthesiology review*, ed 3, London, 2002, Churchill Livingstone; Robertson KM et al: *Anesthesiology board review*, ed 2, New York, 2006, McGraw-Hill.)

4.23. Correct Answer: **b**
Infusing a narcotic continuously into the epidural space *improves* joint and muscle movement, promotes earlier postoperative activity, and provides consistent, long-term pain relief. Vomiting incidence remains high after both intramuscular and epidural morphine. Other benefits of epidural analgesia include less sedation and anxiety, decreased likelihood of pulmonary infections and deep vein thrombosis, reduced myocardial oxygen demand, and suppressed metabolic and endocrine responses to stress. Risk of respiratory depression and *progressive*, not episodic, sedation increases with epidural narcotics. Adding a local anesthetic to the narcotic solution *can* alter motor strength though, so that walking or upright positions are associated with orthostatic hypotension or muscle weakness. (Drain C, editor:

Perianesthesia nursing: a critical care approach, ed 4, Philadelphia, 2003, Saunders; Rathmell JP, Neal JM, Viscomi CM: *Regional anesthesia: the requisites in anesthesiology*, St. Louis, 2004, Mosby.)

4.24. Correct Answer: **c**
The epidural space is a *potential* space between the dura mater covering the spinal canal and the epidural wall. This space is filled with nerves, lymphatic tissue, and veins enmeshed in fat—but no fluid—and extends from the neck to the sacrum. Blood may appear in fluid aspirated from the epidural space after back surgery when the dura is entered. (Drain C, editor: *Perianesthesia nursing: a critical care approach*, ed 4, Philadelphia, 2003, Saunders; Rathmell JP, Neal JM, Viscomi CM: *Regional anesthesia: the requisites in anesthesiology*, St. Louis, 2004, Mosby.)

4.25. Correct Answer: **b**
Addition of epinephrine prolongs anesthesia and analgesia, *increases* block intensity, limits peak local anesthetic plasma concentrations, acts as a test dose, and provides independent anesthesia and analgesia via alpha-adrenergic stimulation at the spinal cord. (Cole DJ, Schlunt M: *Adult perioperative anesthesia: the requisites in anesthesiology*, St. Louis, 2004, Mosby; Rathmell JP, Neal JM, Viscomi CM: *Regional anesthesia: the requisites in anesthesiology*, St. Louis, 2004, Mosby.)

Set 2

	Answer Key		

4.26.	d	**4.40.**	a
4.27.	b	**4.41.**	d
4.28.	d	**4.42.**	b
4.29.	c	**4.43.**	a
4.30.	d	**4.44.**	d
4.31.	a	**4.45.**	b
4.32.	a	**4.46.**	c
4.33.	a	**4.47.**	d
4.34.	c	**4.48.**	c
4.35.	d	**4.49.**	d
4.36.	b	**4.50.**	c
4.37.	a	**4.51.**	b
4.38.	c	**4.52.**	b
4.39.	d	**4.53.**	c

SET 2

4.26. Correct Answer: **d**
Cocaine prevents norepinephrine uptake at peripheral adrenergic nerve sites. Cocaine also directly stimulates the sympathetic nervous system, which releases catecholamines. Epinephrine (Adrenalin) surge, with severe hypertension, racing tachycardia, and cardiac failure, results. (Cole DJ, Schlunt M: *Adult perioperative anesthesia: the requisites in anesthesiology*, St. Louis, 2004, Mosby; Quinn D, Schick L, editors: *ASPAN's perianesthesia nursing core curriculum: preoperative, Phase I and Phase II PACU nursing*, Philadelphia, 2004, Saunders.)

4.27. Correct Answer: **b**
Pseudocholinesterase is a serine hydrolase capable of hydrolyzing esters including succinylcholine, mivacurium, acetylcholine, and ester-type local anesthetics. Succinylcholine is a depolarizing muscle relaxant that mimics the acetylcholine at the myoneural junction, whereas mivacurium is a nondepolarizing muscle relaxant that competes with the acetylcholine at the myoneural junction. Mivacurium is hydrolyzed by plasma cholinesterase at 80% of the rate of succinylcholine metabolism. Atracurium, another nondepolarizing muscle relaxant, is metabolized chemically by the Hoffman elimination and enzymatically by nonspecific plasma esterases. Rocuronium, another nondepolarizing muscle relaxant, is eliminated via the liver. (Faust RJ, editor: *Anesthesiology review*, ed 3, London, 2002, Churchill Livingstone; Quinn D, Schick L, editors: *ASPAN's perianesthesia nursing core curriculum:*

preoperative, Phase I and Phase II PACU nursing, Philadelphia, 2004, Saunders.)

4.28. Correct Answer: **d**
Metoprolol, a cardioselective beta blocker, is considered as a class 2 antidysrhythmia drug. Indications for use include treatment of hypertension, supraventricular and ventricular dysrhythmias, and acute myocardial infarction. Toxic effects may include hypotension potentiated by volatile anesthetics, bradycardia, bronchospasm, and cardiac failure. Methamphetamine, a central nervous system (CNS) stimulant, causes hypertension by stimulating both alpha and beta adrenergic receptors. Metoprolol prevents beta adrenergic receptors from vasodilating but results in increased vasoconstriction induced by the alpha adrenergic receptor stimulation; therefore patients have increased hypertension. (Leung J: *Cardiac and vascular anesthesia: the requisites in anesthesiology*, St. Louis, 2004, Mosby; McGuinness T: Methamphetamine abuse, *Am J Nurs* 106[12]:54-59, 2006.)

4.29. Correct Answer: **c**
Meperidine causes the least amount of smooth muscle spasm. (Miller RD et al, editors: *Anesthesia* (2-vol set with CD-ROM for Windows & Macintosh), ed 5, London, 2000, Churchill Livingstone.)

4.30. Correct Answer: **d**
Essentially no ventilatory or cardiovascular depression or any effect on the biliary tract is seen with Toradol. Hepatic toxicity may result from NSAID use; therefore the liver transaminase plasma levels increase, not decrease.

Periodic assessment of liver function is recommended in patients on long-term NSAID therapy. (Cole DJ, Schlunt M: *Adult perioperative anesthesia: the requisites in anesthesiology*, St. Louis, 2004, Mosby; Drain C, editor: *Perianesthesia nursing: a critical care approach*, ed 4, Philadelphia, 2003, Saunders; Rathmell JP, Neal JM, Viscomi CM: *Regional anesthesia: the requisites in anesthesiology*, St. Louis, 2004, Mosby.)

4.31. Correct Answer: **a**
Adequate analgesia is not a prerequisite to injecting an NSAID like ketorolac. An NSAID does not act on opiate receptors but may *augment* the pain relief provided by a narcotic. The ketorolac dose is reduced for elderly patients, patients who weigh less than 50 kg, and patients with renal or liver insufficiency. NSAIDs also alter platelet function and so are avoided for patients with "bleeding problems" (coagulopathy), history of gastrointestinal ulcers, and renal or hepatic disease. Cross sensitivity can occur when a patient with an aspirin allergy receives NSAIDs. (Quinn D, Schick L, editors: *ASPAN's perianesthesia nursing core curriculum: preoperative, Phase I and Phase II PACU nursing*, Philadelphia, 2004, Saunders; Skidmore-Roth L: *Mosby's 2006 nursing drug reference*, St. Louis, 2006, Mosby.)

4.32. Correct Answer: **a**
Nalbuphine (Nubain) is a strong analgesic with mixed agonist/antagonist effect at pain receptors. Agonist effects partially stimulate kappa and stimulate sigma receptors. Nalbuphine has *antagonistic* effects at mu pain receptors. Therefore nalbuphine antagonizes (reverses) respiratory depression created by the narcotics that stimulate mu receptors. Nalbuphine also can reverse analgesia produced by other

narcotics and begin withdrawal symptoms in an addicted person. When a patient has received *no* narcotic, nalbuphine's strong analgesic effects are equal to morphine's but with less respiratory depression and less addictive potential. (Drain C, editor: *Perianesthesia nursing: a critical care approach*, ed 4, Philadelphia, 2003, Saunders; McCaffery M, Pasero C: *Pain: clinical manual*, ed 2, St. Louis, 1999, Mosby; St. Marie B, editor: *Core curriculum for pain management nursing*, Philadelphia, 2002, Saunders.)

4.33. Correct Answer: **a**
Magnesium enhances the neuromuscular block produced by both nondepolarizing and depolarizing agents. The principal action of magnesium is that it can enter the nerve terminal and replace or decrease the amount of calcium that enters, which stabilizes the postsynaptic membrane. (Drain C, editor: *Perianesthesia nursing: a critical care approach*, ed 4, Philadelphia, 2003, Saunders; Quinn D, Schick L, editors: *ASPAN's perianesthesia nursing core curriculum: preoperative, Phase I and Phase II PACU nursing*, Philadelphia, 2004, Saunders; Roizen MF, Fleisher LA: *Essence of anesthesia practice*, ed 2, Philadelphia, 2002, Saunders.)

4.34. Correct Answer: **c**
Severe acute alcohol withdrawal produces hallucinations, restlessness, disorientation, and tremors about 2 days after alcohol consumption stops. Concurrent sympathetic nervous system stimulation causes the tachycardia, hypertension, and diaphoresis. If the patient abused cocaine, the nurse would more likely observe increased pulmonary congestion, hyperthermia, excessive talking, and epistaxis. Confusion from local anesthetic toxicity is also associated with tremors, numbness, and tinnitus. Intraspinal bleeding

produces severe back pain at the site of the bleeding, as well as motor and sensory deficits. Consider fat embolism syndrome as another possible contributor to the patient's confusion 2 days after injury. (Drain C, editor: *Perianesthesia nursing: a critical care approach*, ed 4, Philadelphia, 2003, Saunders; Quinn D, Schick L, editors: *ASPAN's perianesthesia nursing core curriculum: preoperative, Phase I and Phase II PACU nursing*, Philadelphia, 2004, Saunders.)

4.35. Correct Answer: **d**
Pseudocholinesterase is the principal enzyme in the metabolism of succinylcholine and ester-type local anesthetics resulting in prolonged paralysis. Patients with deficits in pseudocholinesterase may be frightened but unable to thrash about. The PACU nurse should always determine that the patient breathes adequately before turning to other possible causes! Hypoxic patients first become agitated, though very high pCO_2 levels (hypercarbia) cause sedation. Sedatives, anticholinergic medications, electrolyte imbalances, pain, and a full bladder also can produce central nervous system excitement. The exact incidence of wild agitation, disorientation, and confusion after anesthesia (emergence delirium or excitement) is unknown, but age, surgical procedure, and intraoperative medications are factors. Young children and teens or patients with psychologic depression, significant alcohol use, or preoperative anxiety seem to have a higher likelihood of significant and extended agitation. (Drain C, editor: *Perianesthesia nursing: a critical care approach*, ed 4, Philadelphia, 2003, Saunders.)

4.36. Correct Answer: **b**
Physostigmine, an anticholinesterase medication that penetrates the blood-brain barrier, increases the concentration of acetylcholine in the neuromuscular junction and eases impulse transmission. Small doses of physostigmine titrated to effect can counter emergence delirium. This response to emergence from anesthesia may relate to pain and fear; protection, safety, and emotional support may be all that are needed to "ride out" this excitement phase. (Drain C, editor: *Perianesthesia nursing: a critical care approach*, ed 4, Philadelphia, 2003, Saunders; Skidmore-Roth L: *Mosby's 2006 nursing drug reference*, St. Louis, 2006, Mosby.)

4.37. Correct Answer: **a**
The optic nerve is a brain tract, and it is possible to have an intrathecal injection via the optic nerve sheath resulting in apnea. (Rathmell JP, Neal JM, Viscomi CM: *Regional anesthesia: the requisites in anesthesiology*, St. Louis, 2004, Mosby; Robertson KM et al: *Anesthesiology board review*, ed 2, New York, 2006, McGraw-Hill.)

4.38. Correct Answer: **c**
Bradycardia is one cholinergic response that can occur after physostigmine administration. In effect, cholinergic responses like bradycardia, bronchospasm, nausea, salivation, or incoordination can replace anticholinergic symptoms. (Cole DJ, Schlunt M: *Adult perioperative anesthesia: the requisites in anesthesiology*, St. Louis, 2004, Mosby; Drain C, editor: *Perianesthesia nursing: a critical care approach*, ed 4, Philadelphia, 2003, Saunders.)

4.39. Correct Answer: **d**
Resedation, with reoccurrence of respiratory depression, is the primary potential adverse effect after flumazenil administration. The selected dose of flumazenil may return the patient to a wakeful condition but

be ineffective to completely reverse residual, recurrent effects of large or long-acting doses of benzodiazepines. Flumazenil does not reverse any effects of non-benzodiazepine medications; renarcotization is possible. (Cole DJ, Schlunt M: *Adult perioperative anesthesia: the requisites in anesthesiology*, St. Louis, 2004, Mosby; Kost M: *Moderate sedation/ analgesia: core competencies for practice*, ed 2, Philadelphia, 2004, Saunders; Product information: *Flumazenil (Romazicon)*, Nutley, NJ, 1994, Roche Laboratories; Odom-Forren J, Watson DS: *Practical guide to moderate sedation/analgesia*, ed 2, St. Louis, 2005, Mosby.)

4.40. Correct Answer: **a**
Succinylcholine (Anectine), the only depolarizing muscle relaxant, acts like acetylcholine at the skeletal muscle cell receptor site by binding to the receptor and then depolarizing the membrane. As long as succinylcholine occupies the receptor site, repolarization is blocked and acetylcholine has no effect. Therefore the cell membrane cannot depolarize for the next muscle contraction. Paralysis, usually of short duration, results. Unlike succinylcholine, vecuronium (Norcuron) is a nondepolarizing muscle relaxant with pharmacologically reversible effects. (Burden N et al: *Ambulatory surgical nursing*, ed 2, Philadelphia, 2000, Saunders; Quinn D, Schick L, editors: *ASPAN's perianesthesia nursing core curriculum: preoperative, Phase I and Phase II PACU nursing*, Philadelphia, 2004, Saunders.)

4.41. Correct Answer: **d**
Absolute contraindications to neuraxial anesthesia/analgesia include patient refusal, bacteremia/sepsis, increased intracranial pressure, infection at needle insertion site, shock or severe hypovolemia, and

coagulopathy. Relative contraindications include preexisting neurologic disease, severe psychiatric disease, aortic stenosis, left ventricular outflow tract obstruction, congenital heart conditions, and deformities or previous surgery of the spinal column. Multiple sclerosis is characterized by chronic inflammation, demyelination, and scarring of the myelin sheath of the CNS, and although there is a relative contraindication to spinal anesthesia, it is not an absolute contraindication for patients to have a spinal. (Drain C, editor: *Perianesthesia nursing: a critical care approach*, ed 4, Philadelphia, 2003, Saunders; Faust RJ, editor: *Anesthesiology review*, ed 3, London, 2002, Churchill Livingstone; Rathmell JP, Neal JM, Viscomi CM: *Regional anesthesia: the requisites in anesthesiology*, St. Louis, 2004, Mosby.)

4.42. Correct Answer: **b**
Tinnitus, circumoral tingling, blurred vision, and confusion are among the symptoms of mild local anesthetic toxicity. Though intravascular absorption seldom occurs, the large volume of medication injected for epidural use *is* a potential risk. Symptoms abate with decreasing or discontinuing the infusion rate, increasing oxygen delivery, and providing emotional support. Aspirating the epidural catheter to detect cerebrospinal fluid or blood is *essential* before initiating an epidural infusion. (Cole DJ, Schlunt M: *Adult perioperative anesthesia: the requisites in anesthesiology*, St. Louis, 2004, Mosby; Miller RD et al, editors: *Anesthesia* (2-vol set with CD-ROM for Windows & Macintosh), ed 5, London, 2000, Churchill Livingstone.)

4.43. Correct Answer: **a**
Most pediatric anesthesiologists try to prevent nausea and vomiting by

administering a serotonin antagonist such as ondansetron (0.05 mg/kg to 2 mg) plus dexamethasone (0.5 mg/kg to a maximum of 10 mg). By using propofol rather than inhalation agents, anesthesiology has seen a decrease in PONV. Droperidol has a "black box" warning that indicates decreased usage because of the potential for the development of dysrhythmias including prolongation of the Q-T interval and torsades de pointes. Dexamethasone in conjunction with a serotonin antagonist (ondansetron, dolasetron, Kytril) lowers the incidence and severity of PONV. (Litman RS: *Pediatric anesthesia: the requisites in anesthesiology*, St. Louis, 2004, Mosby.)

4.44. Correct Answer: **d**
After the small anesthetic doses needed for a brief dental extraction, the patient should be quickly conscious and possibly in need of *analgesia*. The surgical procedure was brief, so delayed resedation or muscle weakness from residual, tissue-stored medication is unlikely. If the biochemcal balance is normal, the rocuronium (Zemuron) should clear in less 30 minutesor with reversal medications. Alfentanil (Alfenta) is much less potent than its prototype fentanyl; small doses have an effect for only 20 to 30 minutes. Moist packing occludes the posterior throat during surgery and prevents blood from moving past the mouth; airway obstruction from unremoved throat packing or gauze to provide postoperative gum pressure poses greater risk than vomiting a stomach full of blood. Dysreflexia is unlikely with cerebral palsy. Diffusion hypoxia with *shallow* breathing is a possibility for only 5 to 10 minutes after nitrous oxide is discontinued and so is unlikely in the PACU.

A "*balanced anesthesia technique*" capitalizes on the cumulative effects of an inhalation anesthetic like nitrous oxide, a narcotic or barbiturate, and/or a muscle relaxant. (Burden N et al: *Ambulatory surgical nursing*, ed 2, Philadelphia, 2000, Saunders; Drain C, editor: *Perianesthesia nursing: a critical care approach*, ed 4, Philadelphia, 2003, Saunders; Litman RS: *Pediatric anesthesia: the requisites in anesthesiology*, St. Louis, 2004, Mosby.)

4.45. Correct Answer: **b**
Metoclopramide (Reglan) blocks dopamine receptors in the chemoreceptor trigger zone (CTZ) to decrease emesis; it also increases gastrointestinal motility to decrease gastric volume. Metoclopramide does not alter histamine receptors. (Burden N et al: *Ambulatory surgical nursing*, ed 2, Philadelphia, 2000, Saunders; Skidmore-Roth L: *Mosby's 2006 nursing drug reference*, St. Louis, 2006, Mosby.)

4.46. Correct Answer: **c**
Even though the patient received only one intraoperative dose of morphine, the effects can persist for hours. Researchers report depressed respiratory responses to hypercarbia 6 to 9 hours after epidural morphine dosing. Morphine is a hydrophilic narcotic and moves cephalad through the cerebrospinal fluid toward the respiratory center in the brainstem. Migration takes approximately 3 to 6 hours, with respiratory depression persisting for up to 12 hours. Pruritus from epidural morphine arises from its histamine release and is unassociated with allergic respiratory distress. (Burden N et al: *Ambulatory surgical nursing*, ed 2, Philadelphia, 2000, Saunders; Faust RJ, editor: *Anesthesiology review*, ed 3, London, 2002,

Churchill Livingstone; Litman RS: *Pediatric anesthesia: the requisites in anesthesiology*, St. Louis, 2004, Mosby.)

4.47. Correct Answer: **d**
Succinylcholine is a depolarizing muscle relaxant; Atracurium and Vecuronium are considered intermediate-acting nondepolarizing muscle relaxants with an onset of 3 to 5 minutes and a duration of action of 20 to 35 minutes. Rocuronium has a rapid onset of 1 to 1.5 minutes and a duration of action of 12 to 30 minutes. (Drain C, editor: *Perianesthesia nursing: a critical care approach*, ed 4, Philadelphia, 2003, Saunders; Quinn D, Schick L, editors: *ASPAN's perianesthesia nursing core curriculum: preoperative, Phase I and Phase II PACU nursing*, Philadelphia, 2004, Saunders.)

4.48. Correct Answer: **c**
The seizure activity produced during electroconvulsive therapy stimulates the sympathetic nervous system and increases catecholamine release. Until these subside, the patient often is hypertensive and tachycardic. Most patients have no consequences, but the occasional patient has cardiovascular or cerebral damage from additional oxygen demand. (Burden N et al: *Ambulatory surgical nursing*, ed 2, Philadelphia, 2000, Saunders; Cole DJ, Schlunt M: *Adult perioperative anesthesia: the requisites in anesthesiology*, St. Louis, 2004, Mosby.)

4.49. Correct Answer: **d**
Hypertensive crisis, hyperthermia, seizures, and rigidity have resulted when *meperidine* is given to a patient with circulating MAOIs. The neurologic and vascular excitation can be fatal. Reactions with other narcotics that release histamine such as morphine sulfate are not as severe. MAOI levels remain in the system for 3 to 4 weeks, even after discontinuance. In addition, accumulation of meperidine metabolites after large analgesic doses can produce seizures. (Burden N et al: *Ambulatory surgical nursing*, ed 2, Philadelphia, 2000, Saunders; Cole DJ, Schlunt M: *Adult perioperative anesthesia: the requisites in anesthesiology*, St. Louis, 2004, Mosby.)

4.50. Correct Answer: **c**
Though consciousness is drug depressed, the patient must retain his ability to "independently and continuously maintain a patent airway." A patient under conscious sedation also responds "appropriately" to verbal or touch stimulation. An anesthesia provider need not be present because management and monitoring of the patient during his procedure is within the PACU nurse's scope of practice. (ASPAN: *2006-2008 Standards of perianesthesia nursing practice*, Cherry Hill, NJ, 2006, ASPAN; Burden N et al: *Ambulatory surgical nursing*, ed 2, Philadelphia, 2000, Saunders; Kost M: *Moderate sedation/analgesia: core competencies for practice*, ed 2, Philadelphia, 2004, Saunders; Odom-Forren J, Watson DS: *Practical guide to moderate sedation/analgesia*, ed 2, St. Louis, 2005, Mosby.)

4.51. Correct Answer: **b**
Medications for conscious sedation include medications classified as narcotics and sedatives but not as anesthetics. Sedatives decrease anxiety and discomfort but stop short of obliterating airway control or consciousness. Patients can still breathe and respond appropriately to verbal stimuli. Therefore doses are titrated to response lest they oversedate and anesthetize. Thiopental, propofol, ketamine, and methohexital are classified as

anesthetics. (ASPAN: *2006-2008 Standards of perianesthesia nursing practice*, Cherry Hill, 2006, ASPAN; Burden N et al: *Ambulatory surgical nursing*, ed 2, Philadelphia, 2000, Saunders; Kost M: *Moderate sedation/analgesia: core competencies for practice*, ed 2, Philadelphia, 2004, Saunders; Odom-Forren J, Watson DS: *Practical guide to moderate sedation/analgesia*, ed 2, St. Louis, 2005, Mosby.)

4.52. Correct Answer: **b**
Rapid entry of sodium into nerve cells is blocked by local anesthetics. The cell membrane retains an ongoing resting condition and does not respond to stimuli. The normal resting condition of a cell membrane is actually an ionized charge. Potassium ion (K^+) has free "access" into the nerve cell membrane, whereas access by sodium ion (Na^+) is restricted. Normally, when a depolarizing electrical stimulus alters cell membrane permeability, sodium ions flood in, producing an action potential and muscle contraction. (Burden N et al: *Ambulatory surgical nursing*, ed 2, Philadelphia, 2000, Saunders; Cole DJ, Schlunt M: *Adult perioperative anesthesia: the requisites in anesthesiology*, St. Louis, 2004, Mosby; Drain C, editor: *Perianesthesia nursing: a critical care approach*, ed 4, Philadelphia, 2003, Saunders; Miller RD et al, editors: *Anesthesia* (2-vol set with CD-ROM for Windows & Macintosh), ed 5, London, 2000, Churchill Livingstone; Rathmell JP, Neal JM, Viscomi CM: *Regional anesthesia: the requisites in anesthesiology*, St. Louis, 2004, Mosby; Robertson KM et al: *Anesthesiology board review*, ed 2, New York, 2006, McGraw-Hill; Roizen MF, Fleisher LA: *Essence of anesthesia practice*, ed 2, Philadelphia, 2002, Saunders.)

4.53. Correct Answer: **c**
Usually conservative treatment is indicated for the first day, and after 24 hours the treatment of choice would be an epidural blood patch. Epidural blood patches relieve over 90% to 95% of the cases. (Drain C, editor: *Perianesthesia nursing: a critical care approach*, ed 4, Philadelphia, 2003, Saunders; Quinn D, Schick L, editors: *ASPAN's perianesthesia nursing core curriculum: preoperative, Phase I and Phase II PACU nursing*, Philadelphia, 2004, Saunders; Rathmell JP, Neal JM, Viscomi CM: *Regional anesthesia: the requisites in anesthesiology*, St. Louis, 2004, Mosby.)

Chapter 5

The Spectrum of Perianesthesia Clinical Practice

Scenarios and items in this section represent situations that exemplify perianesthesia nursing practice. This specialty is defined by a set of knowledge and skills related to *anesthetic medications, techniques*, and *surgical manipulations* that significantly alter a patient's organ systems. These concepts are considered together because the perianesthesia clinical nurse:

- Focuses on anesthesia-induced alterations of airway, circulation, consciousness, and neurologic function that require astute nursing consideration, whether for 5 minutes or 5 hours

- Practices this unique body of knowledge for varied and highly individual patient situations
- Synthesizes and applies concepts from multiple clinical disciplines to a diverse clinical population and spectrum, which includes infants, critically-ill patients, elderly individuals, and a vvariety of organ system or musculoskeletal procedures
- Distinguishes priorities from an assortment of wide-ranging and frequently simultaneous concerns

ESSENTIAL CORE CONCEPTS	AFFILIATED CORE CURRICULUM CHAPTERS
Nursing Process	**Chapters 3, 35, 56, 61**
Assessment	
Planning and Implementation	
Evaluation	
Perianesthesia Spectrum	**Chapters 2, 4, 7;**
Situational Applications	**Section 5—Chapters 24-37**
Anesthetics	
Pharmacodynamics	
Pharmacokinetics	
Receptors and Blocks	
Regional, Local, General, or Balanced Conscious Sedation	
Standards and Safety	
Perianesthesia Units and Beyond	
Preanesthesia to Discharge Education	
Priorities: Imminent Need or Remote Potential	
Surgical Manipulations	

Cautery and Blood Loss
Position, Injury, and Pain

Clinical Continuums

Airway: From Patency to Obstruction
Awareness: From Delays to Delirium
Cardiac: From Heartbeat to Heart Failure
Consciousness: From Sedation to Self-
    Awareness
Hemodynamics: From Hemorrhage to
    Hemostasis
From Hypotension to Hypertension
From Vessel Patency to Stagnation
Immunity: From Allergy to Sepsis
Nausea: From Retching to Relief
Neurologic: From Deficit to Function
Oxygenation: From Hypoxia to Toxicity
Pain: From Angst to Comfort
Pulmonary: From Ventilation to Apnea
From Croup to Aspiration
Temperature: From Shivers to Sweats

SET 1

ITEMS 5.1–5.22

5.1. A nurse caring for an ambulatory surgical patient in the main PACU rather than a PACU used exclusively for outpatients understands that this patient is most likely to experience:
a. a positive response to the technical environment.
b. a less stressful environment.
c. care delivered by a nurse who is more experienced in handling emergency treatment protocols.
d. a more rapid reunion with significant others.

5.2. Regular, frequent hand washing is a proven means of preventing cross-contamination in the perianesthesia setting, yet this practice is often overlooked. The best method to change behavior and ensure that hand washing is regularly performed by nursing staff is to:
a. install hand sanitizer dispensers at every bedside.
b. replace hand washing with use of protective gloves.
c. monitor hand washing compliance of personnel.
d. provide regular education regarding the importance of hand washing.

5.3. A PACU nurse accepts a 46-year-old male patient from the operating room. The anesthesia provider reports that a 1% mepivicaine lumbar epidural anesthesia was administered for the 20-minute lower extremity procedure, rather than 1% lidocaine lumbar epidural anesthesia because:
a. mepivicaine has a longer duration of action.
b. the patient is susceptible to hypotension.
c. the patient has a history of cardiac dysrhythmias.
d. mepivicaine has a low level of potency and toxicity.

5.4. A 7-year-old boy is admitted to the PACU after undergoing general anesthesia for orthopedic repair of a congenital foot anomaly. The child has had three prior surgeries related to this anomaly and arrives in the PACU sedate but responding appropriately to simple commands. The nurse applies oxygen, observes symmetric chest expansion, and auscultates the lungs, which are clear. The child exhibits inspiratory and expiratory throat sounds at a rate of 16 breaths per minute, a SpO_2 of 96%, and a heart rate of 114 bpm. It is most important to closely monitor this child's airway because:
a. there is an audible partial obstruction.
b. oropharyngeal suctioning is frequently indicated.
c. there is potential for rapid airway obstruction.
d. he is positioned in a ¾ prone position.

5.5. Family member visitation in the PACU should:
a. be limited to pediatric patients.
b. begin when a pediatric patient is admitted to the PACU.
c. only be determined by the individual nurse caring for a patient.
d. be based on practitioner guidelines developed within their perianesthesia practice setting.

NOTE: Consider the scenario and items 5.6-5.7 together.

An alert, oriented 60-year-old woman arrives in the PACU after a 2½-hour surgery for placement of a right total hip prosthesis. An 8-mg 0.75% bupivacaine (Marcaine) spinal anesthesia was administered 30 minutes preoperatively, and the patient received intraoperative IV doses of 3 mg of midazolam and 8 mg of morphine. Assessment reveals absence of sensation at the T7 dermatome, and she is unable to move both legs.

5.6. The patient tells the nurse that she is worried about being unable to move her legs. The PACU nurse calculates the known residual effects of bupivacaine and advises the patient not to worry because her leg movements:
a. could remain anesthetized for 3 to 6 more hours.
b. will return within 30 to 60 minutes.
c. will return entirely in 90 minutes.
d. should completely return to normal in 2 hours.

5.7. Twenty minutes after PACU admission, the patient verbalizes dizziness and says she is feeling very weak. The nurse examines the patient and notes that her blood pressure has dropped from 128/84 on admission to 90/54. The nurse's next immediate action is to:
a. notify the attending anesthesia provider.
b. assess for surgical bleeding.
c. deliver a bolus of IV fluid.
d. place the patient in Trendelenburg position.

5.8. A male patient has been in the PACU for 30 minutes recovering from general anesthesia for a gastrectomy procedure for malignant tumor. A nasogastric tube is in place with small amounts of bright, bloody drainage present. He is now awake and oriented, lying on his left side, respirations are normal, and the lungs are clear and equal bilaterally. He reports a pain level of 4/10 at the incision area after the nurse administered a total of 3 mg of IV morphine 15 minutes ago for a reported pain level of 8/10. The nurse's next action is to assist the patient with repositioning to a semi-Fowler position to:
a. enhance comfort of the indwelling nasogastric tube.
b. instruct the patient to perform coughing and deep breathing exercises.
c. promote comfort and decrease pressure on the suture lines.
d. check the wound dressing.

5.9. Unless a known contraindication exists, the preferred method of postoperative pain control for a Phase I gastrectomy procedure patient is:
a. patient-controlled analgesia (PCA) in the demand dose mode.
b. a low thoracic epidural analgesia delivery system.
c. PCA with a continuous infusion rate.
d. a mid-thoracic epidural analgesia delivery system.

5.10. A 39-year-old female patient is in Phase I PACU after receiving general anesthesia. Her cardiac monitor shows sinus bradycardia at a rate of 42 bpm. She easily arouses to verbal stimuli and states she feels fine except for 2/10 incision pain from her right breast biopsy site. Her preanesthetic blood pressure assessment was documented as 124/74 and is now 100/62 with a SpO_2 of 98% on oxygen at 4 liters/minute by nasal cannula. The most appropriate action by the nurse caring for this patient is to consult the anesthesiologist and anticipate:
a. an IV fluid bolus of crystalloid solution.
b. administration of a 0.1-mg dose of IV atropine.
c. moving the emergency crash cart closer to the bedside.
d. continued stir-up regimen and observation.

5.11. The PACU nurse performs an assessment on an 80-kg, 72-year-old male patient admitted 10 minutes earlier after general anesthesia for transurethral resection of the bladder tumor, after a failed spinal anesthetic attempt. The nurse observes a very sedate patient who barely responds to loud verbal and touch stimuli with 8 breaths per minute, shallow respirations, clear breath sounds that are diminished throughout both lung fields, and a SpO_2 of 82% on oxygen at 60% by facemask. The nurse confirms airway patency, increases the FiO_2 to 100%, stimulates the patient to take deep breaths, and has a colleague immediately call the attending anesthesiologist. With regard to the respiratory parameters identified during this assessment, the nurse:

a. understands that hypoventilation is a significant postoperative problem.
b. retrieves the intubation tray and prepares to use a size 7.5-mm tube.
c. does not question the placement or accuracy of the pulse oximeter reading.
d. expects the normal tidal volume range for this gentleman to measure between 400 and 560 mL/kg.

5.12. The clinical characteristics of moderate sedation and analgesia include:
a. inability to control secretions, patent airway, and easy arousal.
b. maintenance of protective reflexes, patent airway, and response to verbal or light tactile stimulation.
c. partial loss of protective reflexes, not easily aroused, and patent airway.
d. maintenance of protective reflexes, partial loss of airway, and easy arousal.

5.13. Which of the following statements is *true* regarding assessment of the patient receiving moderate sedation/analgesia?
a. It is not always possible to predict an individual patient's reaction to sedation.
b. It is possible to predict an individual patient's reaction to sedation if following medication guidelines available in the Physician's Desk Reference (PDR).
c. Spontaneous ventilation is frequently inadequate with moderate sedation; therefore the patient requires critical ventilatory assessment.
d. Airway intervention is often required when using moderate sedation.

NOTE: Consider the scenario and items 5.14-5.16 together.

A surgeon refers a 54-year-old female patient with Type 2 diabetes to the preanesthesia evaluation and testing unit for blood work, ECG, preanesthesia evaluation, and education. The preanesthesia nurse reviews the surgeon's preoperative history and physical and related physician orders for this patient and then escorts the patient to a private area and begins the preanesthesia interview. The patient is scheduled for an outpatient laparoscopic cholecystectomy procedure in 7 days, arrives for her preanesthesia appointment alone, and states she lives alone. She follows a diabetic diet and takes daily Glucophage to successfully manage blood sugar readings in the desired range established by her endocrinologist.

5.14. Collaborative nurse and attending surgeon considerations regarding the preparation of a patient for outpatient surgery should include:
a. identifying the responsible adult caregiver for the postoperative period.
b. allowing the preanesthesia nurse to perform specific testing based on the history and physical findings.
c. reporting findings for all preoperative tests performed.
d. standing orders for all consents to be obtained in the preanesthesia unit.

5.15. The patient is closely monitored during the perianesthesia period involving general anesthesia. The perianesthesia nurse understands that in a perianesthesia diabetic patient:
a. glucose-free urine levels are a desired outcome.
b. the target serum glucose level is <200 mg/dL.
c. fluid losses are less significant because of increased cardiac stressors from anesthesia.
d. a preoperative or intraoperative infusion of 5% dextrose IV solution is contraindicated.

5.16. The patient arrives in the PACU awake and oriented with stable vital signs and denies any untoward symptoms. Soon after PACU admission, she has a blood pressure of 108/58 and exhibits shallow breathing, diaphoretic skin, pallor, and vertigo. The nurse notifies the attending anesthesia provider and anticipates:
a. treatment consistent with an impending myocardial infarction.
b. performing a finger-stick blood sugar and obtaining an elevated result on the glucometer.

c. insulin administration to prevent further progression of early diabetic coma.
d. IV intravenous administration of a concentrated dextrose solution.

NOTE: Consider the scenario and items 5.17-5.20 together.

A 45-year-old female patient is admitted to the preoperative holding area for an elective abdominal hysterectomy under general anesthesia. She is a nonsmoker with no significant medical history or problems (American Society of Anesthesiologists [ASA] I). She has had no previous surgeries but does have a history of motion sickness. Postoperative pain management will include IV PCA with fentanyl. Based on the ASPAN *Evidence-Based Clinical Practice Guideline for the Prevention and/or Management of PONV/PDNV*, answer questions 5.17-5.20.

5.17. Based on the presenting risk factors, the patient is at a _____ risk for developing PONV.
a. low
b. moderate
c. severe
d. very severe

5.18. Based on the presenting level of risk for developing PONV, you can expect to work with the anesthesia and surgical team to implement at least _____ prophylactic measure(s).
a. 0
b. 1
c. 2
d. 3

5.19. Based on the patient's presenting factors, which of the following prophylactic combinations are most likely to be administered?
a. Total IV anesthesia (TIVA), dexamethasone, scopolamine patch

b. TIVA, dexamethasone, metoclopramide
c. TIVA, scopolamine patch, metoclopramide
d. TIVA, 5-HT$_3$ receptor antagonist, metoclopramide

5.20. If rescue therapy is indicated, which agent should the PACU nurse administer?
a. Dexamethasone
b. 5-HT$_3$ antagonist
c. Promethazine
d. Metoclopramide

NOTE: Consider the scenario and items 5.21-5.22 together.

An anesthesiologist orders a continuous fentanyl epidural infusion for a 44-year-old female after a total abdominal hysterectomy procedure. The awake patient verbalizes 9/10 pain to the admitting nurse upon arrival in the PACU. The anesthesia provider immediately treats this pain report by administering a 100-mcg bolus dose of epidural fentanyl.

5.21. The PACU nurse expects this patient to experience an onset of pain relief from this fentanyl dosage within:
a. 5 to 10 minutes.
b. 10 to 20 minutes.
c. 15 to 25 minutes.
d. 20 to 30 minutes.

5.22. While connecting the epidural fentanyl infusion, the PACU nurse recognizes that this medication:
a. is less potent than epidural morphine.
b. has few undesirable side effects.
c. requires good catheter placement because of the medication's properties.
d. requires infrequent dosing adjustments.

SET 2

ITEMS 5.23–5.42

NOTE: Consider the scenario and items 5.23-5.24 together.

A male patient is admitted to the preanesthesia unit at 10 AM for a 12 noon surgical procedure. The history and physical documents no known allergies for this patient. The patient is employed as an industrial environmental services worker and frequently wears latex gloves. During the admission interview he tells the nurse he "might be" allergic to latex because his hands have been breaking out in a rash every day lately after wearing the gloves. All operating rooms are actively running cases on this morning, and the hospital does not have a dedicated latex-free operating room.

5.23. The type of latex reaction described by this patient is classified as a:
   a. Type I reaction.
   b. Type II reaction.
   c. Type III reaction.
   d. Type IV reaction.

5.24. Based on the patient's initial self-report, in addition to notifying the surgeon, surgical team, and anesthesia team, the preanesthesia nurse's next most appropriate action is to:
   a. immediately check vital signs using non-latex unit equipment.
   b. collect a more detailed history from the patient.
   c. initiate a latex-free IV infusion.
   d. contact an allergist to examine the patient.

5.25. Which of the following is the most commonly occurring postoperative complication?
   a. Postoperative hypothermia
   b. Sinus tachycardia
   c. Postoperative nausea and vomiting (PONV)
   d. Postoperative wound infection

NOTE: Consider the scenario and items 5.26-5.27 together.

A postoperative femoral-popliteal graft procedure patient met criteria for discharge from the Phase I PACU to a cardiac observation unit. The PACU nurse coordinated the patient's transfer by telephone with the accepting nurse, notified the nurse that this patient required continuous telemetry monitoring, and stated the patient would arrive to the assigned room in 5 to 10 minutes. The two nurses agreed that a verbal hand-off report would take place in person at the patient's bedside.

5.26. To ensure safe transfer of care for this patient, the PACU nurse's most appropriate action is to:
   a. administer only small amounts of opioid medication just before discharge from PACU.
   b. apply supplemental oxygen to prevent hypoxemia during the transport phase.
   c. assign appropriate staff members to transport the patient.
   d. position the portable cardiac monitor in plain view of the unit aide pushing the gurney.

NOTE: The scenario continues.

The PACU nurse arrives on the nursing unit with the patient, notifies the unit clerk of the patient's arrival, requests the accepting nurse's assistance, and then takes the patient directly to the assigned room. After a 9-minute wait and a second request for a relief nurse by the PACU nurse, no telemetry unit nurse has arrived in the room. The PACU nurse is paged to immediately return to the PACU because of limited staffing available in the PACU and the pending arrival of two critical care patients from the operating room.

5.27. The PACU nurse's most appropriate action is to:
   a. wait at the bedside until the accepting unit nurse comes for report.
   b. attach the telemetry, give the alert patient a call light, and leave a written report for the nurse.
   c. request immediate relief from the telemetry unit charge nurse or administrative supervisor.
   d. have an experienced nursing assistant remain with the patient until the nurse can come.

5.28. A patient received a usual dose of succinylcholine during general anesthesia and is admitted to the PACU with previously undiagnosed atypical pseudocholinesterase deficiency. The nurse understands that this patient can have sustained apnea for up to:
   a. 12 hours.
   b. 24 hours.
   c. 36 hours.
   d. 48 hours.

5.29. During preanesthesia screening a 48-year-old female reports that she has been taking Maxzide 25 mg/day for treatment of hypertension for 1 year and *Gingko biloba* extract 120 mg/day for the beneficial antioxidant properties for the past 6 months. The surgery is scheduled for 3 weeks from the date of the preanesthesia appointment. Based on the patient's self-report regarding medication and herbal supplement use, the preanesthesia nurse recognizes that *Gingko biloba:*
   a. increases the platelet count.
   b. should be discontinued for 7 days before surgery.
   c. has no known interactions with thiazide diuretics.
   d. should be discontinued for 2 weeks before surgery.

NOTE: Consider the scenario and items 5.30-5.31 together.

A patient unsuccessfully attempted vaginal birth after a previous cesarean delivery and was taken to the operating room for failure to progress during a difficult 22-hour labor period.

The patient was admitted to the PACU after receiving general anesthesia for cesarean delivery of a healthy 4.2-kg boy. The nurse examines the patient on admission, performs a fundus check, and discovers her uterus is boggy and the perineal pad is completely soaked with blood.

5.30. The nurse most effectively performs external uterine massage by:
   a. supporting the lower uterus.
   b. applying a bimanual compression technique.
   c. asking the patient to simultaneously tighten the abdominal muscles to promote uterine contraction.
   d. instructing the patient to take shallow breaths to prevent increased diaphragmatic pressure during the massage.

NOTE: The scenario continues.

Oxytocin 20 units/1000 mL of normal saline is infusing at 500 mL/hour. Thirty minutes after PACU admission, the second perineal pad is completely soaked with blood and the patient's blood pressure has dropped to 88/52 with the monitor showing sinus tachycardia at 126 bpm. The anesthesia record indicates that the estimated blood loss in surgery was 1050 mL with no blood replacement products administered. The bleeding remains uncontrolled in the PACU and the patient requires massive transfusion therapy.

5.31. While administering repeated units of packed red blood cells, the PACU nurse understands that massive transfusion therapy is defined as:
   a. administering 8 or more units of packed red blood cells in a 24-hour period.
   b. a 50% replacement of blood volume within 3 hours.
   c. an estimated blood loss of more than 4000 mL.
   d. replacing 75% of the patient's circulating blood volume.

5.32. A female patient admitted to the PACU has blockade after spinal anesthesia assessed at the T4 dermatome. During Phase I recovery, this patient is at increased risk to develop:
   a. sympathetic blockade hypertension.

b. deep vein thrombosis caused by venous stasis.

c. respiratory insufficiency.

d. urinary incontinence.

5.33. The most accurate measure of the patient's core temperature in the PACU is made with a:

a. pulmonary artery catheter.

b. oral thermometer.

c. tympanic thermometer.

d. bladder thermometer.

NOTE: Consider the scenario and items 5.34-5.35 together.

During the PACU admission assessment on a barely responsive elderly man, the nurse observes occasional premature ventricular contractions on the cardiac monitor. During the 150-minute surgery, the patient received oxygen with nitrous oxide and thiopental, then Tracrium, fentanyl, halothane, and dolasetron. Blood pressure is 84/50, measured by a noninvasive automatic device. The attending anesthesia provider orders an immediate 200-mL normal saline fluid bolus.

5.34. Considering the inhalation anesthetic used for this patient, the nurse determines that the presence of ventricular ectopy is most likely related to:

a. parasympathetic nervous system stimulation.

b. a decreased rate of SA node discharge.

c. a decrease in bundle of His–Purkinje and ventricular conduction times.

d. decreased ventricular automaticity.

5.35. The medication most likely to cause an increase in cardiac dysrhythmias as a result of pharmacokinetic interaction with the inhalation anesthetic used for this patient is:

a. furosemide.

b. chlorpromazine.

c. epinephrine.

d. gentamycin.

5.36. A patient receives midazolam in the PACU. Which of the following statements is true about midazolam?

a. Midazolam has a rapid onset of action, moderate amnesic effects, faster peak effect in elderly adults, and is contraindicated for patients with acute narrow-angle glaucoma.

b. Midazolam does not inhibit the activity of any known drugs, has excellent amnesic effects, and is water soluble.

c. Midazolam is metabolized by an agent in the blood and excreted through the urine, has excellent amnesic effects, and is contraindicated for patients with acute narrow-angle glaucoma.

d. Midazolam has a rapid onset of action, excellent amnesic effects, is water soluble, and is contraindicated for patients with acute narrow-angle glaucoma.

5.37. A patient received a single injection of 15 mg of extended-release epidural morphine (EREM) after repair of a severe orthopedic trauma to the left lower extremity. While giving a transfer-of-care report to the surgical unit nurse, the PACU nurse states that the patient may have effective pain relief from EREM for how many hours?

a. 24

b. 36

c. 48

d. 60

5.38. The primary investigator of a nursing research project invites perianesthesia staff member participation in data collection. The study's purpose is to compare analgesic effects and patient responses to a nonsteroidal antiinflammatory drug (NSAID) and a narcotic medication. The perianesthesia nurses' role is to document participants' relevant physiologic data and reported pain level based on a 0-10 numeric pain scale before and after the medication is administered. Before participating in data collection, the perianesthesia nurse questions the researcher to ensure that:

a. the steps to collect data are well defined.

b. descriptive statistics will be applied to validate data analysis.

c. reliability testing was performed on the data assessment tool.

d. approval was granted by an institutional review board.

5.39. The optimal postoperative positioning of the bariatric surgery patient is:
a. left side-lying with head of bed elevated 20° to 30°.
b. semi-recumbent.
c. supine until the patient is awake and responding appropriately to commands.
d. right side-lying with head of bed elevated 20° to 30°.

5.40. A visually impaired patient arrives for surgery. The preanesthesia nurse conducts the preoperative interview and facilitates care management while paying special attention to:
a. speaking in a normal tone and volume.
b. guiding the patient to the bathroom for preoperative voiding while giving directions from behind the patient.
c. ambient environmental sounds.
d. witnessing the patient's signature on the surgical consent form.

5.41. A 36-year-old man had surgical repair of an inguinal hernia and is now in Phase II PACU. While performing discharge teaching, the postanesthesia nurse addresses postdischarge pain medication and treatment. The nurse instructs the patient to take pain medication:
a. when his pain level is self-rated at 5/10 to 6/10.
b. every 4 hours around the clock.
c. at early onset to maintain an acceptable pain goal.
d. only after trying other comfort measures.

5.42. Perianesthesia care of the immunosuppressed patient includes:
a. mandatory placement of the patient in protective isolation.
b. assessment for classic signs and symptoms of infection.
c. constant direct visualization of needle puncture and incision sites.
d. cleansing of common-use monitoring items before application.

SET 3

ITEMS 5.43–5.60

NOTE: Consider the scenario and items 5.43-5.44 together.

A 90-kg male is being cared for in the PACU after general anesthesia for a three-level lumbar fusion procedure. The nurse observed sinus rhythm with occasional premature atrial contractions for the first 20 minutes of his PACU course and now responds to a monitor alarm indicating the high heart rate limit has been exceeded at 132 bpm. The nurse examines the patient who is breathing well, shows a blood pressure drop from 128/78 on admission to 108/62, responds to verbal stimuli, is oriented to place, and states he feels sleepy but fine. The nurse obtains and reviews the cardiac monitor strip, immediately notifies the attending anesthesia provider, and performs a 12-lead ECG. The anesthesiologist arrives and identifies the sustained ECG rhythm as supraventricular tachycardia.

5.43. The anesthesiologist orders an immediate dose of IV propranolol. The PACU nurse understands that propranolol:
a. is a beta adrenergic receptor antagonist.
b. dosing for this patient should not exceed a 9-mg total.
c. can be rapidly administered in a 1- to 2-mg IV dose.
d. has a peak action time of 3 minutes.

NOTE: The scenario continues.

The patient has a history of thrombolytic events; therefore the surgeon's postoperative orders request anticoagulant therapy with a heparin-loading dose to be followed by a continuous heparin infusion.

5.44. Regarding the heparin order, the PACU nurse's most appropriate action is to:
a. initiate the order as soon as possible.
b. keenly assess for postoperative bleeding because of increased partial thromboplastin time associated with this anticoagulant therapy.
c. notify the surgeon and anesthesiologist of an associated risk related to this medication.
d. place a "Bleeding Precautions" sign on the patient's bed.

5.45. A normal 7.3-kg infant's total lung capacity is calculated to equal:
a. 438 mL.
b. 475 mL.
c. 511 mL.
d. 548 mL.

5.46. A new anesthesia provider group has recently taken over the contract services for a freestanding surgery center, completely replacing the previous anesthesia providers with new practitioners. The PACU nursing staff note an increased trend of emergence delirium in their pediatric surgical population manifested as thrashing, disorientation, and agitation. The nurses perform a retrospective review of the pediatric anesthesia records, which reveals increased use of which of the following inhalation agents associated with increased incidence of emergence behavioral changes in pediatric cases:
a. sevoflurane.
b. desflurane.
c. isoflurane.
d. halothane.

5.47. The preanesthesia nurse informs the surgical team and PACU staff that a patient has a documented history of reactive airway disease, hepatitis B, and human immunodeficiency virus (HIV) infection. The PACU staff plans to care for this patient in the early post anesthesia period by:
a. placing contaminated needles in a high-risk isolation container.

b. wearing a protective face shield, gown and gloves.

c. wearing gloves.

d. placing contaminated IV tubing in the sharps container after discontinuation.

5.48. When caring for the geriatric patient, the perianesthesia nurse understands that:

a. aging causes an increase in systolic and diastolic blood pressure of 8 to 9 mmHg per decade.

b. renal blood flow and glomerular filtration rates are minimally impacted.

c. the number of drug receptor sites decreases.

d. medication uptake occurs rapidly necessitating smaller dosages.

5.49. In relation to inhalation anesthetic agents, minimum alveolar concentration (MAC):

a. values are higher when the inhalation anesthetic agent is more potent.

b. is the percent of inhalation anesthetic agent breathed that prevents movement during surgical incision in 75% of patients.

c. represents the minimum 21% oxygen required as a carrier gas for inhalation anesthetic agents.

d. is best described as the potency for each inhalation anesthetic agent.

5.50. A 54-year-old male presents to the PACU after an open abdominal aortic aneurysm repair under general anesthesia. Surgical time was 4 hours. Blood loss was 2400 mL with adequate blood and fluid replacement. Risk factors for hypothermia in this patient include all *except:*

a. gender of patient.

b. length and type of surgical procedure.

c. significant fluid shift.

d. general anesthesia.

5.51. The patient presents with a pulmonary artery temperature reading of 35.5° C (95.9° F). The most appropriate warming intervention would be to:

a. apply warmed cotton blankets.

b. apply forced air warming.

c. apply warming lights.

d. increase the ambient room temperature.

5.52. A patient returns to the same-day procedure unit from the anesthesia interventional pain treatment service for recovery after a stellate ganglion block was performed. The postanesthesia nurse understands that stellate ganglion blockade can produce:

a. dilated but reactive pupils.

b. a high spinal anesthesia.

c. reflex sympathetic dystrophy syndrome.

d. irritation of the coughing reflex.

5.53. The recommended amount of electrical energy to deliver for initial pediatric defibrillation is:

a. 1 joule/kg.

b. 2 joules/kg.

c. 3 joules/kg.

d. 4 joules/kg.

5.54. A 22-year-old female is admitted to the preanesthesia unit for a carpal tunnel release procedure. As the nurse explains the process for preparing her for surgery, the patient appears quite anxious and expresses fear and anxiety about needle sticks because of prior negative encounters with venipunctures. The patient is scheduled to go into the operating room in 30 minutes. The preanesthesia nurse understands that lidocaine iontophoresis:

a. is less effective than lidocaine infiltration.

b. is more time consuming than application of a eutectic mixture of local anesthetic (EMLA).

c. may aggravate the needle phobia.

d. is an excellent choice for this patient.

5.55. A patient with extensive metastatic cancer is scheduled for a bowel resection under general anesthesia to relieve an obstruction. The patient arrives in the preoperative holding area with an active "Do Not Resuscitate" order.

The most appropriate way for the nurse to manage this situation is to:

a. explain to the patient that intubation is a requirement for anesthesia during this procedure.
b. support automatic suspension of the DNR order during the perianesthesia period.
c. facilitate a discussion regarding the DNR order with the patient and the surgical care team before surgery.
d. tell the patient the active DNR status is not impacted by a surgical intervention.

5.56. Incorporating culturally competent care for Chinese-American patients in the perianesthesia environment requires the nurse to understand their existing belief structure, which includes:

a. a propensity for resisting blood draws.
b. believing that external causes of disease are rooted in poor familial relationships.
c. believing that internal causes of disease relate to a labile emotional state.
d. believing that illness results from an imbalance in yin and yang.

NOTE: Consider the scenario and items 5.57-5.58 together.

A 19-year-old female is admitted late one evening to the preoperative holding area for an emergency incision and drainage of an infected right 5th finger. The anesthesiologist inserts a femoral IV line after multiple unsuccessful attempts to access a peripheral upper extremity vein. The patient is fully oriented and has a temperature of 38° C (100.4° F), blood pressure of 90/52, and heart rate of 72 bpm. She appears thin, pale, nervous, and jittery with dilated pupils, rhinorrhea, and multiple small, round scars on the inner and outer aspects of both forearms and calves. She says she feels nauseous, repeatedly denies use of any medications or street drugs, and says she has no idea how or why the infection in her finger occurred.

5.57. Based on the initial physical examination, the nurse deduces the patient is most likely:

a. in an acute stage of opiate abstinence.
b. becoming septic.
c. taking a central nervous system sympathomimetic drug.
d. injecting cocaine.

5.58. The patient arrives in the PACU reactive from general anesthesia and is asking for pain medication. She received 12 mg of intraoperative morphine sulfate and rates her operative pain at 10/10. The nurse administers 3 mg of IV morphine sulfate and anticipates that the patient will:

a. require supplemental doses of butorphanol.
b. require liberal opioid doses in the PACU.
c. respond well to this dose.
d. have increased risk for quinine toxicity.

5.59. The perianesthesia nurse recognizes that propofol has many beneficial properties including:

a. rare episodes of pain on injection.
b. adjuvant analgesic properties.
c. less psychomotor impairment.
d. drug clearance equal to hepatic blood flow.

5.60. A 58-year-old male patient weighing 85 kg is intubated on arrival in the PACU. The anesthesia provider asks the nurse to notify her when the patient meets criteria for extubation. Acceptable tidal volume (TV), vital capacity (VC), and negative inspiratory force (NIF) extubation parameters for this patient are:

a. TV = 400 mL, VC = 1290 mL, NIF = 17 cm water pressure.
b. TV = 425 mL, VC = 1175 mL, NIF = 20 cm water pressure.
c. TV = 450 mL, VC = 1290 mL, NIF = 22 cm water pressure.
d. TV = 475 mL, VC = 1150 mL, NIF = 18 cm water pressure.

SET 4

NOTE: Consider the scenario and items 5.61-5.63 together.

5.61. A female patient is receiving a bone marrow test in the procedural area that is currently staffed by PACU. She is 81 years old, weighs 280 pounds, and has a history of hypertension, stable atrial fibrillation, and diabetes. Which of the following monitors is *not* a standard procedure for a patient with this patient's history of:
a. pulse oximeter.
b. capnograph.
c. cardiac monitor.
d. blood pressure monitoring.

5.62. The preadmission history for this patient would be best served with inclusion of:
a. blood glucose level, airway assessment, vital signs, and current medications.
b. vital signs, blood glucose level, current medications, and clotting time.
c. vital signs, airway assessment, hemoglobin and hematocrit (H&H), and discharge planning.
d. vital signs, current medications, thyroid levels, and sleep apnea assessment.

5.63. This patient would be at risk for:
a. hyperglycemia, hypertension, hypothyroidism, and hypercarbia.
b. hypercarbia, hypoxemia, hypertension, and hypoglycemia.
c. sleep apnea, dysrhythmias, hypocarbia, and hypoglycemia.
d. hypercarbia, hypotension, hypoglycemia, and dysrhythmias.

NOTE: The scenario continues.

5.64. Soon after the patient's temperature drops to 96° F, the nurse also notes that the pulse oximeter is now reading 91% saturation. She calls this immediately to the attention of the physician even though alarm limits are set below 90% because the:
a. oxygen saturation level is not adequate for this patient because of her obesity.
b. patient's hypothermia has contributed to a right shift of the oxygen-hemoglobin disassociation curve causing the hemoglobin to have a decreased affinity for hemoglobin; therefore the oxygen saturation level is lower than the pulse oximeter reading.
c. patient's hypothermia has contributed to a left shift of the oxygen-hemoglobin disassociation curve causing the hemoglobin to have an increased affinity for hemoglobin; therefore the oxygen saturation level is lower than the pulse oximeter reading.
d. patient needs increased oxygenation because of her history of atrial fibrillation.

NOTE: Consider the scenario and items 5.65-5.66 together.

A 35-year-old male patient arrives in the preoperative unit for jointly scheduled surgical procedures. The patient will undergo a right knee arthroscopy to be performed by the orthopedic surgeon and a left forearm scar revision procedure to be performed by the plastic surgeon.

5.65. The perianesthesia nurse understands that risk factors for wrong site surgery:
a. are not related to site verification policies and procedures.
b. are minimized by adherence to a preoperative verification checklist.
c. expand with effective surgical team communication.
d. are marginally related to preanesthesia patient assessment.

5.66. In response to related sentinel events, The Joint Commission (TJC) developed a universal protocol to prevent wrong site, wrong procedure, wrong person surgery. This TJC patient safety protocol includes all the following steps *except:*
   a. operative site marking.
   b. a preoperative verification process.
   c. a "time out" period taken immediately before the patient is brought to the operating room.
   d. the operative site is marked in a manner that allows clear visualization after the patient has been draped in the operating room.

5.67. The following properties are true about fentanyl:
   a. hydrophilic, slow onset, and minimal histamine release.
   b. lipophilic, slow onset and no effect on histamine release.
   c. lipophilic, rapid onset and minimal histamine release.
   d. hydrophilic, rapid onset and minimal histamine release.

5.68. The surgeon decides to use propofol for sedation on a patient and requires the use of a certified registered nurse anesthetist (CRNA) or anesthesiologist (MDA). The reason(s) may be that propofol:
   a. is an anesthetic agent and your state board of nursing has not approved nurse-administered propofol sedation.
   b. is a sedative and your state board of nursing has not approved nurse-administered propofol sedation.
   c. is not approved for use in the elderly.
   d. has a slow effect on the patient.

5.69. The American Society of PeriAnesthesia Nurses in its statement on the role of the RN in management of patients undergoing sedation includes all *except:*
   a. ACLS and/or PALS provider status recommended.
   b. presedation evaluation must be conducted.
   c. airway assessment using Mallampati scoring system is required.
   d. the RN should have no other responsibilities that leave the patient unattended or would compromise monitoring.

SET 1

ANSWER KEY

5.1.	c		**5.12.**	b
5.2.	d		**5.13.**	a
5.3.	b		**5.14.**	a
5.4.	c		**5.15.**	b
5.5.	d		**5.16.**	d
5.6.	a		**5.17.**	d
5.7.	b		**5.18.**	d
5.8.	c		**5.19.**	a
5.9.	b		**5.20.**	b
5.10.	d		**5.21.**	a
5.11.	a		**5.22.**	c

SET 1

5.1. Correct Answer: **c**
Ambulatory surgical patients cared for in a main PACU rather than in a PACU used exclusively for outpatients receive care delivered by a nurse who is more experienced in handling emergency treatment protocols. Although there are cost-effective advantages to combining inpatient and outpatient postanesthesia care units, the less sedate outpatients often experience increased fear and a negative response to noises from monitors, alarms, more traffic, and ventilators. In addition to a more stressful environment, the ambulatory patient frequently experiences a delay in reuniting with significant or responsible others when the Phase I inpatient and outpatient PACU is combined. (Burden N, editor: *Ambulatory surgical nursing*, ed 2, Philadelphia, 2000, Saunders.)

5.2. Correct Answer: **d**
Although regular and frequent hand washing is a proven means of preventing cross-contamination in the perianesthesia setting, the practice is often overlooked when caring for multiple patients in this busy practice setting. Although the installation of hand-sanitizer dispensers at every bedside, the use of protective gloves, and monitoring of compliance can improve hand-washing adherence by personnel, these do not change human behavior. The best method to change behavior and ensure that nursing staff habitually wash their hands is to provide regular education regarding the importance of hand cleansing in the prevention of cross-contamination and the spread of microorganisms. Patients should also be encouraged to ask their caregivers if they washed their hands. (Sandlin D: Too busy to wash your hands in PACU? *J PeriAnesth Nurs* 19[4]:263-264, 2004.)

5.3. Correct Answer: **b**
Mepivicaine's 1- to 2-hour duration of action is longer than lidocaine's 0.75- to 1.5-hour duration of action, so lidocaine would be a more appropriate selection for a 20-minute procedure and for a patient with a history of cardiac dysrhythmias. Lidocaine, a vasodilator, is associated with a higher incidence of hypotension, dizziness, and sleepiness. The 1% mepivicaine, with a medium level of potency and toxicity, does not cause vasodilation to the degree that lidocaine does and is a better selection for lumbar epidural anesthesia in patients susceptible to hypotension. (Quinn D, Schick L, editors: *ASPAN's perianesthesia nursing core curriculum: preoperative, Phase I and Phase II PACU nursing*, Philadelphia, 2004, Saunders.)

5.4. Correct Answer: **c**
It is most important to closely monitor this child's airway because there is potential for rapid airway obstruction. Although there is an audible partial obstruction, the child's admission respiratory parameters are satisfactory. After extubation, posterior oropharyngeal suctioning should be avoided if possible because it can cause additional trauma to laryngeal musculature. To prevent laryngospasm, the ¾ prone position is preferred in children for promoting oral secretions drainage away from the vocal chords. (Drain C, editor: *Perianesthesia nursing: a critical*

care approach, ed 4, Philadelphia, 2003, Saunders.)

5.5. Correct Answer: **d**
As a result of advances in anesthesia management, the use of more regional anesthetic techniques, and more research to document PACU visitation practices, postanesthesia care units have increasingly supported the integration of family member/caregiver visitation policies. Although wide-ranging institutional practices and varied concerns among individual nurses regarding visitation exist, research reveals that visitation in the Phase I level of care benefits patients and families. Pediatric postanesthesia patients are frequently reunited with parents once reacted from anesthesia, but PACU visitation is not always extended to adult patients. To ensure a consistent approach to PACU visitation practices within a facility, perianesthesia nurses should develop guidelines suitable for their specific practice setting and work with hospital administration to establish an organized visitation program based on those guidelines. (ASPAN: A position statement on visitation in Phase I level of care in *2006-2008 Standards of perianesthesia nursing practice*, Cherry Hill, NJ, 2006, ASPAN.)

5.6. Correct Answer: **a**
Bupivacaine is a highly potent, long-acting amino-amide. An 8-mg, 0.75% bupivacaine spinal dosage can demonstrate residual anesthetic effects for 3 to 10 hours after the initial medication administration. It is important to educate the patient on physiologic effects of the medication and to reassure the patient that a lack of movement is expected but will resolve over time. (Drain C, editor: *Perianesthesia nursing: a critical care approach*, ed 4, Philadelphia,

2003, Saunders; Quinn D, Schick L, editors: *ASPAN's perianesthesia nursing core curriculum: preoperative, Phase I and Phase II PACU nursing*, Philadelphia, 2004, Saunders.)

5.7. Correct Answer: **b**
Postoperative hypotension from a sympathetic blockade and the resultant venous dilation is usually encountered in the first 30 minutes after PACU admission. This results in a decreased venous return and a lower cardiac output. Another common cause of postoperative hypotension is bleeding. Therefore the nurse's next immediate action is to assess for surgical bleeding to rule out this causative factor. If bleeding is present, the nurse should immediately notify the attending surgeon and the attending anesthesia provider. In the absence of bleeding, the nurse should notify the attending anesthesia provider and initiate treatment that includes administration of 500 mL of IV crystalloid and elevation of the legs. (Drain C, editor: *Perianesthesia nursing: a critical care approach*, ed 4, Philadelphia, 2003, Saunders.)

5.8. Correct Answer: **c**
To prevent aspiration, abdominal surgery patients are frequently placed in a side-lying position in the immediate postoperative period until the laryngeal reflexes are restored. Once the patient is awake and respiratory effort is adequate, repositioning to a semi-Fowler position is desirable to decrease pressure on the suture lines and to enhance respiratory effort. In the scenario described, with the patient in a side-lying position, a nurse could effectively check the wound dressing, instruct the patient to perform coughing and deep-breathing exercises, and

monitor function and comfort of the indwelling nasogastric tube. The repositioning action taken by this nurse best serves to address respiratory and incision pressure considerations for this patient. (Drain C, editor: *Perianesthesia nursing: a critical care approach*, ed 4, Philadelphia, 2003, Saunders; Quinn D, Schick L, editors: *ASPAN's perianesthesia nursing core curriculum: preoperative, Phase I and Phase II PACU nursing*, Philadelphia, 2004, Saunders.)

5.9. Correct Answer: **b**
High abdominal incisions cause a significant amount of postoperative pain. All the options listed are potentially effective methods of pain control for a gastrectomy patient, but the preferred method of postoperative pain control for a Phase I gastrectomy procedure patient is a low thoracic epidural analgesia delivery system, with PCA as the second option. Pain treatment in this patient population should be liberal yet astute because of a related potential for respiratory system depression. (Quinn D, Schick L, editors: *ASPAN's perianesthesia nursing core curriculum: preoperative, Phase I and Phase II PACU nursing*, Philadelphia, 2004, Saunders; Drain C, editor: *Perianesthesia nursing: a critical care approach*, ed 4, Philadelphia, 2003, Saunders.)

5.10. Correct Answer: **d**
Postoperative sinus bradycardia, defined as a heart rate of less than 60 bpm, occurs frequently in the PACU caused by the depressant effects of anesthetic agents and is often seen in young, healthy individuals. Usually, no aggressive treatment is necessary for sinus bradycardia. In the case of a Phase I PACU patient with minimal symptoms associated with a heart rate of

42 bpm, the nurse caring for the patient will consult with the attending anesthesiologist and anticipate performing continued stir-up regimen techniques while maintaining close observation of the patient. More aggressive interventions are initiated for symptoms of decreased cardiac output, such as profound hypotension, dizziness, nausea, or ventricular escape beats. Pain can cause excessive parasympathetic stimulation leading to bradycardia, but this is an unlikely causative factor at a pain level of 2/10. Moving the emergency crash cart closer to the bedside is a cautious but unessential action. The administration of an IV fluid bolus requires an overall assessment of the perioperative fluid balance for this patient, and administration of a 0.01-mg dose of IV atropine is below the therapeutic IV dose range of 0.05 to 1 mg. (Drain C, editor: *Perianesthesia nursing: a critical care approach*, ed 4, Philadelphia, 2003, Saunders.)

5.11. Correct Answer: **a**
The post–general anesthesia respiratory parameters identified during the assessment of this 80-kg, 72-year-old gentleman are consistent with hypoventilation. In addition to airway obstruction, atelectasis, and aspiration, hypoventilation is a significant postoperative respiratory problem requiring early detection and treatment to restore adequate respiratory function. The normal respiratory rate is 12 to 20 breaths per minute with normal tidal volume range of 5 to 8 mL/kg. The shallow respirations are indicative of continued depression from opioid or anesthetic medications administered, so the patient's anesthesia record should be reviewed to assess this causative factor and guide treatment. Should the anesthesia provider determine

that reintubation is required, a size 8.0- to 8.5-mm tube is most appropriate for this male patient. Examining and ensuring proper sensor placement and accuracy of the pulse oximetry reading is always an appropriate differential diagnosis measure for the PACU nurse. Calculation of an expected normal tidal volume for this patient would measure between 400 and 640 mL/kg. (ASPAN: *Redi-Ref 2004: ambulatory/PACU/pediatric*, Cherry Hill, NJ, 2004, ASPAN; Drain C, editor: *Perianesthesia nursing: a critical care approach*, ed 4, Philadelphia, 2003, Saunders.)

5.12. Correct Answer: **b**
Clinical characteristics of a patient undergoing moderate sedation and analgesia include maintenance of protective reflexes, independent and continuous maintenance of patent airway, appropriate response to physical stimulation and/or verbal command, easy arousal (responds to verbal or light tactile stimulation), and cardiovascular status usually maintained. (Odom-Forren J, Watson D: *Practical guide to moderate sedation/ analgesia*, ed 2, St. Louis, 2005, Mosby; Amercan Society of Anesthesiologists, Task Force on Sedation and Analgesia by Non-anesthesiologists: Practice guidelines for sedation and analgesia by non-anesthesiologists: an updated report, *Anesthesiology* 96:1004-1017, 2002.)

5.13. Correct answer: **a**
It is not always possible to predict an individual patient's reaction to sedation. That is why the American Society of Anesthesiologists and The Joint Commission state that persons administering moderate sedation and/or analgesia should be capable of rescuing patients who move to the next level of sedation

beyond that intended. (Odom-Forren J, Watson D: *Practical guide to moderate sedation/ analgesia*, ed 2, St. Louis, 2005, Mosby; American Society of Anesthesiologists, Task Force on Sedation and Analgesia by Non-anesthesiologists: Practice guidelines for sedation and analgesia by non-anesthesiologists: an updated report, *Anesthesiology* 96:1004-1017, 2002.; Joint Commission on Accreditation of Healthcare Organizations: *Hospital accreditation standards*, Oakbrook Terrace, Ill, JCAHO, 2005.)

5.14. Correct Answer: **a**
Collaborative preanesthesia nurse/ attending surgeon considerations regarding the preparation of a patient for outpatient surgery must include the identification of a responsible adult caregiver for the postoperative period, which is a fundamental requirement for performing outpatient surgery. Surgeons and anesthesia providers are responsible for establishing specific policy and procedure agreements for how preoperative patients are handled within a health care system. The main responsibility for preanesthetic screening belongs to the attending surgeon, who also is responsible for obtaining the operative consent. Therefore when performing the preoperative history and physical and related physician orders for a patient, the surgeon must consider each patient's medical and social situation to determine if the patient needs consultation by an appropriate medical specialist, diagnostic or laboratory testing, or referral for preanesthesia evaluation and teaching. Ideally, all outpatients should be seen in the preanesthesia evaluation unit for evaluation and education. (Quinn D, Schick L, editors: *ASPAN's perianesthesia nursing*

core curriculum: preoperative, Phase I and Phase II PACU nursing, Philadelphia, 2004, Saunders; Burden N, editor: *Ambulatory surgical nursing*, ed 2, Philadelphia, 2000, Saunders.)

5.15. Correct Answer: **b**
Diabetes is a chronic metabolic disease associated with insulin insensitivity or deficiency, hyperglycemia, and glycosuria. Throughout the perianesthesia period, severe fluid losses and hypoglycemia should be avoided with a maintenance goal of < 200 mg/dL for serum glucose levels observed. Use of a preoperative and intraoperative infusion of 5% dextrose IV solution is indicated to prevent hypoglycemia, but this intervention warrants close monitoring for related hyperglycemia requiring treatment with insulin. The PACU nurse's objective is to maintain mild hyperglycemia over hypoglycemia. Urine glucose levels do not directly reflect the current serum glucose level in a diabetic patient, and mild glycosuria is considered to be more desirable than glucose-free urine levels. The patient's overall fluid and electrolyte balance should be closely monitored and treated to prevent potential complications resulting from imbalances. (Drain C, editor: *Perianesthesia nursing: a critical care approach*, ed 4, Philadelphia, 2003, Saunders.)

5.16. Correct Answer: **d**
A sudden onset of symptoms, such as shallow breathing, confusion, combativeness, incoherence, diaphoretic skin, pallor, weakness, and vertigo are associated with a hypoglycemic reaction. After the nurse notifies the attending anesthesia provider, the nurse can anticipate performing a finger-stick blood sugar accompanied by IV administration of a concentrated

dextrose solution to raise the serum glucose level. Diabetic coma is rarely seen in the PACU, and the obvious symptoms differ from those described in this patient. (Quinn D, Schick L, editors: *ASPAN's perianesthesia nursing core curriculum: preoperative, Phase I and Phase II PACU nursing*, Philadelphia, 2004, Saunders.)

5.17. Correct Answer: **d**
The patient presents with four risk factors: female gender, nonsmoker, history of motion sickness, and use of postoperative opioids. These risk factors place the patient at a very severe level of risk with an 80% or greater chance of experiencing PONV. (ASPAN's evidence-based clinical practice guideline for the prevention and/or management of PONV/PDNV, *J PeriAnesth Nurs* 21[4]: 230-250, 2006.)

5.18. Correct Answer: **d**
Prophylactic plans for PONV should be based on the patient's risk factor assessment. The number of recommended prophylactic interventions increases with the level of risk. Because this patient presents with an 80% or greater chance of developing PONV, three or more prophylactic interventions are recommended. (ASPAN's evidence-based clinical practice guideline for the prevention and/or management of PONV/PDNV, *J PeriAnesth Nurs* 21[4]: 230-250, 2006.)

5.19. Correct Answer: **a**
The use of a combination of TIVA, dexamethasone, and a scopolamine patch work together in a cost-effective manner to prevent PONV by depressing and/or antagonizing three different emetic trigger sites. Propofol (used in TIVA) depresses antiemetic triggers in the chemoreceptor trigger zone (CTZ),

vagal nuclei, and other centers associated with PONV. Dexamethasone is thought to antagonize prostaglandins or release endorphins. The scopolamine patch is particularly relevant because of the patient's history of motion sickness and antagonizes muscarinic and histamine receptors. This prophylactic combination attacks multiple receptors while maintaining the 5-HT$_3$ and NK1 receptors' availability for rescue therapy should the need arise. (ASPAN's evidence-based clinical practice guideline for the prevention and/or management of PONV/PDNV, *J PeriAnesth Nurs* 21[4]: 230-250, 2006.)

5.20. Correct Answer: **b**
Based on the rationale just mentioned, the most effective receptors available for rescue treatment are the 5-HT$_3$ and NK1 receptors. Dexamethasone is not effective for rescue therapy because of delayed onset, and promethazine and metoclopramide have not been shown to be as effective for PONV rescue treatment. (ASPAN: Evidence-based clinical practice guideline for the prevention and/or management of PONV/PDNV, *J PeriAnesth Nurs* 21[4]: 230-250, 2006.)

5.21. Correct Answer: **a**
Lipid-soluble fentanyl exhibits a rapid onset of action within 4 to 10 minutes after epidural administration. The peak epidural effect can occur in less than 30 minutes, and the effective duration may be as long as 3 to 8 hours. (Drain C, editor: *Perianesthesia nursing: a critical care approach*, ed 4, Philadelphia, 2003, Saunders.)

5.22. Correct Answer: **c**
Lipid-soluble medications such as fentanyl and sufentanil rapidly bind to lipid molecules causing absorption into the epidural fat, thus limiting their spread from the epidural site of injection. This binding factor makes accurate placement of the epidural catheter tip essential for efficacy with this medication administration method. Because of the variation in absorption, fentanyl can increase the amount of nursing care required for a patient because of required dosage adjustments. Fentanyl is an mu receptor agent that is 100 times more potent than morphine. It has several untoward side effects including: pruritus, somnolence, increased risk of respiratory depression, nausea, and urinary retention. (Miaskowski C: Patient-controlled modalities for acute postoperative pain management, *J PeriAnesth Nurs* 20[4]:255-267, 2005; Quinn D, Schick L, editors: *ASPAN's perianesthesia nursing core curriculum: preoperative, Phase I and Phase II PACU nursing*, Philadelphia, 2004, Saunders.)

Set 2

Answer Key

5.23.	d		**5.33.**	a
5.24.	b		**5.34.**	b
5.25.	c		**5.35.**	c
5.26.	c		**5.36.**	d
5.27.	c		**5.37.**	c
5.28.	d		**5.38.**	d
5.29.	d		**5.39.**	b
5.30.	a		**5.40.**	a
5.31.	b		**5.41.**	c
5.32.	c		**5.42.**	d

Set 2

5.23. Correct Answer: **d**
The patient in this scenario described symptoms occurring after latex exposure that are consistent with those in a type IV reaction. There are four categories of latex hypersensitivity reactions. A type I reaction is the most severe and is an immediate, local or systemic reaction caused by immunoglobulin gamma E antibodies, which can cause anaphylaxis. A type II reaction is cytotoxic in nature and targets a specific organ system, such as the kidneys. The type III reaction is an immune complex response to a foreign substance. A type IV reaction involves a local skin response manifested by a rash, swelling, pruritus, and redness. (Burden N, editor: *Ambulatory surgical nursing*, ed 2, Philadelphia, 2000, Saunders.)

5.24. Correct Answer: **b**
In a facility lacking a dedicated latex-free operating room, early notification of a suspected latex allergy is necessary for the surgical and anesthetic team to facilitate surgery schedule revisions or to accommodate safe preparation of a previously latex-exposed environment. An operating room generally requires at least 1 hour of ventilation to clear ambient latex particles circulating in the air. Based on the patient's initial self-report of symptoms related to latex exposure, in addition to notifying the surgical and anesthesia team of this previously undocumented allergy, a next most appropriate preanesthesia nursing action is to collect a more detailed history from the patient regarding any history of allergy to foods, especially tropical fruits. The nurse must question the

patient about any history of asthma or prior respiratory reaction to rubber products to include itchy or teary eyes, coughing, swelling, hives, chest tightness, runny nose, or wheezing. When assessing any patient for latex sensitivity, the nurse must specifically ask if the patient has ever experienced swelling of the lips after a visit to the dentist or any local irritation after use of a diaphragm or condom. The latex-sensitive patient should immediately be identified with an allergy band noting the sensitivity, and all equipment used to care for the patient throughout the perianesthesia period must be composed of a non-latex product. (Burden N, editor: *Ambulatory surgical nursing*, ed 2, Philadelphia, 2000, Saunders.)

5.25. Correct Answer: **c**
Postoperative nausea and vomiting is the most common postoperative complication, affecting at least one third of the surgical population or at least 75 million people per year. (ASPAN's evidence-based clinical practice guideline for the prevention and/or management of PONV/PDNV, *J PeriAnesth Nurs* 21[4]: 230-250, 2006.)

5.26. Correct Answer: **c**
Postanesthesia patient transportation policies are developed to ensure safe transfer of care for surgical patients. Based on specific patient needs, the professional nurse is charged with determining the number of staff members required to safely transport a patient, the appropriate competency level of accompanying transport personnel, and the mode of patient transportation. In this scenario, the patient has an order for

continuous telemetry monitoring; therefore cardiac monitoring must be maintained at all times during the transport phase of care. The PACU nurse's most appropriate action is to assign an appropriate mix of staff members to transport the patient, which in this case necessitates positioning the portable cardiac monitor in plain view of a licensed professional nurse who can perform the cardiac monitoring, not the unit aide pushing the gurney. Although supplemental oxygen may be indicated for a patient to prevent hypoxemia during the transport phase and appropriate administration of opioids in the PACU may help to better control pain during transport and movement, the details provided in the descriptive scenario do not support those responses. (ASPAN: Resource 10: "Safe Transfer of Care" in *2006-2008 Standards of perianesthesia nursing practice,* Cherry Hill, NJ, 2006, ASPAN.)

5.27. Correct Answer: **c**
The American Nurses Association *Code of Ethics* serves to guide perianesthesia nurses' ethical decisions and actions. A nurse has a professional responsibility to protect the well-being of a patient by consistently upholding safe practices and by ensuring the patient is cared for by a professional nurse. The PACU nurse's most appropriate action is to request immediate relief from the unit charge nurse or administrative supervisor. Although the nurse could elect to wait at the bedside until the unit's accepting nurse came for report, this does not solve the dilemma of inadequate unit staffing or a pressing demand for nursing care in the PACU and on the telemetry unit. Notification of the administrative personnel responsible for ensuring adequate staffing levels is a prudent action

in this scenario. The remaining choices violate the recommended standard of safe perianesthesia transfer of care. (ASPAN: "Perianesthesia Standards for Ethical Practice" *2006-2008 Standards of perianesthesia nursing practice,* Cherry Hill, NJ, 2006, ASPAN; ASPAN: Resource 10: "Safe Transfer of Care" in *2006-2008 Standards of perianesthesia nursing practice,* Cherry Hill, NJ, 2006, ASPAN.)

5.28. Correct Answer: **d**
The patient with atypical pseudocholinesterase deficiency receiving a usual dose of succinylcholine during general anesthesia can remain apneic for up to 48 hours. Atypical pseudocholinesterase, an inherited disorder, occurs in approximately 1 in 2800 people. Patients with atypical pseudocholinesterase have a succinylcholine resistance and should receive nondepolarizing muscle relaxants that can be reversed instead of an irreversible depolarizing neuromuscular blocking agent such as succinylcholine. (Drain C, editor: *Perianesthesia nursing: a critical care approach,* ed 4, Philadelphia, 2003, Saunders.)

5.29. Correct Answer: **d**
Because patients' use of herbal supplements is steadily increasing, perianesthesia nurses must be familiar with possible adverse reactions and potentially dangerous drug interactions associated with the use of all herbal supplements. *Gingko biloba* is reportedly used for memory improvement and treatment of dementia and peripheral vascular disease. Patients ingesting 120 mg per day or more of *Gingko biloba* appear to have a greater incidence of prolonged bleeding time, and this supplement may potentiate anticoagulants. Therefore the patient

must be instructed to discontinue *Gingko biloba* for 2 weeks before surgery. There exists a potential for untoward reactions with thiazide diuretics and sedative medications, and although it is recommended that *Gingko biloba* not be taken in combination with a thiazide diuretic or a sedative, more studies are required to validate these negative drug interactions. (Messina BA: Herbal supplements: facts and myths, *J PeriAnesth Nurs* 21[4]:268-278, 2006.)

5.30. Correct Answer: **a**
After cesarean delivery the fundus requires frequent checks to assess for firm contraction status. Uterine atony involves a failure of the uterus to contract after delivery of the placenta, which can lead to excessive bleeding. To stimulate uterine contraction, the nurse performs external uterine massage while always supporting the lower uterus during the massage. Because fundus checks and uterine massage are uncomfortable procedures for cesarean patients with a lower abdominal incision, the patient should be instructed to perform slow, deep breathing and to relax the abdominal muscles as much as possible. A bimanual compression technique is performed by the physician and involves placing one fist inside the vagina with the other hand externally massaging the uterus through the abdomen. (Chichester M: When your patient is from the obstetric department: postpartum hemorrhage and massive transfusion, *J PeriAnesth Nurs* 20[3]:167-176, 2005; Drain C, editor: *Perianesthesia nursing: a critical care approach*, ed 4, Philadelphia, 2003, Saunders.)

5.31. Correct Answer: **b**
Massive transfusion therapy is defined as a 50% replacement of

blood volume within 3 hours, administering 10 or more units of packed red blood cells in a 24-hour period, an estimated blood loss of more than 5000 mL, and replacing a patient's entire circulating blood volume. (Chichester M: When your patient is from the obstetric department: postpartum hemorrhage and massive transfusion, *J PeriAnesth Nurs* 20[3]:167-176, 2005.)

5.32. Correct Answer: **c**
The landmark assessment point for the T4 dermatome is at the nipple line. A patient with a high spinal blockade may exhibit objective symptoms such as diaphragmatic breathing with absence of intracostal muscle action; hypotension; urinary retention; and difficulty verbalizing. The potential for respiratory insufficiency exists with a high spinal blockade. This risk requires close observation by the nurse because the patient's inspiratory capacity is weakened while clinical signs including ventilatory effort, respiratory rate, and SpO_2 may be satisfactory on initial assessment. The patient might express anxiety over a perceived inability to breathe because the chest wall sensation is blocked. Nursing actions include patient education regarding the effects of the anesthetic, reassurance that the blockade will resolve over time, and administration of appropriate comfort measures. Sympathetic blockade causes hypotension, not hypertension. While deep vein thrombosis caused by venous stasis is a concern, this is addressed with lower extremity compression stockings worn throughout the perioperative and postoperative period. (Drain C, editor: *Perianesthesia nursing: a critical care approach*, ed 4, Philadelphia, 2003, Saunders.)

5.33. Correct Answer: **a**
Core temperature can be directly measured in the pulmonary artery, distal esophagus, and nasopharynx. Infrared tympanic thermometry studies have shown mixed results regarding accuracy, and oral and bladder sites can only estimate a core temperature. (ASPAN's evidence-based clinical practice guideline for the prevention and/or management of PONV/PDNV, *J PeriAnesth Nurs* 21[4]: 230-250, 2006.)

5.34. Correct Answer: **b**
Approximately 60% of patients undergoing anesthesia will experience cardiac dysrhythmias; therefore continuous cardiac monitoring is performed in the PACU. Inhalation anesthetics, such as halothane, isoflurane, and enflurane, slow the rate of SA node discharge and prolong bundle of His–Purkinje and ventricular conduction times. These inhalation agents can also increase ventricular automaticity, evoke nodal rhythms, or cause both effects. Cardiac dysrhythmias may also result from anticholinergic and catecholamine effects, which alter autonomic nervous system balance in the sympathetic and parasympathetic nervous system. Perianesthesia cardiac dysrhythmias are also related to medications that alter sympathetic activity and light anesthesia during emergence in the immediate postoperative period. Many postanesthesia patients do not require treatment for transient anesthesia-related dysrhythmias but require continuous monitoring to ensure stability of the cardiovascular system in the perianesthesia period. (Drain C, editor: *Perianesthesia nursing: a critical care approach*, ed 4, Philadelphia, 2003, Saunders.)

5.35. Correct Answer: **c**
Epinephrine is the medication most likely to cause an increase in cardiac dysrhythmias because of a pharmacokinetic interaction with halothane, the inhalation anesthetic used for this patient. All volatile inhalation anesthetics can sensitize the heart to sympathomimetic amines like epinephrine. Halothane, with its lasting residual effect, is particularly likely to cause dysrhythmias from a pharmacokinetic interaction with epinephrine or other sympathomimetic amines administered in the PACU. In the event that epinephrine administration is essential for producing vasoconstriction in a patient, the concentration should be no greater than 1:100,000 to 1:200,000 and the total dose should not exceed 30 mL of a 1:100,000 solution over 60 minutes. Furosemide interacts with halothane to produce hypotension. Chlorpromazine interacts with nondepolarizing skeletal muscle relaxants by enhancing neuromuscular blockade. Aminoglycosides, such as gentamycin, reportedly interact with skeletal muscle relaxants and some anesthetic agents but do not necessarily impact cardiac ectopy. (Drain C, editor: *Perianesthesia nursing: a critical care approach*, ed 4, Philadelphia, 2003, Saunders.)

5.36. Correct Answer: **d**
Midazolam has a rapid onset of action, has excellent amnesic effects, is water soluble, and is contraindicated for patients with acute narrow-angle glaucoma and untreated open-angle glaucoma. Midazolam has a slower peak effect in elderly adults, inhibits activity of the cytochrome P-450 microsomal enzyme system (e.g., cimetidine and warfarin), and is metabolized by the liver. (Odom-Forren J, Watson D: *Practical*

guide to moderate sedation/analgesia, ed 2, St. Louis, 2005, Mosby; Drain C, editor: *Perianesthesia nursing: a critical care approach*, ed 4, Philadelphia, 2003, Saunders.)

5.37. Correct Answer: **c**
A patient receiving extended-release epidural morphine (EREM) may have effective pain relief after major surgery for up to 48 hours after injection. EREM is delivered as a single bolus dose in the lumbar epidural space with usual doses of 15 mg after lower extremity orthopedic procedures and 10 to 15 mg after pelvic or lower abdominal procedures. Adverse effects are similar to those of any opioid, with nausea and pruritus ranking the highest in incidence and hypotension noted as a fairly common occurrence. (Pasero C, McCaffery M: Extended-release epidural morphine [DepoDur®], *J PeriAnesth Nurs* 20[5]:345-350, 2005.)

5.38. Correct Answer: **d**
Ethical concerns are of primary interest to every nurse participating in data collection for a research study. Before data collection involving human subjects, the researcher must obtain written consent from the institutional review board (IRB) or human subjects committee, and this is the primary question a data collection participant must confirm before participating in the study. The IRB renders an independent judgment regarding ethical implications and study methodology of the proposed research project. Ethical research activities include honesty and integrity of process, protection of patients from harmful effects while ensuring benefits prevail over risks, and adherence to institutional guidelines. The IRB also establishes written or verbal informed consent requirements for a research study.

(Quinn D, Schick L, editors: *ASPAN's perianesthesia nursing core curriculum: preoperative, Phase I and Phase II PACU nursing*, Philadelphia, 2004, Saunders.)

5.39. Correct Answer: **b**
The optimal postoperative positioning of the bariatric patient is semi-recumbent, and this position should be achieved immediately post-operatively providing the patient has hemodynamic stability. The semi-recumbent position has been shown to increase pulmonary functional residual capacity, improve ventilation effort, and optimize oxygenation in morbidly obese postoperative abdominal surgery patients. The supine position can worsen obstructive sleep apnea, which is prevalent in the morbidly obese population, caused by posterior displacement of the tongue. The head of the bariatric patient's bed ideally should be elevated to a 30° to 45° angle. (Marley RA, Hoyle B, Ries C: Perianesthesia respiratory care of the bariatric patient, *J PeriAnesth Nurs* 20[6]:404-431, 2005.)

5.40. Correct Answer: **a**
A visually impaired patient may or may not have other disabilities, so this factor should be identified by a nurse when caring for the patient. Because hearing is often more finely tuned in a visually impaired individual, it is important for the preanesthesia nurse to introduce himself or herself while speaking in a normal volume and tone. The nurse should ask the patient to confirm that he or she can adequately hear the nurse. It is important for the nurse to introduce all staff members in the room and to explain environmental sounds to orient the patient to the environment. Provision of a safe environment includes offering an arm to the

patient while ambulating from one location to another. Ideally, the patient grasps the nurse's arm right above and behind the elbow and walks just slightly behind the nurse to anticipate an approaching step. Instructions and consents should be provided in a form the patient can use independently, such as on audiotape or in a Braille version. (Quinn D, Schick L, editors: *ASPAN's perianesthesia nursing core curriculum: preoperative, Phase I and Phase II PACU nursing*, Philadelphia, 2004, Saunders.)

5.41. Correct Answer: **c**
The nurse instructing a patient on post-discharge pain medication and treatment understands that once they are sensitized, pain receptors become increasingly irritated and are subsequently harder to control. Pain medication should be taken at the early onset of pain to better control and maintain pain levels within the patient's established postoperative functional pain goal. Waiting to medicate until a pain level is self-rated at 5/10 to 6/10 will likely contribute to pain receptor irritability, and ingesting pain medication every 4 hours around the clock may not be necessary. Complementary therapies and relaxation techniques can enhance a patient's comfort status and are intended to be supportive of pain control but are not intended to replace medication treatment for acute postoperative pain. (Quinn

D, Schick L, editors: *ASPAN's perianesthesia nursing core curriculum: preoperative, Phase I and Phase II PACU nursing*, Philadelphia, 2004, Saunders; Burden N, editor: *Ambulatory surgical nursing*, ed 2, Philadelphia, 2000, Saunders.)

5.42. Correct Answer: **d**
Perianesthesia care of the immunosuppressed patient necessitates strict aseptic technique to include cleansing of common-use perianesthesia monitoring items before application to prevent cross-contamination. Opinions on the use of protective isolation for the immunosuppressed patient differ, but any patient with a peripheral leukocyte count below 2000 cells/mm will likely benefit from placement in protective isolation. An immunosuppressed patient may not exhibit classic symptoms of infection. Close temperature monitoring is indicated, and a temperature of 38° C (100.4° F) or greater must be immediately reported to the attending physician. All needle-puncture and incision sites should be cleansed and treated with appropriate antimicrobial ointments and then dressed appropriately, so constant direct visualization may not always be possible. However, puncture and incision sites should be examined daily to assess for possible infection. (Drain C, editor: *Perianesthesia nursing: a critical care approach*, ed 4, Philadelphia, 2003, Saunders.)

SET 3

ANSWER KEY

5.43.	b		**5.52.**	b
5.44.	c		**5.53.**	b
5.45.	c		**5.54.**	d
5.46.	a		**5.55.**	c
5.47.	b		**5.56.**	d
5.48.	c		**5.57.**	a
5.49.	d		**5.58.**	b
5.50.	a		**5.59.**	c
5.51.	b		**5.60.**	c

Set 3

RATIONALES AND REFERENCES

5.43. Correct Answer: **b**
Propranolol (Inderal) is an alpha adrenergic receptor antagonist that can interact with inhalation anesthetics to produce bradycardia and hypotension but is effectively used to treat supraventricular tachycardia associated with catecholamine surge from anesthesia, pheochromocytoma, and hyperthyroidism. The maximum recommended propranolol dose is 0.1 mg/kg, so for this 90-kg patient the cumulative dose should not exceed a 9 mg total. IV doses of propranolol should not exceed 1 mg/minute, and peak action time is 1 minute with 1- to 6-hour duration of action. The PACU nurse should monitor the heart rate and blood pressure closely after administration of each propranolol dose, and the anesthesia provider should use this medication with caution in patients with a known history of COPD and asthma. (ASPAN: *Redi-Ref 2004: ambulatory/PACU/ pediatric*, Cherry Hill, NJ, 2004, ASPAN; Drain C, editor: *Perianesthesia nursing: a critical care approach*, ed 4, Philadelphia, 2003, Saunders; Quinn D, Schick L, editors: *ASPAN's perianesthesia nursing core curriculum: preoperative, Phase I and Phase II PACU nursing*, Philadelphia, 2004, Saunders.)

5.44. Correct Answer: **c**
Although the other responses to this question appear prudent in a postoperative patient with a significant preexisting condition that warrants anticoagulant therapy, the postanesthesia nurse's most appropriate action regarding the heparin order is to notify the surgeon and anesthesiologist of an associated risk related to use of this medication. This patient is being actively treated with propranolol for supraventricular tachycardia, and heparin and propranolol have a known drug interaction that causes myocardial depression. Heparin displaces propranolol from plasma protein-binding sites by increasing the number of free fatty acids, thus increasing free propranolol. (Drain C, editor: *Perianesthesia nursing: a critical care approach*, ed 4, Philadelphia, 2003, Saunders; Quinn D, Schick L, editors: *ASPAN's perianesthesia nursing core curriculum: preoperative, Phase I and Phase II PACU nursing*, Philadelphia, 2004, Saunders.)

5.45. Correct Answer: **c**
A normal infant's total lung capacity is measured at 70 mL/kg. Therefore a 7.3-kg infant with no structural or physiologic abnormalities has a calculated total lung capacity of 511 mL. The total lung capacity for a normal adult is calculated at 80 mL/kg. (Quinn D, Schick L, editors: *ASPAN's perianesthesia nursing core curriculum: preoperative, Phase I and Phase II PACU nursing*, Philadelphia, 2004, Saunders.)

5.46. Correct Answer: **a**
Sevoflurane has quickly replaced halothane as the inhalation agent of choice for the pediatric surgical population although sevoflurane is associated with increased incidence of emergence behavioral changes in pediatric cases. The benefits of sevoflurane use in children include rapid induction and emergence, decreased airway irritation, and a non-pungent odor that lends itself to easier mask induction

with children. Knowledge of emergence behavioral changes related to sevoflurane use allows the PACU nurse to assess for and rule out other causes of postoperative agitation while focusing on delivery of supportive care during the transient emergence period. (Moos DD: Sevoflurane and emergence behavioral changes in children, *J PeriAnesth Nurs* 20[1]:13-18, 2005.)

5.47. Correct Answer: **b**
Standard Precautions, formerly called *Universal Precautions*, must be implemented across the health care delivery setting. This scenario involves a patient with a history of reactive airway disease, hepatitis B, and HIV infection. All staff members must care for this patient by wearing personal protective equipment (PPE) appropriate for the contact or procedure being performed. A history of reactive airway disease predisposes this patient to coughing after extubation with potential for droplet transmission, so appropriate PPE for the nurse includes wearing a protective face shield, gloves, and gown. Gloves are changed and hands washed after each patient contact. In lieu of a needleless delivery system, discontinued contaminated needles must be immediately placed in a puncture-resistant biohazard container and IV tubing can be disposed of in a biohazard waste receptacle. (Drain C, editor: *Perianesthesia nursing: a critical care approach*, ed 4, Philadelphia, 2003, Saunders.)

5.48. Correct Answer: **c**
The geriatric population is increasing as life expectancy has lengthened, so more elderly patients are undergoing surgical procedures and anesthesia. The nurse must understand effects of the aging process and the accompanying special perianesthesia considerations related to geriatric patients. The correct answer to the question is related to pharmacodynamics. In an elderly patient, the number of drug receptor sites decreases along with decreased albumin levels, which results in unbound available drugs, thus creating an amplified pharmacologic effect. The progressive decline of the hepatic and renal systems impacts medication metabolism and clearance. Renal blood flow and glomerular filtration rates decrease, and the renal system exhibits decreases in tissue mass and function, which can impact the effectiveness of homeostatic fluid balance and drug clearance. IV medication onset is slowed by decreased circulation, which can lead to repeat dosing and potential medication overdose. Aging causes an increase in systolic blood pressure of 6 to 7 mmHg per decade with little measurable change in the diastolic levels. (Monarch S, Wren K: Geriatric anesthesia implications, *J PeriAnesth Nurs* 19[6]:379-384, 2004.)

5.49. Correct Answer: **d**
Minimum alveolar concentration (MAC) is a commonly used term that best describes the potency for each inhalation anesthetic agent. MAC is the percent of inhalation anesthetic agent breathed that prevents movement during surgical incision in 50% of patients. Because movement is not desired during standard surgical incision, the inhalation anesthetic concentration is usually delivered at 1.5 to 2.5 MAC to ensure absence of movement. MAC values are lower when the inhalation anesthetic agent is more potent. MAC is used as a general guideline for anesthetic administration; therefore the concentration must be titrated on an individual basis. MAC can also

vary by age; it is slightly higher in children than in adults and decreases with advancing age. Oxygen is almost always delivered as an adjuvant carrier gas for inhalation anesthetic agents along with a combination of nitrous oxide and air. (Drain C, editor: *Perianesthesia nursing: a critical care approach*, ed 4, Philadelphia, 2003, Saunders; Burden N, editor: *Ambulatory surgical nursing*, ed 2, Philadelphia, 2000, Saunders.)

5.50. Correct Answer: **a**
Contributing risk factors for perioperative hypothermia include extremes of ages, female gender, ambient room temperature, length and type of surgical procedure, cachexia, preexisting conditions (e.g., peripheral vascular disease, endocrine disease, pregnancy, burns, open wounds), significant fluid shifts, use of cold irrigants, use of general anesthesia, and use of regional anesthesia. (ASPAN's evidence-based clinical practice guideline for the prevention and/or management of PONV/PDNV, *J PeriAnesth Nurs* 21[4]: 230-250, 2006.)

5.51. Correct Answer: **b**
The only active warming measure that has been shown by research studies to be effective is forced air warming devices. All other choices are considered passive or preventive measures and may maintain a patient's temperature but will not increase the patient's temperature. (ASPAN's evidence-based clinical practice guideline for the prevention and/or management of PONV/PDNV, *J PeriAnesth Nurs* 21[4]: 230-250, 2006.)

5.52. Correct Answer: **b**
A stellate ganglion block is usually performed under local anesthesia to treat reflex sympathetic dystrophy and to manage upper extremity

circulatory insufficiency. The post-anesthesia nurse should be familiar with the common side effects and dangerous complications from this block. Usual unpleasant side effects seen in the recovery phase of care include the sensation of a lump in the throat; temporary hoarseness or dysphagia; Horner's syndrome marked by miosis (contraction of the pupil), ptosis (drooping of eyelids), and anhidrosis (inability to sweat); flushing of the skin and conjunctiva; increased temperature in the ipsilateral (same side of the block, i.e. right or left) arm and hand; hematoma; and ipsilateral nasal congestion. The injection of anesthetic for stellate ganglion blockade must be precise or it can produce a high spinal anesthesia, pneumothorax, laryngeal nerve paralysis, and blockade of the cardioaccelerator fibers. (ASPAN: *Redi-Ref 2004: ambulatory/PACU/ pediatric*, Cherry Hill, NJ, 2004, ASPAN; Quinn D, Schick L, editors: *ASPAN's perianesthesia nursing core curriculum: preoperative, Phase I and Phase II PACU nursing*, Philadelphia, 2004, Saunders.)

5.53. Correct Answer: **b**
The recommended amount of electrical energy to deliver for initial pediatric defibrillation is 2 joules/kg of body weight. If this amplitude is ineffective, progression to 4 joules/ kg is advisable. Pediatric cardioversion is performed using 0.5 to 1 joule/ kg of body weight. (ASPAN: *Redi-Ref 2004: ambulatory/PACU/pediatric*, Cherry Hill, NJ, 2004, ASPAN; Quinn D, Schick L, editors: *ASPAN's perianesthesia nursing core curriculum: preoperative, Phase I and Phase II PACU nursing*, Philadelphia, 2004, Saunders.)

5.54. Correct Answer: **d**
Lidocaine iontophoresis is an excellent choice for a patient who is

anxious and expressing fear and anxiety about needle sticks because of prior negative venipuncture encounters. Iontophoresis involves a controller system, an active drug reservoir, and low-voltage electrical current applied by patch to skin contact to deliver medication via the transdermal route. The analgesic effect from lidocaine iontophoresis delivery can be achieved in 10 minutes and is no less effective than lidocaine infiltration via injection. Lidocaine injection can aggravate the patient's needle phobia. Application of a eutectic mixture of local anesthetic (EMLA) is not feasible because this method requires an extended application time of 60 to 120 minutes and the patient in this scenario is scheduled to go into the operating room in 30 minutes. (Pasero C: Lidocaine iontophoresis for dermal procedure analgesia, *J PeriAnesth Nurs* 21[1]:48-52, 2005.)

5.55. Correct Answer: **c**
The most appropriate way for a nurse to manage the situation described in this scenario is to facilitate a discussion regarding the parameters of the DNR order with the patient and the surgical care team before surgery. The 1990 Patient Self-determination Act states that patients must be made aware of the right to prepare advance directives related to life-prolonging treatment. Opinions and policies surrounding DNR orders and the perianesthesia/perioperative period differ by institution, although health care providers have an ethical responsibility to support the patient's right to self-determination. For any patient with an existing DNR order who requires anesthesia and surgery, the American Society of Anesthesiologists, the American College of Surgeons, and the Association of peri-Operative

Registered Nurses support the policy of "required reconsideration," and the American Society of PeriAnesthesia Nurses recommends that the patient reconsider and clarify directives regarding resuscitation. The most ethical solution to this situation is to provide the patient with a choice to maintain, suspend, or modify the DNR order by outlining specific goal-directed or procedure-directed orders to be put in writing before anesthesia induction. (ASPAN: "A Position Statement on the Perianesthesia Patient with a Do-Not-Resuscitate Advance Directive" in *2006-2008 Standards of Perianesthesia Nursing Practice,* Cherry Hill, NJ, 2006, ASPAN; Guarisco KK: Managing do-not-resuscitate orders in the perianesthesia period, *J PeriAnesth Nurs* 19[5]:300-307, 2004.)

5.56. Correct Answer: **d**
Incorporating culturally competent care for all patients in the perianesthesia environment is the responsibility of every nurse, and this requires the study of cultural belief structures in diverse populations. Cultural competence includes care delivery strategies based on the behaviors, beliefs, attitudes, and cultural heritage of a client. The nurse caring for Chinese-American patients understands their cultural belief structure holds that illness results from imbalance in yin and yang or the balance in positive and negative energy forces involving physical and spiritual harmony and balance with nature. Internal causes of disease relate to either absent or excessive emotions, and external causes of disease are rooted in exposure to the physical elements of nature. Chinese-Americans have a deep respect for and adherence to traditional Chinese medicine, may be wary of highly technical Western medical care, and view

removing large amounts of blood from the body as a disruption in vitality. It is also essential to appreciate that variability exists with cultural groups. (Quinn D, Schick L, editors: *ASPAN's perianesthesia nursing core curriculum: preoperative, Phase I and Phase II PACU nursing*, Philadelphia, 2004, Saunders.)

5.57. Correct Answer: **a**
Based on the initial physical examination, the nurse deduces this patient is most likely in an acute stage of opiate abstinence. The physical symptoms (thin, pale, nauseous, nervous and jittery with dilated pupils, rhinorrhea, and multiple small, round scars on the inner and outer aspects of both forearms and calves) are consistent with heroin addiction and early opioid withdrawal. Although the patient denies use of any medications or street drugs, her skin shows classic scarring from subcutaneous "skin popping" of a drug, bilateral arm veins are collapsed, and the finger infection may be related to drug injection with a dirty needle. Central nervous system sympathomimetic drugs would create symptoms different from those exhibited by this patient, such as tachycardia, hypertension, palpitations, dysrhythmias, and temperature regulation changes. (Burden N, editor: *Ambulatory surgical nursing*, ed 2, Philadelphia, 2000, Saunders; Drain C, editor: *Perianesthesia nursing: a critical care approach*, ed 4, Philadelphia, 2003, Saunders.)

5.58. Correct Answer: **b**
The nurse anticipates that this patient will require liberal opioid doses in the PACU. A nurse should maintain a nonjudgmental attitude while caring for any patient. The perioperative period is not the appropriate time to withhold opioids from an addicted patient, because that could precipitate a severe withdrawal episode. This patient received 12 mg of intraoperative morphine sulfate during a 1-hour procedure and rates her operative pain at 10/10 on admission to PACU, so she may not respond well to an initial 3-mg dose in PACU. Butorphanol and nalbuphine should be avoided because their agonist/antagonist properties can promote acute withdrawal symptoms. (Burden N, editor: *Ambulatory surgical nursing*, ed 2, Philadelphia, 2000, Saunders; Drain C, editor: *Perianesthesia nursing: a critical care approach*, ed 4, Philadelphia, 2003, Saunders.)

5.59. Correct Answer: **c**
Propofol's beneficial properties include less psychomotor impairment; rapid and alert emergence; rapid onset, metabolism, and elimination; less nausea, vomiting, and anesthesia hangover effect; and shorter recovery and discharge time. Drug clearance is greater than hepatic blood flow. The incidence of pain on injection is approximately 40% for peripheral veins and 10% for larger veins. This drug has no adjuvant analgesic properties. (Quinn D, Schick L, editors: *ASPAN's perianesthesia nursing core curriculum: preoperative, Phase I and Phase II PACU nursing*, Philadelphia, 2004, Saunders.)

5.60. Correct Answer: **c**
Extubation criteria include restoration of muscle strength after administration of muscle relaxants, the ability to lift the head off the bed for at least 5 seconds, appropriate responses to commands, presence of the swallow reflex, and these measurable respiratory parameters: tidal volume (TV) of at least 5 mL/kg; vital capacity (VC) of at least

15-20 mL/kg; and negative inspiratory force of 20 to 25 cm water pressure. For an 85-kg patient, the measured TV should exceed 425 mL and the VC should be 1275 to 1700 mL. (Quinn D, Schick L, editors: *ASPAN's perianesthesia nursing core curriculum: preoperative, Phase I and Phase II PACU nursing*, Philadelphia, 2004, Saunders.)

SET 4

ANSWER KEY

5.61.	b		**5.66.**	c
5.62.	a		**5.67.**	c
5.63.	b		**5.68.**	a
5.64.	c		**5.69.**	c
5.65.	b			

SET 4

5.61. Correct Answer: **b**
Although it is imperative that the nurse assess and monitor the patient's ventilatory status, it is not a standard that a capnograph is used for that purpose. The nurse may simply ask the patient to take deep breaths and use a stethoscope to gauge the depth of ventilation. It is a standard to use a pulse oximeter on all patients undergoing moderate sedation to assess oxygenation, and a cardiac monitor must be used at a minimum on patients with a history of cardiac dysrhythmias. (Odom-Forren J, Watson D: *Practical guide to moderate sedation/analgesia*, ed 2, St. Louis, 2005, Mosby; American Society of Anesthesiologists, Task Force on Sedation and Analgesia by Non-anesthesiologists: Practice guidelines for sedation and analgesia by non-anesthesiologists: an updated report, *Anesthesiology* 96:1004-1017, 2002.)

5.62. Correct Answer: **a**
The key items of importance to this patient include vital signs (hypertension, atrial fibrillation), airway assessment (obesity), blood glucose level (what is her blood sugar before procedure because of the patient's NPO status), and current medications (because of prior existing medical conditions and were the medications taken the morning of surgery). (Odom-Forren J, Watson, D: *Practical guide to moderate sedation/analgesia*, ed 2, St. Louis, 2005, Mosby.)

5.63. Correct Answer: **b**
Although many of the conditions listed were possible risks, **b** contained all current possibilities for this patient given her history.

The patient is at risk for hypercarbia and hypoxemia because of her obesity and age, and hypertension and hypoglycemia because of her medical history. The patient is not likely to have hypocarbia (low carbon dioxide level) because respiratory depression results in hypercarbia; hypothyroidism because thyroid problems are not part of her medical history; or hypotension because of the patient's history of hypertension. (Odom-Forren J, Watson, D: *Practical guide to moderate sedation/analgesia*, ed 2, St. Louis, 2005, Mosby.)

5.64. Correct Answer: **c**
The oxyhemoglobin curve is shifted to the left with increased pH, decreased temperature, PCO_2, and 2,3-DPG levels. This shift to the left causes increased affinity of hemoglobin for oxygen, which results in less oxygen saturation levels (oxygen levels available to the tissues.) (Odom-Forren J, Watson, D: *Practical guide to moderate sedation/analgesia*, ed 2, St. Louis, 2005, Mosby; Nagelhout JJ, Zaglaniczny KL: *Nurse anesthesia*, ed 2, Philadelphia, 2001, Saunders.)

5.65. Correct Answer: **b**
Wrong site, wrong side surgeries are more frequently found in orthopedic, podiatric, neurosurgical, urological, and general surgery specialties. The risk factors for wrong site surgery include emergent procedures; multiple simultaneous procedures performed and multiple surgeon involvement; communication breakdowns among the patient, surgical team, and patient family members; unusual patient characteristics; cultural and language barriers; incomplete patient

assessment; and staffing issues. Inappropriate abbreviations and illegible handwriting are not related to site verification policies and procedures. Development of and adherence to a preoperative checklist standardizes and structures correct surgical site verification and minimizes the risk of a sentinel event. (Dunn D: Surgical site verification: A through Z, *J PeriAnesth Nurs* 21[5]:317-331, 2006.)

5.66. Correct Answer: **c**
The Joint Commission's "Universal Protocol for Preventing Wrong Site, Wrong Procedure, Wrong Person Surgery™" includes the following steps: a preoperative verification process to ensure all relevant documents and studies are reviewed and confirmation that these match each other and the patient's and surgical team's understanding of the procedure; operative site marking that, when possible, actively includes the patient during the site verification process; and the operative site marked in a manner that allows it to be visualized in the operating room after the patient has been prepped and draped. A "time out" period is taken immediately before the procedure is begun to conduct the final verification of the correct patient, procedure, site, and implants if applicable. (Joint Commission on Accreditation of Healthcare Organizations: *Universal protocol for preventing wrong site, wrong procedure, wrong person surgery™*. Website: www.jointcommission.org/ PatientSafety/UniversalProtocol. Accessed January 20, 2007.)

5.67. Correct Answer: **c**
Fentanyl is lipophilic, has a rapid onset (1-2 minutes), and has a minimal histamine release.

Odom-Forren J, Watson, D: *Practical guide to moderate sedation/analgesia*, ed 2, St. Louis, 2005, Mosby; Drain C, editor: *Perianesthesia nursing: a critical care approach*, ed 4, Philadelphia, 2003, Saunders.

5.68. Correct Answer: **a**
Propofol is currently classified as an anesthetic agent. Controversy exists as to whether propofol should be administered by educated and competent RNs or restricted to use by an anesthesia provider, as the insert now dictates. A few boards of nursing have released position statements that state administration of propofol is within the realm of RN administration, and other boards of nursing have issued statements saying that it is not within the scope of practice for an RN. (Odom-Forren J, Watson, D: *Practical guide to moderate sedation/analgesia*, ed 2, St. Louis, 2005, Mosby; Odom-Forren J: The evolution of nurse monitored sedation, *J PeriAnesth Nurs* 20[6]:385-398, 2005.)

5.69. Correct Answer: **c**
The ASPAN statement on role of the RN in management of the patient undergoing sedation recommends that ACLS and/or PALS is maintained, a presedation evaluation is completed, and the RN is to have no other responsibilities that would leave the patient unattended or compromise continuous monitoring. Certainly an airway assessment is a key component of a presedation evaluation, but ASPAN does not require a specific method or scoring system to achieve that goal. (ASPAN: *2006-2008 Standards of perianesthesia nursing,* Cherry Hill, NJ, 2006, ASPAN.)

Chapter 6

Cardiac, Vascular, and Pulmonary Systems

Scenarios and questions in this section focus on the *cardiac, vascular, and pulmonary* systems. These concepts are considered together because of their interconnectedness and interdependence. The concepts reviewed in the context of this body system include:

- Pharmacology
- Pathophysiology
- Technology
- Nursing process and standards

ESSENTIAL CORE CONCEPTS	AFFILIATED CORE CURRICULUM CHAPTERS
Nursing Process	**Chapter 3**
Assessment	
Planning and Implementation	
Evaluation	
Preexisting Medical Conditions	**Chapter 19**
Cardiovascular Diseases	
Pulmonary Diseases	
Obesity	
Immediate Preoperative Preparation	**Chapter 23**
Medication Protocol	
Acid-Base Balance	**Chapter 25**
Anesthetic Agents and Adjuncts	**Chapter 26**
Anesthesia Continuum	
Anesthesia Options	
Regional Techniques	
IV Anesthetic Induction Agents	
IV Opioid Anesthetics	
IV Anesthetic Adjuncts	
Gaseous and Volatile Inhalational Anesthetics	

Depolarizing and Nondepolarizing Muscle
  Relaxants
Reversal Agents

Moderate Sedation/Analgesia   **Chapter 27**

Thermoregulation   **Chapter 28**

Thermoregulation
Malignant Hyperthermia

Hemodynamic Monitoring   **Chapter 30**

Physiologic Variables
Pressure Monitoring and Troubleshooting

Respiratory Care   **Chapter 31**

Postoperative Oxygen Therapy
Airway Management
Postoperative Mechanical Ventilation
Difficult Airway
Administration of Aerosolized Medications
Select Postoperative Respiratory Care Issues

Cardiovascular Care   **Chapter 32**

Anatomy and Physiology
Assessment and Management
Cardiovascular Operative Procedures
Cardiac Complications
Cardioactive Drugs

Neurologic Care   **Chapter 33**

Neurologic Assessment
Dynamics of Increased Intracranial Pressure
  (ICP)
Neurologic Complications

Immediate Postoperative Assessment   **Chapter 35**

Respiratory Adequacy
Circulatory Adequacy
Fluid and Electrolyte Balance
Temperature Regulation
Level of Consciousness
Peripheral Circulation

Perianesthesia Complications   **Chapter 36**

Critical Postanesthesia Assessments
Airway Integrity
Cardiovascular Stability

SET 1

6.1. In the preoperative setting, a patient states that he always gets antibiotics before dental procedures. Which of the following items in the patient's history would explain his statement?
   a. Pacemaker placed 2 years ago
   b. Coronary artery bypass graft (CABG) 2 years ago
   c. Atrial septal defect (ASD) repair as a child
   d. Prosthetic repair of mitral valve

6.2. The nurse should be aware that recommendations for the prevention of subacute bacterial endocarditis (SBE) are based on which of the following pieces of information?
   a. Prophylaxis always includes a regimen of multiple antibiotics.
   b. Antibiotic regimen is usually based on procedural/patient risk assessments.
   c. Antibiotics for SBE prophylaxis are effective only if given pre-procedure.
   d. Vancomycin is usually not given for prophylaxis because of its side-effect profile.

6.3. Which of the following procedures would *not* require SBE prophylaxis?
   a. Cranial wound abscess drainage under general anesthesia
   b. Insertion of myringotomy tubes under moderate sedation
   c. Cystoscopy with bladder fulguration under general anesthesia
   d. Circumcision with local anesthetic

NOTE: Consider the scenario and items 6.4-6.5 together.

A 62-year-old woman 10 days post–triple CABG presents to the PACU after an uncomplicated débridement of her infected sternal incision. She begins to complain of dyspnea and sharp, stabbing chest pain. There is ST segment elevation on her ECG. The pain subsides when the patient sits upright.

6.4. Upon auscultation, the perianesthesia nurse hears a pericardial friction rub. The priority nursing intervention after notifying a physician is to:
   a. assess for signs and symptoms of cardiovascular compromise.
   b. position and medicate the patient to adequate comfort level.
   c. prepare for immediate pericardiocentesis.
   d. Begin ACLS algorithm depending on cardiac dysrhythmia.

6.5. The patient becomes increasingly hemodynamically unstable. The nurse suspects cardiac tamponade from which of the following assessments?
   a. Central venous pressure (CVP) reading of 6 mmHg
   b. No output from mediastinal chest tubes
   c. Bradycardia
   d. Distinct S1/S2 heart sounds

6.6. A patient in the preoperative setting has a history of congestive heart failure (New York Heart Association functional classification type II). Which of the following observations are most concerning?
   a. The only patient weight noted was from 2 weeks ago.
   b. The patient was short of breath after walking to the bathroom.
   c. The patient's maintenance IV has infiltrated.
   d. The patient's ankles are noted to be edematous.

NOTE: Consider the scenario and items 6.7-6.9 together.

A moderately obese male patient, recently extubated after a left-sided thoracotomy, continues to be sedate and occasionally has desaturations of his oxygen saturation levels despite stimulation and encouragement to cough and deep breathe.

The patient is wearing a simple facemask with a flow of 8 L/min. Arterial blood gases are drawn, and the values are as follows:

pH	7.32	Normal 7.35-7.45
$PaCO_2$	50	Normal 35-45 mmHg
HCO_3	25	Normal 22-26 mEq/L
PaO_2	65	Normal 80-100 mmHg

6.7. These laboratory results indicate:
a. metabolic acidosis.
b. metabolic alkalosis.
c. respiratory acidosis.
d. respiratory alkalosis.

6.8. Which of the following could be ruled out as a risk factor for this particular acid-base imbalance?
a. Obesity
b. Thoracic surgical procedure
c. Potential for obstructive sleep apnea
d. Residual endotracheal tube irritation

6.9. In this situation, the nurse would first:
a. prepare for immediate reintubation.
b. reposition the patient's head and give a jaw thrust/support.
c. do a full cardiovascular assessment.
d. consider narcotic reversal.

6.10. A patient arrives to the PACU hypothermic. The patient's last set of arterial blood gases indicates metabolic alkalosis. Physiologically, these factors would:
a. increase oxygen's affinity to the hemoglobin molecule.
b. lead to a decrease in cardiac oxygen demand.
c. eventually initiate aerobic cellular processes.
d. decrease the risk of cardiac ischemia.

6.11. A partial pressure of oxygen below 60 to 100 mmHg generally indicates that a patient is experiencing:
a. a myocardial infarction.
b. rapid dissociation of oxygen from hemoglobin.
c. hypercapnia.
d. a drop in systolic blood pressure.

NOTE: Consider the scenario and items 6.12-6.14 together.

An extubated patient awakens in the PACU and realizes that no major surgical procedure has occurred, leading the patient to believe that he probably has a grave diagnosis and an inoperable tumor. The patient immediately begins to hyperventilate and is inconsolable.

6.12. Hyperventilation and the panicked state of the patient can lead to which of the following acid-base imbalances?
a. Metabolic acidosis
b. Metabolic alkalosis
c. Respiratory acidosis
d. Respiratory alkalosis

6.13. The perianesthesia nurse's primary intervention is to:
a. coach the patient to assist in reducing respirations.
b. provide airway support with a bag-valve-mask set up.
c. provide emotional support and coach breathing.
d. apply limb restraints.

6.14. Which of the following set of arterial blood gas (ABG) values indicates that the anxiolytic sedative that was given is beginning to be effective?
a. pH = 7.45 CO_2 = 34 HCO_3 = 22
b. pH = 7.34 CO_2 = 47 HCO_3 = 26
c. pH = 7.32 CO_2 = 31 HCO_3 = 24
d. pH = 7.45 CO_2 = 30 HCO_3 = 23

6.15. Which of the following statements is true regarding the impact of sedation level on the cardiac and respiratory systems?
a. Moderate sedation may require airway intervention.
b. Spontaneous ventilation is maintained for a moderately sedated patient.
c. Minimal sedation should not alter cardiac function but will alter respiratory function.
d. Cardiac function is not impaired by general anesthesia.

6.16. A healthy 58-year-old male patient with no cardiovascular health history presents

to the PACU after a radical retropubic prostatectomy done under spinal anesthesia. The patient begins to exhibit progressive hypotension and tachycardia. Which of the following might the nurse suspect as the cause?
a. Tumor compression of the spinal cord
b. Sympathetic blockage from the spinal block
c. Onset of diabetes insipidus
d. Delayed reaction of intraoperative beta blockers

6.17. An anesthesiologist rushes to the PACU to put an epidural into a patient who is having intractable pain from a thoracoabdominal procedure. Other attempts have been made to insert an epidural, and the physician decides to try to place one at what he believes to be the T3 level. The nurse observes for which of the following complications?
a. Blunted consciousness
b. Tachycardia or bradycardia
c. Parasympathetic blockade
d. Complete cardiopulmonary collapse

NOTE: Consider items 6.18-6.20 together.

6.18. An elderly patient not receiving optimal pain relief, despite treatment with the recommended dose of narcotics, has ketamine additionally ordered. Which of the following interventions would the nurse anticipate to be carried out first?
a. Preparing for insertion of nasal trumpet/airway
b. Inserting and adjusting the patient's hearing aids and warning of side effects
c. Administering a premedication fluid bolus
d. Warning the patient that it may take some time for the medication to work

6.19. The patient becomes agitated and confused and is attempting to climb off the cart. Pharmacologic intervention will most likely entail:
a. naloxone (Narcan).
b. flumazenil (Romazicon).
c. diphenhydramine (Benadryl).
d. midazolam (Versed).

6.20. The patient quickly grows calm but then becomes apneic and unresponsive. What would be considered as the **primary** cause of this effect?
a. Inadequate reversal of administered medications
b. Synergistic effect of administered medications
c. Delayed onset of ketamine
d. Expected side effect of ketamine

6.21. A patient's arterial line is showing a dampened waveform and readings that are 50 mmHg higher than the measurement with the blood pressure cuff. Which of the following interventions is most appropriate?
a. Move the blood pressure cuff to the arm with the arterial line.
b. Inject 20 mL of normal saline directly into the arterial line.
c. Discontinue the arterial line.
d. Reposition the patient's wrist.

6.22. Mean arterial pressure (MAP) is an important clinical indicator of:
a. perfusion of both vital and non-vital organs.
b. perfusion of only vital organs.
c. perfusion of only nonvital organs.
d. vascular muscle disinhibition.

6.23. Which of the following statements is correct regarding the placement of a central venous catheter?
a. Radiographic verification is not needed if hemodynamic readings are normal.
b. The transducer should be zeroed 3 above the phlebostatic access point.
c. Auscultation of lung sounds is necessary to rule out pneumothorax.
d. Full inflation of the wedge pressure balloon must be verified.

6.24. Capnography can be a potentially helpful tool in the PACU because:
a. it is an excellent indicator of a patient's inspired oxygen levels.
b. a large increase in readings can help identify malignant hyperthermia.
c. increased readings may indicate hyperventilation.

d. increased readings may indicate blood loss.

NOTE: Consider items 6.25-6.27 together.

A 35-year-old African-American woman is admitted to the PACU after an open cholecystectomy that was complicated by extensive bleeding. The postoperative hemoglobin was 7.5 g/dL. The nurse is having difficulty seeing a clear plethysmographic (pleth) wave and is getting pulse oximetry readings of 65% to 90% that are inconsistent with the nurse's visual assessment of the patient and stability of the patient's hemodynamics.

6.25. Which of the following might the nurse rule out as a potential cause of the wide range of readings?
a. The patient's anemia
b. The patient's dark skin
c. The patient's clear acrylic nails
d. The probe being attached to the patient's ear

6.26. Considering the patient's oxygen saturations and a poor pleth waveform, the nurse's primary intervention is to:
a. call the anesthesiologist.
b. apply oxygen per unit protocols.
c. relocate the probe until a satisfactory waveform is seen.
d. prepare to insert a nasal airway to assist with breathing.

6.27. What does the nurse need to consider when caring for this patient, after considering the oxyhemoglobin dissociation curve?
a. Pulse oximetry measures arterial oxygen saturation.
b. Pulse oximetry should be considered separately from direct patient assessment.
c. Pulse oximetry can be used to determine anemia.
d. Oxygen saturation percent (SpO_2) is always a good indicator of oxygenation.

6.28. Which of the following oxygen delivery devices offers the highest concentration of oxygen (FiO_2)?

a. Venturi mask (Venti mask)
b. Partial non-rebreather mask
c. Non-rebreather mask
d. Simple facemask

6.29. A patient with severe chronic obstructive pulmonary disease (COPD) requires both humidification of oxygen and a tightly controlled flow rate. Which of the following would be the **best** choice for oxygen therapy?
a. Venturi mask (Venti mask)
b. Partial non-rebreather mask
c. Non-rebreather mask
d. Simple facemask

6.30. An intubated patient with a central line has a sudden drop in blood pressure. Which of the following would reflect a priority intervention?
a. Check a CVP reading
b. Give a 200-mL normal saline fluid bolus
c. Run an ECG strip
d. Give a breath with a bag-valve-mask/Ambu bag

6.31. For which of the following patients would insertion of a nasopharyngeal airway be a safe intervention?
a. Facial trauma
b. Post–tonsillectomy/adenoidectomy
c. Diagnosed clotting disorder
d. Wired jaw

6.32. Which of the following would be an **unexpected** complication seen in a patient with a newly created tracheostomy?
a. Mediastinal subcutaneous emphysema
b. Pleural effusion
c. Pneumothorax
d. Feeling of shortness of breath despite adequate oxygenation

6.33. A patient with a newly created tracheostomy continues to have difficulty keeping her oxygen saturations greater than 90% with oxygen flow at 10 L/min per tracheostomy collar. Despite reminders to cough and deep breath, the patient is growing lethargic and continues to have difficulty maintaining her oxygen saturation greater

than 90%. Which of the following is the *lowest* priority for the nurse?
a. Auscultate lung sounds and assess respiratory effort.
b. Ensure that tracheostomy tube is inflated and correctly positioned.
c. Contact the physician for possible blood draw of arterial blood gases.
d. Hyper-oxygenate and suction the patient if warranted.

6.34. A patient has an intra-aortic balloon pump (IABP) inserted for treatment of cardiogenic shock. The perianesthesia nurse knows that:
a. the patient may lie prone or on the left side.
b. the catheter is generally inserted through the chest wall.
c. patients must be sedated while the IABP is functioning.
d. the IABP increases both stroke volume and myocardial perfusion.

6.35. Which of the following assessments should indicate to the nurse that an IABP balloon/catheter has migrated out of the descending aorta?
a. Carotid bruit heard upon auscultation
b. Patient complaint of blurred vision
c. Absent radial pulses
d. Increase in cardiac output

6.36. Which of the following could be ruled out as a cause of hypertension in a post-surgical patient?
a. Presence of endotracheal tube
b. Full bladder
c. High pressure ventilation
d. Sympathetic nervous system stimulation

6.37. A patient with a diagnosis of COPD presents postoperatively after bronchoscopy with worsening dyspnea and respiratory distress. Which modality of care might be considered to avoid intubation?
a. Continuous positive airway pressure (CPAP) or noninvasive nasal mask ventilation
b. Coughing and deep breathing every 5 minutes with oxygen per nasal cannula at 4 L/min

c. Close-fitting facemask with oxygen at 10 L/min
d. Nasal cannula with oxygen at 4 L/min

6.38. The perianesthesia nurse needs to be aware of which of the following in care of obese patients?
a. These patients are at a decreased risk of aspiration related to faster gastric emptying.
b. These patients experience an increase in the duration of action for highly lipid-soluble drugs.
c. Dose calculations for minimally lipophilic drugs are based on actual weight for this patient population.
d. This patient population has a low incidence of deep vein thrombosis (DVT).

6.39. The PACU nurse assesses a recently intubated patient and notes that lung sounds are not equal bilaterally nor does the chest rise and fall. After notifying the physician, the nurse immediately:
a. removes the endotracheal tube.
b. gives three large-volume breaths via anesthesia/Ambu bag.
c. pulls the endotracheal tube back 1 cm.
d. administers albuterol nebulizer treatment via endotracheal tube.

6.40. All the following can be used to evaluate a patient's preload *except:*
a. right atrial pressure (RAP).
b. systemic vascular resistance (SVR).
c. central venous pressure (CVP).
d. pulmonary capillary wedge pressure (PCWP).

6.41. In comparing the use of cardiac index (CI) measurements with the use of cardiac output (CO) in the clinical setting, the nurse knows that:
a. CI takes into account a patient's body size and vascular flow.
b. CI takes into account systemic vascular resistance.
c. CI and CO are equally valuable indicators.
d. CI is a more reliable indicator of readiness for extubation.

6.42. Which of the following symptoms would be indicative of the early symptoms of compartment syndrome?
   a. Absent pulses in operative extremity
   b. Blackened toes or fingers
   c. Hypersensitivity in operative extremity
   d. Extreme pain in extremity despite analgesics

NOTE: Consider items 6.43-6.44 together.

After repair of a congenital tibial bone disorder requiring osteotomy, a patient has been receiving narcotics for almost 3 hours in the PACU. The following laboratory results were obtained:

Laboratory Test	Result	Normal
White blood cell (WBC) count	18,000	5,000-10,000
Blood urea nitrogen (BUN)	35 mg/dL	5-25 mg/dL
Potassium	4.8 mEq/L	3.5-5.3 mEq/L
Creatinine kinase MM-isoenzyme	40 mcg/mL	5-25 mcg/mL

6.43. The nurse suspects:
   a. malignant hyperthermia.
   b. muscle necrosis.
   c. myocardial infarction.
   d. hemorrhage.

6.44. Which co-morbidity would be of greatest concern for this patient?
   a. A past history of a difficult intubation
   b. COPD requiring home oxygen therapy
   c. Type-II diabetes
   d. A history of schizophrenia

6.45. A patient with severe facial trauma presents to the PACU after a motorcycle accident. In the OR the patient received 20 mg IV morphine and 300 mcg Fentanyl total and is now showing signs of an obstructive respiratory pattern. Initial airway management includes:
   a. suctioning to clear secretions and insertion of an oral airway.

b. suctioning to clear secretions and insertion of a nasal airway.
   c. preparing for oral intubation.
   d. preparing for percutaneous tracheostomy.

6.46. When preparing to extubate a patient, the endotracheal tube is removed:
   a. at the end of inspiration.
   b. at the end of expiration.
   c. as the patient coughs.
   d. at the end of either inspiration or expiration.

6.47. A patient with an implanted cardioverter defibrillator (ICD) goes into ventricular fibrillation upon transfer into the PACU. Which of the following statements is *true* about an ICD?
   a. Patients with an ICD will never require external defibrillation.
   b. Cardiopulmonary resuscitation (CPR) should be interrupted when the ICD fires.
   c. Defibrillation paddles/pads should be placed directly over the ICD to override it.
   d. Defibrillation paddles/pads should not be placed directly over the ICD.

NOTE: Consider items 6.48-6.50 together.

6.48. After above-the-knee amputation, a patient grows progressively bradycardic and hypotensive and begins to complain of shortness of breath. The lowest priority of care would be:
   a. increasing IV fluids unless contraindicated.
   b. increasing or applying supplemental oxygen.
   c. checking surgical dressings and drains.
   d. ordering stat chest x-ray and ABGs.

6.49. As the patient's condition worsens, which of the following interventions, including transcutaneous pacing, would the nurse expect for treatment of the bradycardia?
   a. Amrinone and phenylephrine
   b. Ephedrine and dopamine

c. Phenylephrine and atropine
d. Fentanyl, midazolam, and atropine

6.50. During transcutaneous pacing, the nurse notes that not all pacer spikes are accompanied by a QRS complex. Which of the following is the ***most*** immediate intervention?
a. Adjust sensitivity
b. Increase milliamp output
c. Switch to asynchronous mode
d. Change battery in device

SET 2

6.51. Tachycardia and tachypnea in the presence of rapidly rising expired carbon dioxide levels in a patient with a clenched jaw should cause the nurse to immediately suspect:
a. malignant hyperthermia.
b. thyroid storm.
c. seizure.
d. hypoglycemia.

6.52. A patient with an acute exacerbation of his asthma complains of tremors while receiving nebulized albuterol treatment. The nurse should:
a. offer a warm blanket or apply an active warming device.
b. switch over to nebulized racemic epinephrine.
c. explain to the patient that this is a normal side effect.
d. immediately discontinue the treatment.

NOTE: Consider items 6.53-6.54 together.

6.53. A 3-year-old child who has just undergone adenotonsillectomy presents to the perianesthesia nurse with a high-pitched, barky cough and oxygen saturations ranging from 85% to 92%. The nurse should suspect:
a. an acute exacerbation of asthma.
b. post-extubation laryngeal edema.
c. hemorrhage in tonsil/adenoid vascular bed.
d. aspiration of gastric contents into the lungs.

6.54. Primary interventions for this child should include:
a. nasopharyngeal airway and oral suctioning.
b. high-Fowler position with oxygen at 10 L/min per close-fitting mask at 10L.

c. positioning to child's comfort and NSAIDs.
d. humidified oxygen and racemic epinephrine.

6.55. The PACU nurse is preparing to extubate a patient with a known difficult airway. Which of the following would be the *least* likely choice for airway intervention if a problem did arise?
a. Airway exchange catheter
b. Laryngeal mask airway
c. Fiberoptic bronchoscope
d. Venturi mask

6.56. After an abdominal hysterectomy, a patient with a known history of malignant hyperthermia begins to have dark, cola-colored urine output. Which of the following should the nurse be most concerned about?
a. Hypocalcemia
b. Shock-like vasodilation
c. Metabolic alkalosis
d. Renal failure

6.57. In a patient with a new onset of atrial fibrillation, which of the following would *least* likely be the cause?
a. Alcohol or drug use
b. Sepsis
c. Obstructive sleep apnea
d. Hyperthyroidism

6.58. In comparing therapy for a patient with new onset, unstable atrial fibrillation (less than 48 hours) with therapy for a patient who has had atrial fibrillation longer than 48 hours, the nurse knows that:
a. cardioversion may be attempted without long-term anticoagulation for new onset.
b. therapeutic international normalized ratio (INR) levels must first be

achieved before treatment in either circumstance.

c. transesophageal echocardiogram is first required in either circumstance.

d. rate control is a higher priority in new onset.

6.59. A Phase II patient, after carpal tunnel repair under moderate sedation, has abnormal pleth-wave tracings. Upon atta-ching ECG leads the nurse recog-nizes the patient is in atrial fibrillation. Which of the following statements made by this patient should come as a surprise to the nurse?

a. "I feel short of breath and have a funny feeling in my chest."

b. "Where am I and why does my chest hurt?"

c. "I feel like I am about to have a seizure."

d. "I feel just fine."

6.60. In a patient experiencing laryngospasm, the nurse would expect to find which of the following after doing a complete respiratory assessment?

a. Patient states that it is hard to breath and is visibly dyspneic

b. Audible wheezes and use of accessory muscles

c. Pink, frothy sputum

d. Inspiratory stridor with tracheal tug

NOTE: Consider items 6.61-6.62 together.

A 68-year-old patient with complications from colon cancer and a prolonged ICU stay presents to the PACU intubated and sedated requiring ventilator assistance after a 4-hour procedure to resect a portion of his colon.

6.61. The patient begins to breathe rapidly over the set rate of the ventilator, is diaphoretic, and has poor oxygen satura-tion readings despite an increase in the FiO_2 level. The nurse should immediately:

a. increase the amount of sedation and analgesic administered.

b. contact the physician to consider a chest x-ray and 12-lead ECG.

c. remove the ventilator and administer breaths via bag-valve-mask.

d. move the patient to the left lateral position.

6.62. The decision is made to extubate the patient. The extubation occurs without difficulty, but the patient is noted to have poor respiratory effort and weak, floppy movements. The nurse should prepare to administer:

a. anxiolytics and intubation supplies.

b. narcotic and benzodiazepine reversal agents.

c. Benadryl and anticholinergics.

d. phenobarbital or valium.

6.63. Phenylephrine and ephedrine are both administered to patients experiencing hypotension in the perioperative period. Which of the following statements about these medications is *true?*

a. Both drugs act as vasoconstrictors with arterial effect greater than venous effect.

b. Phenylephrine and ephedrine are potent alpha-agonists.

c. The indirect action of ephedrine limits the quantity that can be used.

d. Phenylephrine must always be ad-ministered as a continuous infusion.

6.64. The most important indicator of extuba-tion readiness is:

a. hand squeeze to command.

b. sustained head lift for longer than 5 seconds.

c. tongue protrusion to command.

d. tidal volumes greater than 5mL/kg.

6.65. Which of the following patients could potentially be at greatest risk for compli-cations from delayed tracheal tube extubation?

a. 78-year-old patient after removal of acoustic neuroma

b. 42-year-old patient after high esti-mated blood loss (EBL) during radi-cal retropubic prostatectomy

c. 19-year-old patient after LeFort I osteotomy with wired jaw

d. 36-year-old patient after closure of dehisced abdominal wound

6.66. A hypertensive patient (150-180 systolic blood pressure) who recently underwent right carotid endarterectomy begins to vomit. The nurse should:
a. hold pressure to the patient's neck dressing when the patient vomits.
b. consider a vasoactive drip if vomiting is not controlled with antiemetics.
c. monitor for episodes of severe bradycardia.
d. place nasogastric tube for decompression of the stomach.

6.67. In evaluating a patient who recently had a right carotid endarterectomy, the nurse notices that the patient's trachea is slightly deviated to the left. The nurse knows that:
a. this is a normal finding with this surgery.
b. crepitus or subcutaneous air can cause this finding.
c. this could indicate an emergent threat to the patient's airway.
d. this is not a concern as long as neurologic function is intact.

6.68. A patient who has just arrived after a left-sided thoracotomy begins to show odd electrical signals on her ECG and is pulseless. The nurse, in attempting to rapidly determine the cause, should first check:
a. indwelling urinary catheter output.
b. chest tube output.
c. pulses in lower extremities.
d. heart and lung sounds.

6.69. Which of the following assessments is a low priority when caring for a patient who has just undergone a left-sided carotid endarterectomy?
a. Cranial nerve XII (hypoglossal)
b. Cranial nerve VIII (acoustic)
c. Blood pressure (invasive and/or noninvasive)
d. Glasgow Coma Scale

NOTE: Consider items 6.70-6.72 together.

6.70. An 85-year-old hypothermic patient has arrived after total knee arthroplasty under general anesthesia with oral intubation. He had a myocardial infarction (MI) with percutaneous transluminal coronary angioplasty (PTCA) when he was 75 years old. Which of the following factors puts him at increased risk for MI?
a. Surgical procedure
b. Distant cardiac history
c. Age
d. Hypothermia

6.71. Which of the following clinical manifestations is the *least* characteristic of an acute myocardial infarction?
a. ST depression or elevation on a 12-lead ECG with elevated serum lipase
b. Elevated CK-MB and troponin levels with appearance of U wave
c. Hypoglycemia and pericardial friction rub
d. S3/S4 heart sounds and diaphoresis

6.72. The nurse prepares to assist with interventions to reduce further myocardial ischemia. The nurse should be surprised if the physician requested:
a. fibrinolytic therapy.
b. active warming.
c. reintubation.
d. nitroglycerin drip.

6.73. Which of the following would most concern the nurse caring for a patient who has been in the PACU for 2 hours after an open repair of an abdominal aortic aneurysm?
a. Urine output of 50 ml/hr
b. Pulses in bilateral lower extremities attainable only by Doppler
c. Pain rating of 7/10 over the past 2 hours
d. Central line with a right atrial (RA) reading of 3 mmHg

6.74. A nurse prepares to "shoot" a cardiac output reading using the central line. The nurse is not familiar with this procedure and asks for help. Their preceptor should stop them right before they attempt to:
a. inflate the balloon at the end of the distal port.

b. aspirate the contents of the proximal port.

c. use a syringe with 10 mL of iced injectate.

d. inject the proximal port more than once with the injectate.

6.75. The waveform after "shooting" a cardiac output is noted to be dampened. Which of the following would be considered a possible cause of the abnormal reading?

a. Tight connections and a lack of air bubbles in the line and transducer

b. Flush solution pressure is at 100 mmHg

c. Distal port balloon is deflated

d. Patient is in a side-lying position

6.76. The PACU nurse would understand which of the following to be true in caring for a patient with a ventricular ejection fraction (EF) of less than 40%?

a. The patient should be expected to have a cough and shortness of breath.

b. A greater percent of oxygenated and unoxygenated blood will be mixing.

c. Crackles and S3/S4 heart sounds would be expected.

d. High-dose NSAIDs are generally well-tolerated.

6.77. A patient with a difficult airway where facemask ventilation is hampered by a receding chin and redundant neck tissue is soon to be extubated in the PACU. Which of the following would be anticipated strategy to reduce complications?

a. Cricothyrotomy

b. Fiberoptic bronchoscope used to guide extubation

c. Placement of large-bore oral airway

d. Use of Combitube during the procedure

NOTE: Consider items 6.78-6.81 together.

An 18-year-old patient who was the unrestrained driver in a motor vehicle crash presents to the PACU nurse intubated and sedated after evacuation of a subdural hematoma. The neurosurgical team indicates in their orders that short episodes of hyperventilation via the ventilator are acceptable.

6.78. Which of the following is the best reason the therapeutic hyperventilation might be theoretically indicated?

a. To allow for respiratory adjustment in case of acid-base imbalance

b. As a means of decreasing intracranial pressure

c. To decrease blood pressure by increasing intrathoracic pressures

d. For recruitment of deflated alveoli as a means of increasing oxygenation

6.79. Which of the following cares would be *contraindicated* in this patient?

a. Cranial nerve assessment and frequent Glasgow Coma Scale evaluations

b. High-dose barbiturates for heavier sedation

c. Monitoring of intracranial pressure (ICP) via external device

d. Frequent endotracheal (ET)/oral suctioning to clear secretions

6.80. Which of the following reflects accurate information about cerebral perfusion pressure (CPP)?

a. CPP reflects both the intracranial pressure and the mean arterial pressure.

b. It will not hurt the patient to keep CPP elevated (>100 mmHg).

c. ICP does not directly influence CPP.

d. CPP can be determined by noninvasive means.

6.81. The patient's respiratory pattern becomes extremely irregular, the pulse pressure begins to widen, and his heart rate drops into the 40s. The patient is unresponsive when the nurse attempts to wake him. The PACU nurse would immediately:

a. administer narcotics to further sedate the patient.

b. turn the patient to his side.

c. hyperventilate the patient with the Ambu bag.

d. raise the head of the bed to 90°.

NOTE: Consider items 6.82-6.83 together.

A 100-kg patient who is being mechanically ventilated because of flail chest, pneumothorax, and widespread atelectasis has just had a chest X-ray that shows that the atelectasis has not improved.

6.82. The PACU nurse should expect which of the following changes to the patient's ventilator settings?
   a. Addition of positive end-expiratory pressure (PEEP) or continuous positive airway pressure (CPAP)
   b. An increase in the FiO_2 to 75%
   c. An increase of the tidal volume to 1200 mL
   d. Adjust the inspiratory:expiratory (I:E) ratio to 4:1

6.83. The high pressure alarm on the ventilator begins to go off. Which of the following interventions would be most appropriate?
   a. Lower the pressure support setting
   b. Locate any tubing leaks and reco-nnect
   c. Determine if the patient is apneic
   d. Place a bite block in the patient's mouth

NOTE: Consider items 6.84-6.85 together.

A patient experiences poor quality and depth of respirations as well as an uncoordinated respiratory pattern. The nurse suspects that it might be residual neuromuscular blockade.

6.84. Which of the following would signal that this was indeed the source of the patient's difficulties?
   a. Train-of-four measurement with peripheral nerve stimulator showing two strong twitches
   b. Sustained head lift for longer than 5 seconds
   c. Sticks out tongue for longer than 5 seconds
   d. Tidal volumes of at least 5 mL/kg

6.85. Residual neuromuscular blockage can put a patient at risk for:
   a. unplanned/accidental extubation.
   b. pulmonary edema.
   c. aspiration.
   d. cor pulmonale.

NOTE: Consider items 6.86-6.89 together.

A patient newly diagnosed with sepsis is rushed from his ICU bed to the preoperative holding area for placement of a tracheostomy tube and drainage of abdominal abscess.

6.86. In assisting with this patient, the nurse should place top priority on:
   a. placement of indwelling urinary catheter.
   b. initiation of antibiotics as ordered.
   c. placement of a central line.
   d. drawing arterial blood gases.

6.87. Post-procedure, the patient arrives to the PACU intubated and mechanically ventilated. Which of the following would the PACU nurse verify as he or she continues caring for this septic patient?
   a. Initiation of high-dose corticosteroids
   b. Light sedation
   c. Sequential compression devices and TED stockings
   d. High-pressure jet ventilation through the tracheostomy site

6.88. The patient continues to be unstable, and a dopamine drip is ordered. The *lowest* priority for the PACU nurse related to the infusion of this medication is:
   a. careful monitoring of vital signs and the ECG.
   b. vigilance of the peripheral IV site where it is infusing.
   c. determination of fluid volume status before and during administration.
   d. close monitoring of blood glucose levels.

The patient begins to show signs of acute respiratory distress syndrome (ARDS), and the care team has decided to allow for permissive hypercapnia as a means of lowering tidal volumes and decreasing the risk of lung trauma. To determine if this is safe, arterial blood gases are drawn.

pH	7.20	Normal 7.35-7.45
PaCO$_2$	55	Normal 35-45 mmHg
HCO$_3$	18	Normal 22-26 mEq/L
PaO$_2$	70	Normal 80-100 mmHg

6.89. Which of the following actions are indicated considering the above ABG results?
a. Call for an order of sodium bicarbonate and calcium gluconate
b. Call for an order of sodium bicarbonate and an insulin sliding scale
c. Call for an order of magnesium sulfate and lidocaine per weight
d. Advocate for plasmapheresis

6.90. A patient who has just undergone femoral-popliteal artery bypass is receiving a nitroglycerin drip. The patient has a history of frequent sublingual nitroglycerin use because of poorly controlled angina. The PACU nurse knows that:
a. nitrate administration may lead to refractory hypertension.
b. nitrates have both a vasoconstrictive and antithrombic/antiplatelet effect.
c. the patient may not experience the full benefits and efficacy of the drip because of tolerance.
d. the patient may complain of bladder spasms while the infusion is running.

6.91. While flushing and capping the lumen on a newly placed central line, the perianesthesia nurse should:
a. clamp the line and have the patient bear down, if able, while the cap is off.
b. treat the capping and flushing as a "clean" procedure.
c. establish keep-vein-open (KVO) fluids to run at all times to keep lines clear of clots.
d. dress the site, especially if it is a tunneled central line with an implanted cuff.

NOTE: Consider items 6.92-6.93 together.

6.92. A patient with a spinal cord injury arrives after colonoscopy for suspected diverticula. He is hypertensive and sweating profusely, and as he begins to rouse, he has a grand mal seizure. Which of the following physician telephone orders should the nurse question?
a. Raise the head of the bed.
b. Deliver oxygen via bag-valve-mask.
c. Administer anticonvulsant and antihypertensive.
d. Administer epinephrine per weight.

6.93. To stabilize this patient's blood pressure, oral nifedipine is given but seems to have little effect. The physician orders a nitroprusside drip to be started. Which of the following is true about nitroprusside?
a. Quickly becomes toxic to a patient so it should run only for a few hours
b. Should be considered along with bowel and bladder assessment
c. Reduces only preload and has no effect on afterload
d. Can alter sensorium and lead to refractory hypertension

6.94. The difference between bilevel positive airway pressure (BiPAP) and CPAP is:
a. CPAP allows for timed breaths much like a ventilator.
b. both deliver different pressures triggered by inhalation and exhalation.
c. both deliver pressure support and PEEP.
d. BiPAP may be considered in patients who cannot tolerate CPAP.

6.95. A patient with a complicated cardiac history has a syncopal episode followed by a rapid decline in blood pressure. The rhythm on the monitor appears to be a third-degree block. A code is called in the PACU. The nurse would be seen doing which of the following *first?*
a. Drawing up multiple doses of atropine
b. Placing paddles/patches on the patient's chest
c. Determining if there is any relation between the QRS cycles and t waves
d. Call for a 12-lead ECG

6.96. A patient who has undergone placement of an arteriovenous (A-V) fistula in his left arm is resting comfortably. Which of the following care personnel would the nurse stop from doing his or her job?

a. A patient care assistant who places a blood pressure cuff on the right arm

b. A laboratory technician who wants to draw blood from the left arm

c. An infectious disease nurse who wants to give the patient his flu shot in the right arm

d. A student nurse who asks to listen and feel for the bruit on the left arm

6.97. Ramipril works by:

a. causing a direct blockade of beta-1 and beta-2 receptors.

b. decreasing production of angiotensin II.

c. altering cellular calcium re-uptake.

d. stimulating aldosterone secretion.

6.98. Which of the following would be the best intervention for a patient with known acute renal failure requiring an extended Phase II stay because of pain and extensive blood loss?

a. Calling the anesthesiologist for approval to administer Lasix

b. Administering 10 mEq potassium IV bolus over a 30-60 minute period

c. Canceling or delaying scheduled computed tomography (CT) with contrast appointment

d. Administering a renal-dose dopamine infusion and second ketorolac dose

NOTE: Consider items 6.99-6.100 together.

6.99. After placement of a femoral sheath for embolization of a cranial arteriovenous malformation (AVM), the patient complains, "My right foot feels funny." Which of the following would be *least* helpful in ruling out possible non-neurologic causes of the sensation?

a. Measure thigh girth

b. Inspect range of motion on bilateral lower extremities

c. Palpate bilateral dorsalis pedis and posterior tibialis pulses

d. Flush sheath site with prescribed heparin dosage

6.100. The nurse determines that there are no abnormalities at the femoral sheath insertion site or in the surrounding tissue and calls the surgical team to alert them of the deficit. Which of the following orders should the PACU nurse question?

a. Up to bathroom ad lib

b. Neurologic/neurovascular checks every 15 minutes for the first 2 hours post-op

c. Apply TED stockings and sequential compression device

d. Discontinue arterial line

SET 3

NOTE: Consider items 6.101-6.102 together.

An obese man who just awakened from a 2-hour total hip arthroplasty begins to complain of tightness and pain in his non-operative leg. The nurse notes that the leg is edematous and highly suspicious for a deep vein thrombosis (DVT), a problem noted to have occurred with his past two surgeries.

6.101. How many risk factors for a DVT does the patient have?
   a. 2
   b. 3
   c. 4
   d. 5

6.102. Which of the following nursing actions would be most appropriate in this situation?
   a. Call for an order to initiate IV infusion of unfractionated heparin
   b. Apply cold packs to leg and massage site
   c. Place leg in dependent position
   d. Encourage ambulation

6.103. An intubated patient receiving his third infusion of packed red blood cells after complicated removal of a small bowel obstruction presents to the PACU. Thirty minutes later, the nurse notes that pink, frothy sputum is in the ET tube and course rhonchi and crackles can be heard throughout the lung fields. After suctioning the patient, the best nursing action(s) would be to:
   a. call for albuterol treatment.
   b. stop the infusion and KVO site with normal saline.
   c. order stat chest x-ray film.
   d. call for Lasix order and stop blood infusion.

6.104. The PACU nurse is caring for a patient who weighs 70 kg and is on a ventilator with the following ventilator settings and ABGs (see table). Which of the following adjustments to the ventilator would be most appropriate?
   a. Increase respiratory rate to 14
   b. Increase PEEP to 10 cm H_2O
   c. Increase FiO_2 to 70%
   d. Increase tidal volume to 700 mL

Arterial Blood Gases			Ventilator Settings	
pH	7.31	Normal 7.35-7.45	Mode	Assist Control
$PaCO_2$	69	Normal 35-45 mmHg	FiO_2	50%
HCO_3	23	Normal 22-26 mEq/L	Tidal Volume	500 mL
PaO_2	75	Normal 80-100 mmHg	Rate	10/min
			PEEP	5 cm H_2O

6.105. When considering the anatomy of the lungs and how its anatomy might impact post-anesthesia care, which of the following statements is *correct?*
   a. Aspiration is more common into the left rather than the right lobe of the lung.
   b. Ventilation is generally greater in the left than the right lobe of the lung.
   c. The left bronchus turns at a sharper angle toward the lung than the right bronchus.
   d. Decreased or absent lung sounds are a more common finding on the left than the right after intubation.

NOTE: Consider items 6.106-6.108 together.

6.106. After free flap reconstruction of the right breast, the PACU nurse should be most concerned with which of the following?
a. White to light-gray coloration of flap site
b. Jackson-Pratt wound drain to thumb-print suction
c. Order for subcutaneous heparin
d. Core body temperature of 35.2° C (95.4° F)

6.107. The patient begins to complain of back pain and asks the nurse to help her reposition for comfort. Which of the following would be the *correct* option for the nurse?
a. Position in a right side-lying position
b. Allow the patient to lie prone
c. Adjust the head of the bed until a comfortable position is achieved
d. Allow the patient to stretch her arms and rest with her hands behind her head

6.108. The patient has now been in the PACU for 2 hours because of poor pain control, hypothermia, and hypotension. Which of the following assessments would be *unexpected* in this scenario and require a prompt call to the surgical team?
a. Blanching of the skin within 4 seconds
b. Flap site warm to the touch
c. Pulses faint but obtainable by Doppler over flap site
d. Purple/blue color to flap site

NOTE: Consider items 6.109-6.110 together.

6.109. After a traumatic motor vehicle crash, the nurse in the preoperative holding area stabilizes a patient before she is about to go to surgery. The preoperative nurse notes that a chest tube has been placed for blood in the pleural space. The nurse should expect that the tube(s) would be placed:
a. at the second intercostal space on the injured side.
b. at the seventh intercostal space on the injured side.
c. mediastinally at the nipple line.
d. at both the second and seventh intercostal spaces.

6.110. A new graduate nurse assisting that day asks the preoperative nurse about the chest tube drainage device that is attached. Which of the statements made by the new nurse is *correct?*
a. "Attaching the drainage system to wall suction does directly suck air and fluid out of the chest."
b. "The up-and-down motion of the fluid in the water seal column means that the system is working incorrectly."
c. "Bubbles in the suction chamber indicates there is no air leak."
d. "Bubbles in the water seal column indicate there is an air leak."

6.111. After endovascular stenting of a thoracic aneurysm, the patient complains of nagging chest and back pain. The surgical team and anesthesiologist are called, and cardiac origin of the pain is ruled out. There is discussion of an endoleak at the graft site. Which of the following should the nurse prepare for in this scenario?
a. Discharging the patient to CT
b. Fluid resuscitation
c. Application of direct pressure at femoral sites
d. Administration of nitroglycerin as needed

6.112. In reviewing an anesthesia record with a patient as the patient prepares to be discharged from the outpatient surgical center, the patient asks why lidocaine was given to him before he went to sleep. Which of the following would be an *incorrect* answer?
a. It decreases the urge to cough.
b. It counteracts increased pressure in the brain during intubation.
c. It sometimes limits the effect of induction on the heart.
d. It lowers the risk of pulmonary edema and aspiration.

6.113. Rapid sequence induction (intubation) would be *contraindicated* in which of the following patients?
a. Pediatric patient having minor outpatient procedure

b. Stabbing victim with uncertain NPO status

c. Patient with history of fiberoptic intubations

d. Woman with an uncomplicated pregnancy

6.114. Which of the following actions taken by the nurse anesthetist best demonstrate a safe rapid sequence induction (intubation)?

a. Preoxygenation and then administration of succinylcholine

b. Preoxygenation and then administration of etomidate

c. Etomidate and succinylcholine followed by gently bagging with 100% oxygen

d. Preoxygenation followed by simultaneous administration of etomidate and succinylcholine.

6.115. After a 15-second grand mal seizure in a post-craniotomy patient, the immediate priority of care is:

a. reintubation with midline cervical stabilization.

b. removal of bite block and order for padded side rails.

c. oral suctioning and side-lying position.

d. schedule for immediate CT scan.

6.116. Calcium is frequently given to patients with potentially poor cardiac function because of which cardiac effect?

a. Positive inotropic effect

b. Coronary artery vasodilation

c. Slowed AV node conduction

d. Increased diastolic filling

NOTE: Consider items 6.117-6.120 together.

6.117. What are the perianesthesia cardiac implications for an elderly man in atrial fibrillation with a known history of mitral valve regurgitation?

a. Left ventricular hypertrophy and increased risk for myocardial infarction

b. Pulmonary hypertension and fluid overload

c. Renal insufficiency with oliguria and hematuria

d. Aortic calcification and lack of murmur with auscultation of heart sounds

6.118. Which of the following would represent a safe nursing action in caring for this patient?

a. Administration of therapeutic doses of furosemide (Lasix)

b. Fluid bolus to manage decreased cardiac output

c. Delay extubation until patient is highly awake and responsive

d. Hold anticoagulants until patient is ambulatory

6.119. The patient grows somnolent and exhibits left-sided weaknesses of the upper and lower extremities. Considering the patient's health history and the signs and symptoms, the nurse should suspect which of the following?

a. Arteriovenous malformation

b. Myocardial infarction

c. Pulmonary emboli

d. Cerebral emboli

6.120. Which of the following would be the nursing action with the *lowest* priority in this scenario?

a. High-flow oxygen at 10 L/min by mask

b. Elevate head of bed to 30°

c. Aggressive treatment of systolic blood pressure in the 150s

d. Neurologic assessment every 15 to 30 minutes

NOTE: Consider items 6.121-6.122 together.

6.121. A patient who has had a repair of a torn shoulder ligament has had a cardiac ischemic event, and there is concern about the functioning of his kidneys. Which of the following would be the least helpful to the nurse and the care team in determining kidney functioning and extent of damage?

a. Reviewing mean arterial pressures to ensure they were greater than 60 to 75 mmHg

154

b. Determining if urine output has been greater than 0.5 mL/kg/hr
c. Ordering a bedside bladder ultrasound
d. Reviewing intake and output

6.122. In anticipation of treating this episode of acute renal failure, the nurse would expect to:
a. administer vancomycin as prophylaxis and treatment of renal infection.
b. infuse albumin and isotonic saline.
c. prepare patient for placement of temporary dialysis catheter.
d. start renal-dose dopamine infusion for renal vasodilation.

NOTE: Consider the scenario and items 6.123-6.124 together.

A 42-year-old Hispanic male with pelvic and tibial fractures after an on-the-job crush injury presents to the PACU. He becomes progressively short of breath, confused, and febrile and has dropping oxygen saturations unresponsive to supplemental oxygen. The ECG shows tachycardia with multiple PVCs.

6.123. The highest priority for this patient with suspected fat embolus is to:
a. prepare patient for pulmonary angiography.
b. sit patient in high-Fowler position.
c. immediately prepare for intubation.
d. administer corticosteroids.

6.124. The PACU nurse knows that fat embolus can be prevented through:
a. stabilization of fractured extremities and oxygen administration.
b. corticosteroid therapy preoperatively and postoperatively.
c. administration of statin drugs to pull lipids out of the bloodstream.
d. close monitoring of oxygen saturation and ECG.

6.125. After a 6-hour thoracic-lumbar rodding and removal of tumor in the prone position, the patient presents to the PACU supine and intubated with spontaneous respirations. Which of the following

presents the greatest concern to the perianesthesia nurse?
a. Skin breakdown noted on the patient's chest and thighs
b. Edema noted around the eyelids and sclera of both eyes
c. Excessive fluid buildup in face and neck
d. Two surgical drains from the back dressing with a total of 300 mL bloody drainage

6.126. Which of the following findings in a patient who has undergone lower extremity vascular surgery would **not** be attributed to hypothermia?
a. Hypotension
b. Difficulty in palpating pulses
c. Increased patient report of anxiety
d. Capillary refill of 4 seconds

6.127. In considering how the pathophysiology of vascular disease and basic vascular physiology impact perianesthesia care, it is important for the nurse to know that:
a. low fluid volumes increase peripheral vascular resistance.
b. baroreceptors may decrease in function with age.
c. lower systemic vascular resistance will cause vessel hypertrophy.
d. loss of elasticity in the blood vessel wall decreases blood pressure.

6.128. After laparoscopic nephrectomy, a patient in the PACU complains of back pain and shortness of breath and is growing increasingly anxious. Upon taking the patient's blood pressure, the nurse notes that the blood pressure has been trending downward. Which of the following assessments would be **most** helpful in assisting the nurse to determine the cause?
a. Have the patient turn on his side and visually/manually inspect back
b. Have the patient cough and deep breathe 10 times
c. Order hemoglobin and hematocrit, and administer anxiolytics
d. Auscultate for bowel sounds

6.129. A healthy 22-year-old female patient presents after an open appendectomy.

The patient is tachycardic but still somewhat sedate and verbalizes that she is comfortable. The nurse might consider which of the following as the cause?

a. Hypothyroidism
b. Hypervolemia
c. Residual effect of reversal agent
d. Stimulation of baroreceptors

6.130. Which of the following assessments of a patient after bronchoscopy should be of the greatest concern to the perianesthesia nurse?

a. Prolonged, nonproductive cough
b. Difficulty swallowing
c. Occasional premature atrial contractions
d. Fever of 38.8° C (101.8° F)

6.131. How does care and assessment of a patient after bronchoscopy differ from that of a patient after mediastinoscopy?

a. Pneumothorax generally does not occur after mediastinoscopy.
b. Both are generally for gathering biopsies and inspecting the lung.
c. Mediastinoscopy requires only local anesthetic.
d. Subcutaneous emphysema is more common with mediastinoscopy.

6.132. Immediately after video-assisted thoracoscopy and removal of emphysematous tissue in the right lung, the nurse should be most concerned about which of the following?

a. Complaints of numbness and tingling in the right hand
b. Absent lung sounds in the right lower lobe of the lung
c. End-tidal CO_2 levels of 50 mmHg
d. Minimal chest tube air leak

6.133. For which of the following patients would beta blockers be *least* concerning as a means of treating hypertension?

a. Diabetic patient after bronchoscopy with washings
b. Patient with Raynaud's phenomenon after amputation of multiple fingers
c. Asthmatic patient noted to have minimal expiratory wheeze

d. Patient who has also received a dose of verapamil (calcium channel blocker)

6.134. After moderate sedation for magnetic resonance imaging (MRI), an infant with a known congenital heart defect presents to the PACU. Which of the following observations made by the nurse would be most concerning?

a. No in-line air filter on the IV tubing
b. Heat lamp above the bed
c. Tachypnea
d. Baseline oxygen saturations ranging from 70% to 80%

6.135. For which patient scenario should the PACU nurse advocate for ECG monitoring?

a. A 58-year-old patient with American Society of Anesthesiologists (ASA) I classification
b. A severely developmentally disabled patient who is restless and agitated
c. A patient who has received QT-prolonging drugs such as erythromycin or clarithromycin
d. 10-month-old patient after a cleft palate repair

6.136. Which of the following facts about QT prolongation is *true*?

a. Antipsychotic drugs are one of the few classes with low risk of QT prolongation.
b. QT prolongation can lead to torsades de pointes.
c. QT prolongation is indicated by a QTc of more than 0.3 second.
d. Monitoring for QT interval lengthening is impossible without a 12-lead ECG.

6.137. The best way to determine the appropriate-size nasopharyngeal airway is to approximate the distance between:

a. chin to the edge of the jaw line.
b. nostril to epiglottis.
c. edge of teeth to epiglottis.
d. naris to earlobe.

156

6.138. Ease of insertion of the nasopharyngeal airway is facilitated by all the following *except*:
a. lubricating the catheter.
b. spraying numbing agent such as oxymetazoline into naris.
c. withdrawing and rotating if resistance is met.
d. inserting in an anterior and lateral direction.

6.139. Which of the following is true about right versus left bundle branch blocks?
a. A left bundle branch block is always indicative of heart disease of some type.
b. A right bundle branch block is more severe than left bundle branch block.
c. Both indicate that there is a mismatch in the timing of atrial depolarization.
d. These blocks are never benign or asymptomatic.

NOTE: Consider the following scenario and items 6.140-6.142 together.

A 54-year-old morbidly obese female presents to the PACU after total abdominal hysterectomy. She is complaining of intense abdominal pain and is struggling to keep her oxygen saturations above 90% with oxygen at 3 L/min per nasal cannula.

6.140. The nurse is concerned about atelectasis and frequently coaches the patient through coughing and deep-breathing exercises. Which of the following does not explain why this practice is beneficial?
a. Promotes loosening and clearing of airway secretions
b. Promotes redistribution of lung surfactant
c. Promotes increased bronchiole perfusion
d. Recruits deflated alveoli to promote oxygenation

6.141. The patient begins to have ventricular ectopy and goes into respiratory and cardiac arrest. What kinds of preparations are not needed by the nurse in advance to facilitate resuscitative efforts in a morbidly obese patient?

a. Appropriate-size care items such as blood pressure cuffs and sequential compression devices (SCDs)
b. Advocating for placement of invasive arterial line for blood draws and pressure monitoring
c. Acquiring defibrillator that can deliver higher-than-usual levels of electrical discharge to convert lethal rhythms in this patient population
d. Fitting the patient for CPAP/BiPAP mask

6.142. It is determined that the patient is bleeding into her abdomen. In considering the possibility of fluid resuscitation and blood administration, which following statement is true?
a. Survival rates are improved with albumin versus saline.
b. Fluid infusion can be as fast as can be handled by the IV access and the patient.
c. Multiple units of hetastarch and dextran can be administered without complication.
d. Respiratory difficulties associated with fluid resuscitation occur only in patients with lung disease.

6.143. In which of the following patients would a Cheyne-Stokes respiratory pattern be *unexpected?*
a. Patient after cerebrovascular accident (CVA)
b. Patient with exacerbation of congestive heart failure (CHF)
c. Patient with traumatic brain injury diagnosis with increasing intracranial pressure
d. Over-sedated patient with suspected pseudocholinesterase deficiency

6.144. When applying CPAP, the nurse needs to be most concerned about:
a. recent acetylcholine blocking medication.
b. recent open heart surgery.
c. shape of the face and the presence of facial hair.
d. seizure history.

6.145. After thoracotomy for removal of left lung mass, the patient is extubated and breathing comfortably. The nurse and physician collaboratively review the patient's chest x-ray film, which shows that a small area of the patient's left lung is not completely inflated. The nurse should expect to:
   a. prep the patient's side for chest tube insertion.
   b. apply supplemental oxygen by nasal cannula at 4 L/min.
   c. prepare for immediate intubation.
   d. use bag-valve-mask to assist the patient's respiratory effort.

6.146. Vital capacity measurements of the lungs can help the perianesthesia nurse to:
   a. differentiate between obstructive and restrictive lung conditions.
   b. determine how diffusion is occurring across the alveoli.
   c. determine the amount of air left in the lungs after expiration.
   d. estimate the severity of atelectasis.

6.147. A nurse anesthetist is giving report on a patient with a pacemaker. The nurse anesthetist states that the settings are DDI. The nurse assuming care knows that this means:
   a. both the atria and ventricles are being paced and sensed.
   b. neither the atria nor the ventricles are being paced or sensed.
   c. the atria and ventricles are not paced with spontaneous beats.

   d. both of the ventricles are being paced and sensed.

6.148. The best way to differentiate between paroxysmal supraventricular tachycardia (PSVT) and ventricular tachycardia is to note:
   a. the length of the QRS complex.
   b. the estimated beats per minute (bpm).
   c. the presence or absence of a P wave.
   d. how well the patient is tolerating the rhythm.

6.149. A patient who cannot be stimulated and has no pulse shows what appears to be wide fibrillation waves on the ECG monitor. The nurse's first action would be to:
   a. administer 6 mg adenosine.
   b. prepare to shock at 200 joules (J) or biphasic equivalent.
   c. deliver a precordial thump to the chest.
   d. call for 12-lead ECG and ABGs.

6.150. What should the nurse warn the patient of before administration of adenosine for PSVT?
   a. "We will need to have you take a deep breath and bear down."
   b. "You may feel like your heart has stopped beating for a couple of seconds."
   c. "A common side effect of this medication is a pounding headache."
   d. "This medication can be taken orally or through the IV."

SET 1

ANSWER KEY

6.1.	d		**6.26.**	b
6.2.	b		**6.27.**	a
6.3.	c		**6.28.**	c
6.4.	a		**6.29.**	a
6.5.	b		**6.30.**	d
6.6.	a		**6.31.**	d
6.7.	c		**6.32.**	b
6.8.	d		**6.33.**	c
6.9.	b		**6.34.**	d
6.10.	a		**6.35.**	c
6.11.	b		**6.36.**	c
6.12.	d		**6.37.**	a
6.13.	c		**6.38.**	b
6.14.	a		**6.39.**	c
6.15.	b		**6.40.**	b
6.16.	b		**6.41.**	a
6.17.	b		**6.42.**	d
6.18.	b		**6.43.**	b
6.19.	d		**6.44.**	c
6.20.	b		**6.45.**	a
6.21.	d		**6.46.**	a
6.22.	a		**6.47.**	d
6.23.	c		**6.48.**	d
6.24.	b		**6.49.**	d
6.25.	c		**6.50.**	b

SET 1

6.1. Correct Answer: **d**
The American Heart Association publishes clear sub-bacterial endocarditis (SBE) prophylaxis guidelines that list the high- and moderate-risk categories for patients who have had particular cardiac diseases or procedures. In general, the high-risk categories include most valvular diseases and placement of a prosthetic valve or a history of bacterial endocarditis. A history of ASD repair, CABG, or pacemaker placement is not considered to be a risk factor necessitating prophylaxis. The complete guide can be viewed in multiple locations including the original article cited here. (Dajani AS et al: Prevention of bacterial endocarditis: recommendations by the American Heart Association, *JAMA* 277[22]:1794-1801, 1997.)

6.2. Correct Answer: **b**
The American Heart Association guidelines on SBE prophylaxis include a listing of standard-, high-, and moderate-risk patients, the appropriate medications and dosing, and treatment options for those patients with allergies. Prophylaxis may consist of one or two antibiotics including vancomycin (namely for those patients with allergies to penicillin). Prophylactic antibiotic coverage can still be administered within 2 or 3 hours of the procedure. (Dajani AS et al: Prevention of bacterial endocarditis: recommendations by the American Heart Association, *JAMA* 277[22]:1794-1801, 1997; Golembiewski JA: Antibiotic prophylaxis for preventing surgical site infection, *J PeriAnesth Nurs* 19[2]:111-113, 2004; Horstkotte D et al: Guidelines on prevention, diagnosis, and treatment of infective endocarditis executive summary; the task force on infective endocarditis of the European Society of Cardiology, *Eur Heart J* 25[3]:267-276, 2004.)

6.3. Correct Answer: **c**
SBE prophylaxis is generally indicated only for invasive oral/maxillofacial, gastrointestinal, genitourinary, and respiratory procedures. The procedures could be as simple as dental extraction or tonsillectomy-adenoidectomy and as complicated as prostate surgery or sclerotherapy of esophageal varices. (Dajani AS et al: Prevention of bacterial endocarditis: recommendations by the American Heart Association, *JAMA* 277[22]:1794-1801, 1997; Quinn D, Schick L, editors: *ASPAN's perianesthesia nursing core curriculum: preoperative, Phase I and Phase II PACU nursing*, Philadelphia, 2004, Saunders.)

6.4. Correct Answer: **a**
A pericardial effusion is a complication in which fluid fills the parietal and visceral layers of the pericardium, potentially hampering normal heart muscle functioning. Rapid fluid filling of the pericardial layers can lead to tamponade, which can severely limit the volume of blood that can be effectively pumped. A case of cardiac tamponade may require pericardiocentesis or an open sternotomy but would be indicated only if this was indeed occurring. Assessing for and ruling out tamponade is the priority of care. It is correct to sit a patient upright and treat pain using NSAIDs, but it is not the top priority care item here. Although atrial

fibrillation is common in cases of chronic pericarditis, no lethal rhythm was indicated and therefore initiation of ACLS would not yet be appropriate. (Ignatavius DD et al: *Medical-surgical nursing: critical thinking for collaborative care*, ed 4, Philadelphia, 2002, Saunders; Prince SE et al: Postpericardiotomy syndrome, *Heart Lung* 26[2]: 165-168, 1997.)

6.5. Correct Answer: **b**
The backup and decreased performance of the heart would occur as a result of tamponade and would lead to decreased, not increased, cardiac output. Other classic signs and symptoms of cardiac tamponade include increased CVP pressures, muffled heart sounds, jugular venous distention, and pulsus paradoxus. (Quinn D, Schick L, editors: *ASPAN's perianesthesia nursing core curriculum: preoperative, Phase I and Phase II PACU nursing*, Philadelphia, 2004, Saunders; Baltimore JJ: Perianesthesia care of cardiac surgery patients: a CPAN review, *J PeriAnesth Nurs* 16[4]:246-254, 2001; Ignatavius DD et al: *Medical-surgical nursing: critical thinking for collaborative care*, ed 4, Philadelphia, 2002, Saunders.)

6.6. Correct Answer: **a**
The New York Heart Association Functional Classification has four subjective levels for congestive heart failure with level I being the mildest class and level IV being the most severe class. A patient with a level II designation would normally have dyspnea on exertion and the edema described. Although a concern, an infiltrated IV, especially in the preoperative setting, is not life-threatening and can easily be cared for and replaced. Not knowing if the patient has had a gain or loss of weight in the past 2 weeks is a large concern, since it can be telling as to

whether the patient is having an exacerbation of symptoms or is in a worsening congestive state. At the very least, a weight is needed as a baseline for later on in the hospitalization and is essential for calculation of fluid levels and medication dosages. (Gilmore JC: Heart failure and treatment: part I, *J PeriAnesth Nurs* 18[2]:83-90, 2003; Quinn D, Schick L, editors: *ASPAN's perianesthesia nursing core curriculum: preoperative, Phase I and Phase II PACU nursing*, Philadelphia, 2004, Saunders.)

6.7. Correct Answer: **c**
Respiratory acidosis is one of the more common acid-base imbalances encountered in the postoperative setting and is characterized by the laboratory studies shown. An important consideration is that the patient's health history, condition, and surgery put him at risk for hypoxia, which is directly linked to blood acidity. (Quinn D, Schick L, editors: *ASPAN's perianesthesia nursing core curriculum: preoperative, Phase I and Phase II PACU nursing*, Philadelphia, 2004, Saunders.)

6.8. Correct Answer: **d**
Obesity is often linked with obstructive sleep apnea, which is strongly suggested in this scenario. Any type of thoracic or upper abdominal surgery can interfere with normal respiratory functioning because of pain, bleeding, or compromise of respiratory anatomy and physiology. Residual endotracheal tube irritation is more commonly associated with laryngospasm and coughing. (Hurst S et al: Bariatric implications of critical care nursing, *Dimens Crit Care Nurs* 23[2]:76-83, 2004; Quinn D, Schick L, editors: *ASPAN's perianesthesia nursing core curriculum: preoperative, Phase I and Phase II PACU nursing*, Philadelphia, 2004, Saunders.)

6.9. Correct Answer: **b**
Although the blood gas findings are abnormal and concerning, they would not necessarily warrant reintubation from the evidence in this scenario. Reversal of narcotics may be considered if the patient continues to deteriorate, but this may actually exacerbate the situation if the patient has too much pain to breath adequately. Cardiovascular assessment is important but not a top priority in this scenario. Reestablishing or supporting the patient's airway may allow for more adequate oxygenation and may determine what further interventions may be necessary. (Quinn D, Schick L, editors: *ASPAN's perianesthesia nursing core curriculum: preoperative, Phase I and Phase II PACU nursing*, Philadelphia, 2004, Saunders.)

6.10. Correct Answer: **a**
A patient who is hypothermic and alkalotic may be at risk for alterations of oxygenation. Alkalosis and hypothermia cause oxygen to have a higher affinity for the hemoglobin molecule, which translates to decreased delivery of oxygen to the body. Less oxygenation of tissues translates to hypoxia that eventually leads to anaerobic energy process, an inefficient means for the development of cellular energy. Cardiac demand for oxygen will increase as will the risk for ischemia. (Quinn D, Schick L, editors: *ASPAN's perianesthesia nursing core curriculum: preoperative, Phase I and Phase II PACU nursing*, Philadelphia, 2004, Saunders; Drain C, editor: *Perianesthesia nursing: a critical care approach*, ed 4, Philadelphia, 2003, Saunders; Hsia CC: Respiratory function of hemoglobin, *N Engl J Med* 338[4]:239-247, 1998; McCance KL, Huether SE: *Pathophysiology: the biologic basis for disease in adults and children*, ed 4, St. Louis, 2002, Mosby; McQuillan KA et al: *Trauma nursing: from resuscitation through rehabilitation*, ed 3, Philadelphia, 2002, Saunders.)

6.11. Correct Answer: **b**
The affinity of oxygen for hemoglobin determines whether the patient is being adequately oxygenated. If the partial pressure of oxygen drops below 60 mmHg, saturation of hemoglobin with oxygen will be inadequate as a result of the unloading of oxygen from hemoglobin (decreased affinity). A drop in blood pressure or a myocardial infarction may result or cause this change but cannot be directly implied by a decrease in partial pressure of oxygen. Although an increase in carbon dioxide can be a factor in the shifting of a patient into a state of hypoxemia, carbon dioxide is quickly diffused into the lungs so hypoxemia does not always imply hypercapnia. (Quinn D, Schick L, editors: *ASPAN's perianesthesia nursing core curriculum: preoperative, Phase I and Phase II PACU nursing*, Philadelphia, 2004, Saunders; Drain C, editor: *Perianesthesia nursing: a critical care approach*, ed 4, Philadelphia, 2003, Saunders; Hsia CC: Respiratory function of hemoglobin, *N Engl J Med* 338[4]:239-247, 1998; McCance KL, Huether SE: *Pathophysiology: the biologic basis for disease in adults and children*, ed 4, St. Louis, 2002, Mosby; McQuillan KA et al: *Trauma nursing: from resuscitation through rehabilitation*, ed 3, Philadelphia, 2002, Saunders.)

6.12. Correct Answer: **d**
Hyperventilation in a patient with or without an artificial airway is a classic cause of respiratory alkalosis. The condition can be further exacerbated by a patient who is under great emotional stress or

pain or is dealing with immense anxiety. (Quinn D, Schick L, editors: *ASPAN's perianesthesia nursing core curriculum: preoperative, Phase I and Phase II PACU nursing*, Philadelphia, 2004, Saunders.)

6.13. Correct Answer: **c**
One of the most influential roles the PACU nurse can have is providing emotional support and reassurance to a patient such as this. Coaching the patient to reduce respiratory rate will help bring the metabolic system back to a normal state. Although sedatives may be used as a means of assisting this process, reintubation or assisting the patient's breathing may further exacerbate the problem at this point in time. (Moser DK et al: Critical care nursing practice regarding patient anxiety assessment and management. *Intensive Crit Care Nurs* 19[5]:276-288, 2003; Quinn D, Schick L, editors: *ASPAN's perianesthesia nursing core curriculum: preoperative, Phase I and Phase II PACU nursing*, Philadelphia, 2004, Saunders.)

6.14. Correct Answer: **a**
The interventions described should bring the blood pH to a more normal state even if the patient's carbon dioxide level is not perfectly normal as we see in the correct choice, option **a**. Respiratory acidosis would not be expected in a patient who was just in an alkalotic state, although it may have occurred from oversedation with the anxiolytic/sedative. Option **c** is another acidotic state that would not be expected in this scenario. Option **d** represents a corrected state, but the patient's carbon dioxide levels continue to be low, compared with option **a,** in which they are near normal. (Quinn D, Schick L, editors: *ASPAN's perianesthesia nursing core curriculum: preoperative, Phase I and Phase II*

PACU nursing, Philadelphia, 2004, Saunders.)

6.15. Correct Answer: **b**
Minimal sedation, by definition, should alter only responsiveness, and moderate sedation should not alter cardiovascular or airway/ventilation functioning. General anesthesia should blunt awareness and has a high potential for altering cardiovascular/respiratory functioning to the point that intervention is required (i.e., intubation). (Quinn D, Schick L, editors: *ASPAN's perianesthesia nursing core curriculum: preoperative, Phase I and Phase II PACU nursing*, Philadelphia, 2004, Saunders.)

6.16. Correct Answer: **b**
Sympathetic blockade can cause the hypotension and tachycardia seen in this patient, especially since spinal rather than epidural analgesia was provided. Other findings could include reduced venous tone and venous return to the heart and a subsequent decrease in cardiac filling and output. A large volume of blood loss also can occur in the patient who has had a radical retropubic prostatectomy and may also play a role in the symptoms seen. (Quinn D, Schick L, editors: *ASPAN's perianesthesia nursing core curriculum: preoperative, Phase I and Phase II PACU nursing*, Philadelphia, 2004, Saunders.)

6.17. Correct Answer: **b**
Only an epidural placed above the T1 level would cause cardiopulmonary collapse. Generally, hypotension is the most common side effect of epidural placement that may require monitoring and intervention by nursing personnel. Bradycardia may be seen with blocks higher than T3, whereas tachycardia may occur with sympathetic blockage. Either can occur depending on where the epidural

was actually placed. Blunted consciousness and parasympathetic blockage would not be expected side effects of the epidural placement. (Quinn D, Schick L, editors: *ASPAN's perianesthesia nursing core curriculum: preoperative, Phase I and Phase II PACU nursing*, Philadelphia, 2004, Saunders.)

6.18. Correct Answer: **b**
Ketamine is well known for its ability to produce hallucinations and delirium. By ensuring that the patient can hear the nurse to receive reassurance may assist in preventing some of these side effects or perhaps reduce their effect. Although hypotension is considered a side effect, it generally does not warrant prophylactic administration of fluids. Onset is quick and, in general (unless a patient has been overdosed), there is no expectation of respiratory effect requiring airway intervention. (ASPAN: ASPAN pain and comfort clinical guideline, *J PeriAnesth Nurs* 18[4]:232-236, 2003; Pasero C et al: Pain control: ketamine—low doses may provide relief for some painful conditions, *Am J Nurs* 105[4]:60-64,72, 2005; Quinn D, Schick L, editors: *ASPAN's periAnesthesia nursing core curriculum: preoperative, Phase I and Phase II PACU nursing*, Philadelphia, 2004, Saunders.)

6.19. Correct Answer: **d**
Older patients are at a higher risk of delirium associated with ketamine, which may require restraints and/or medication with a benzodiazepine. Naloxone is a narcotic reversal agent and flumazenil is a benzodiazepine reversal agent. Benadryl is generally for sedation, as a sleep aid, or for treating an allergic reaction. (Pasero C et al: Pain control: ketamine—low doses

may provide relief for some painful conditions, *Am J Nurs* 105[4]:60-64, 72, 2005; Quinn D, Schick L, editors: *ASPAN's perianesthesia nursing core curriculum: preoperative, Phase I and Phase II PACU nursing*, Philadelphia, 2004, Saunders.)

6.20. Correct Answer: **b**
The scenario indicated that the patient was not getting adequate pain control with narcotics. Benzodiazepines and narcotics can have a powerful synergistic effect, even with the addition of only small amounts of benzodiazepines. The nurse should not expect any of the effects to be related to ketamine unless the patient had been overdosed, nor would reversal have been appropriate. (Quinn D, Schick L, editors: *ASPAN's perianesthesia nursing core curriculum: preoperative, Phase I and Phase II PACU nursing*, Philadelphia, 2004, Saunders.)

6.21. Correct Answer: **d**
The arterial line and the blood pressure cuff will not always be directly correlated. The blood pressure cuff is a noninvasive, periodic reading, whereas the arterial line is an invasive, continuous evaluation of blood pressure. There is no reason to discontinue the line unless further troubleshooting demonstrates that it is occluded or has migrated from the artery. Moving the blood pressure cuff to the same arm will cause periodic dampening of the arterial line reading when the blood pressure cuff inflates. Injection of anything into the arterial line is generally contraindicated. Repositioning the patient's wrist and allowing a small bolus of the saline or heparin solution used to maintain patency of the system may help. (Quinn D, Schick L, editors: *ASPAN's perianesthesia nursing core curriculum: preoperative, Phase I and Phase II PACU*

nursing, Philadelphia, 2004, Saunders.)

6.22. Correct Answer: **a**
Mean arterial pressure (MAP) is an important indicator of the perfusion of both vital and nonvital organs. Generally, as hypoxia sets in, nonvital organ perfusion is sacrificed for the perfusion of vital organs. (McQuillan KA et al: *Trauma nursing: from resuscitation through rehabilitation*, ed 3, Philadelphia, 2002, Saunders; Drain C, editor: *Perianesthesia nursing: a critical care approach*, ed 4, Philadelphia, 2003, Saunders.)

6.23. Correct Answer: **c**
A central venous catheter offers the nurse many monitoring and interventional tools, but its position also needs to be verified radiographically post-placement regardless of hemodynamic readings. Pneumothorax is a complication of the central venous catheter being placed improperly and should be assessed for by CXR and listening to breath sounds. Leaving the balloon on the wedge port inflated can be extremely dangerous. Zeroing should be done directly at the phlebostatic access point, not above or below, because this can artificially raise or lower hemodynamic readings. (Intravenous Nurses Society: *Infusion nursing standards of practice*, *J Intraven Nurs* [23]:6S, 2000; Masoorli S: Legal issues related to vascular access devices and infusion therapy, *J Infus Nurs* 28:S18-21, S33-36, 2005; Quinn D, Schick L, editors: *ASPAN's perianesthesia nursing core curriculum: preoperative, Phase I and Phase II PACU nursing*, Philadelphia, 2004, Saunders.)

6.24. Correct Answer: **b**
Capnography, the measure of end-tidal carbon dioxide levels, gives an excellent view of trends and momentary views of respiratory and physiologic functioning. Increases in levels may indicate that insufficient carbon dioxide is being expired from the lungs or that overproduction is occurring (as is the case in malignant hyperthermia). Decreased levels may indicate blood loss or hypotension. (Drain C, editor: *Perianesthesia nursing: a critical care approach*, ed 4, Philadelphia, 2003, Saunders; Redmond MC: Malignant hyperthermia: perianesthesia recognition, treatment, and care, *J PeriAnesth Nurs* 16[4]:259-270, 2001.)

6.25. Correct Answer: **c**
Colored nail polish, not clear acrylic nails, will alter pulse oximetry readings. A patient with severe anemia or hypoxemia or who has dark skin may have altered oximetry readings. In this situation, having the probe on the patient's finger is superior to having it placed on the patient's ear or over their nose. (Quinn D, Schick L, editors: *ASPAN's perianesthesia nursing core curriculum: preoperative, Phase I and Phase II PACU nursing*, Philadelphia, 2004, Saunders.)

6.26. Correct Answer: **b**
In the case of patients with dark skin, readings taken from their fingernail beds are superior to those taken from their ear, so the probe should not be moved. Although it is unclear what the patient's oxygen saturation is, it is better to treat it as low than to ignore the level and continue to attempt to get a good reading. There is no indication listed for the insertion of a nasal airway. (Drain C, editor: *Perianesthesia nursing: a critical care approach*, ed 4, Philadelphia, 2003, Saunders; Quinn D, Schick L, editors: *ASPAN's perianesthesia nursing core curriculum: preoperative, Phase I and Phase II PACU*

nursing, Philadelphia, 2004, Saunders.)

6.27. Correct Answer: **a**
Pulse oximetry needs to be considered along with other assessments of the patient's oxygenation status (level of consciousness, respiratory quality and effort, skin color). A patient who is anemic may still have high SpO_2 levels but may not be adequately oxygenated. Insufficient hemoglobin, even when fully saturated, may not be able to carry sufficient oxygen to organs and tissue. The partial pressure of oxygen dissolved in the blood helps determine how well tissues and organs are oxygenated and is not related in a linear manner to the SpO_2 (which measures the other percentage of oxygen that is attached to hemoglobin). (Quinn D, Schick L, editors: *ASPAN's perianesthesia nursing core curriculum: preoperative, Phase I and Phase II PACU nursing*, Philadelphia, 2004, Saunders; Drain C, editor: *Perianesthesia nursing: a critical care approach*, ed 4, Philadelphia, 2003, Saunders; McCance KL, Huether SE: *Pathophysiology: the biologic basis for disease in adults and children*, ed 4, St. Louis, 2002, Mosby; McQuillan KA et al: *Trauma nursing: from resuscitation through rehabilitation*, ed 3, Philadelphia, 2002, Saunders.)

6.28. Correct Answer: **c**
The non-rebreather mask can deliver an FiO_2 of 80% to 95% depending on the brand. Close monitoring is required because a patient could suffocate if the oxygen tubing is kinked or if there is an alteration in oxygen delivery (e.g., if a disconnect occurs or if oxygen delivery is at insufficient levels). The remaining options offer FiO_2 delivery of Venturi mask, 24% to 55%; simple facemask, 40% to 60%; and the partial rebreather, 60% to 75%. (Quinn D, Schick L, editors: *ASPAN's perianesthesia nursing core curriculum: preoperative, Phase I and Phase II PACU nursing*, Philadelphia, 2004, Saunders; Drain C, editor: *Perianesthesia nursing: a critical care approach*, ed 4, Philadelphia, 2003, Saunders; Kozier B et al: Oxygenation. In Kozier B et al: *Fundamentals of nursing: concepts, process, and practice*, ed 7, Upper Saddle River, NJ, 2004, Pearson Education.)

6.29. Correct Answer: **a**
A Venturi mask allows for well-controlled titration of FiO_2. It can also be adapted to allow for humidification. (Drain C, editor: *Perianesthesia nursing: a critical care approach*, ed 4, Philadelphia, 2003, Saunders; Kozier B et al: Oxygenation. In Kozier B et al: *Fundamentals of nursing: concepts, process, and practice*, ed 7, Upper Saddle River, NJ, 2004, Pearson Education; Quinn D, Schick L, editors: *ASPAN's perianesthesia nursing core curriculum: preoperative, Phase I and Phase II PACU nursing*, Philadelphia, 2004, Saunders.)

6.30. Correct Answer: **d**
A rapid drop in blood pressure can indicate many things. Airway evaluation is the primary assessment that should occur in an intubated patient. Quality of respirations, oxygenation status, and evaluation of general ventilatory effort should be considered next. The evaluation of the patient's ECG for ischemia or dysrhythmia would be followed by a determination of his or her fluid status. See Cowling and Haas' hypotension algorithm for a good overview of treatment priorities. (Cowling GE et al: Hypotension in the PACU: an algorithmic approach, *J PeriAnesthes Nurs* 17[3]:159-163, 2002.)

6.31. Correct Answer: **d**
A nasopharyngeal airway is an excellent short-term solution for a patient with soft tissue airway obstruction. Because of potential for injury and damage, it is contraindicated in patients with tonsillectomy/adenoidectomy, cleft palate repair, basilar skull fracture, facial trauma that may have resulted in damage to the cranial vault, nasal septal deformity, or a coagulopathy disorder. (Drain C, editor: *Perianesthesia nursing: a critical care approach*, ed 4, Philadelphia, 2003, Saunders; McQuillan KA et al: *Trauma nursing: from resuscitation through rehabilitation*, ed 3, Philadelphia, 2002, Saunders; Quinn D, Schick L, editors: *ASPAN's perianesthesia nursing core curriculum: preoperative, Phase I and Phase II PACU nursing*, Philadelphia, 2004, Saunders.)

6.32. Correct Answer: **b**
Creation of a percutaneous tracheostomy, whether in an operating room or on an emergency basis in the PACU, carries a certain set of expected complications. These complications include subcutaneous emphysema, pneumothorax, hemorrhage, and post-placement obstruction. Many patients report feeling like they are short of breath despite adequate oxygenation, which is often because of their new "airway" that has a smaller diameter and because of anxiety. Pleural effusion is not a complication that a nurse should prepare for or anticipate in this patient population. (Drain C, editor: *Perianesthesia nursing: a critical care approach*, ed 4, Philadelphia, 2003, Saunders; Fikkers BG et al: Emphysema and pneumothorax after percutaneous tracheostomy: case reports and an anatomic study, *Chest* 125[5]:1805-1814, 2004; McQuillan KA et al: *Trauma*

nursing: from resuscitation through rehabilitation, ed 3, Philadelphia, 2002, Saunders; Woodrow P: Managing patients with a tracheostomy in acute care, *Nurs Stand* 16[44]:39-46, 2002.)

6.33. Correct Answer: **c**
Although an analysis of arterial blood gases may give a clinical view of what is occurring, the patient needs immediate airway intervention that requires immediate nursing assessment and intervention. Patients with new tracheostomies will have a large amount of secretions that require frequent suctioning. Another source of concern could be the tracheostomy tube itself. If not properly inserted or malfunctioning, it could contribute to a patient's respiratory difficulties. (Drain C, editor: *Perianesthesia nursing: a critical care approach*, ed 4, Philadelphia, 2003, Saunders; Russell C: Providing the nurse with a guide to tracheostomy care and management, *Br J Nurs* 14[8]:428-433, 2005.)

6.34. Correct Answer: **d**
The IABP device helps reduce afterload, increase cardiac output, and will increase perfusion to the coronary arteries while, as a rule, reducing the work of the heart. It is generally inserted through the femoral artery, requiring that the patient lie flat with the head of the bed only slightly elevated. It is not a requirement that patients are sedated while the pump is running. (Krau SD: Successfully weaning the intra-aortic balloon pump patient: an algorithm, *Dimen Crit Care Nurs* 18[3]:2-11, 1999; Little C: Your guide to the intra-aortic balloon pump, *Nursing* 34[12]:321-322, 2004; Quinn D, Schick L, editors: *ASPAN's perianesthesia nursing core curriculum: preoperative, Phase I and Phase II*

PACU nursing, Philadelphia, 2004, Saunders.)

6.35. Correct Answer: **c**

It is possible for the balloon and catheter to migrate upstream or downstream from where it was originally supposed to be placed (descending aorta). If it migrates downstream, it can occlude the renal arteries and decrease urine output. Upstream migration can cause occlusion of the left subclavian artery and subsequently an absent radial pulse. One of the more obvious indicators would be a change or lack of support for parameters such as cardiac output and afterload. Neither carotid bruit nor blurred vision would be assessment findings related to IABP use or functioning. (Krau SD: Successfully weaning the intra-aortic balloon pump patient: an algorithm, *Dimen Crit Care Nurs* 18[3]:2-11, 1999; Little C: Your guide to the intra-aortic balloon pump, *Nursing* 34[12]:321-322, 2004; Quinn D, Schick L, editors: *ASPAN's perianesthesia nursing core curriculum: preoperative, Phase I and Phase II PACU nursing*, Philadelphia, 2004, Saunders.)

6.36. Correct Answer: **c**

Generally, high-pressure ventilation can actually lead to hypotension for the intubated patient receiving mechanical ventilation. Multiple factors can lead to or compound hypertension including pain, anxiety, full bladder, respiratory distress, sympathetic nervous system stimulation, renal disease, and myocardial infarct. (Drain C, editor: *Peria-nesthesia nursing: a critical care approach*, ed 4, Philadelphia, 2003, Saunders; Nunnelee JD et al: Assessment and nursing management of hypertension in the perioperative period, *J PeriAnesth Nurs* 15[3]:163-168, 2000; Walker JR:

Antihypertensive agents, *J PeriAnesth Nurs* 14[5]:278-283, 1999.)

6.37. Correct Answer: **a**

A patient with respiratory distress, especially one with COPD, requires prompt and careful intervention. Intubation, though sometimes unavoidable, carries a certain set of risks and complications that can be avoided through the use of aggressive intervention in the form of CPAP or noninvasive nasal mask ventilation. Although not intended for every COPD patient, CPAP or noninvasive nasal mask ventilation can sometimes be considered instead of intubation and may succeed where simple oxygen administration modalities may fail. (Liesching T et al: Acute applications of noninvasive positive pressure ventilation, *Chest* 124[2]:699-713, 2003; Quinn D, Schick L, editors: *ASPAN's perianesthesia nursing core curriculum: preoperative, Phase I and Phase II PACU nursing*, Philadelphia, 2004, Saunders; Vanpee D et al: Effects of nasal pressure support on ventilation and inspiratory work in normocapnic and hypercapnic patients with stable COPD, *Chest* 122[1]:75-83, 2002.)

6.38. Correct Answer: **b**

The obese patient can present a complicated course of care for the perianesthesia nurse. Pharmacologic interventions need to be adjusted because of increased duration of action in highly lipid-soluble drugs. For lipophilic drugs, dosages are based on ideal weight and not on actual weight. Obese patients are at greater risk for aspiration, DVT, and failed or difficult intubation/extubation. These patients may also have many co-morbid cardiopulmonary conditions that can require close care and monitoring. (Hurst S et al: Bariatric implications of critical care nursing, *Dimens Crit Care Nurs* 23[2]:76-83, 2004; Quinn D, Schick L, editors: *ASPAN's perianesthesia nursing core curriculum: preoperative, Phase I and Phase II PACU nursing*, Philadelphia, 2004, Saunders.)

6.39. Correct Answer: **c**
Verification of correct placement of the endotracheal tube (ET) is vitally important when a patient is newly intubated or for the ongoing care of any intubated patient. Breath sounds should be auscultated and assessments should be made of the patient's overall respiratory quality. Gurgling should not be heard (which could indicate intubation of the esophagus), and humidity should be seen in the tube at intervals that are congruent with the patient's respiratory pattern. Use of a commercially available capnography device or capnography monitoring system can also be a valuable tool in evaluating ET placement. Removing the ET would be contraindicated, though pulling the tube back, under order/supervision of physician, at 1-cm intervals with reassessment in between may correct right main stem intubation. Neither giving large breaths nor albuterol therapy will correct right main stem intubation. (Barnes TA et al: AARC clinical practice guideline: management of airway emergencies, *Respir Care* 40[7]:749-760, 1995; Drain C, editor: *Perianesthesia nursing: a critical care approach*, ed 4, Philadelphia, 2003, Saunders.)

6.40. Correct Answer: **b**
Preload, the volume or pressure left in the ventricle at the end of diastole, tells the nurse about the patient's venous return and function of the right side of the heart. The CVP, RAP, and PCWP are the primary means for evaluating preload. Although SVR may influence preload, it is more often associated with, and used as an indicator of, afterload. Afterload is the resistance the heart meets when attempting to eject blood into the body's circulation. (Quinn D, Schick L, editors: *ASPAN's perianesthesia nursing core curriculum: preoperative, Phase I and Phase II PACU nursing*, Philadelphia, 2004, Saunders; Baltimore JJ: Perianesthesia care of cardiac surgery patients: a CPAN review, *J Peri-Anesth Nurs* 16[4]:246-254, 2001.)

6.41. Correct Answer: **a**
Cardiac index and cardiac output are important indicators of the heart's contractility and reflect both heart rate and stroke volume. Cardiac output is calculated by multiplying the heart rate times the stroke volume (CO = HR × SV). Cardiac index takes this value one step further by dividing it by body surface area to incorporate body size and vascular flow. Both values reflect the influence of systemic vascular resistance, and neither is a main indicator of the readiness for extubation, although they may be considered in the larger hemodynamic picture, which may influence extubation decisions. (Quinn D, Schick L, editors: *ASPAN's perianesthesia nursing core curriculum: preoperative, Phase I and Phase II PACU nursing*, Philadelphia, 2004, Saunders; Baltimore JJ: Perianesthesia care of cardiac surgery patients: a CPAN review, *J PeriAnesth Nurs* 16[4]:246-254, 2001; Drain C, editor: *Perianesthesia nursing: a critical care approach*, ed 4, Philadelphia, 2003, Saunders.)

6.42. Correct Answer: **d**
It is vital that compartment syndrome be identified early so as to prevent complications. Early signs

and symptoms include numbness, tingling, pallor, loss of sensation, and severe pain that is difficult to treat and seems out of proportion to the injury or surgery. Although pulselessness would seem like a logical early symptom, it is actually seen in the later stages of compartment syndrome. (Edwards S: Acute compartment syndrome, *Emerg Nurse* 12[3]:32-38, 2004; Quinn D, Schick L, editors: *ASPAN's perianesthesia nursing core curriculum: preoperative, Phase I and Phase II PACU nursing*, Philadelphia, 2004, Saunders; Vaillancourt C et al: Acute compartment syndrome: how long before muscle necrosis occurs? *CJEM* 6[3]:147-154, 2004.)

6.43. Correct Answer: **b**
One of the biggest complications with compartment syndrome, beyond the ischemia in the affected extremity, is the breakdown of muscle tissue, which can lead to renal failure. The laboratory results confirm this suspicion. The nurse would probably also notice dark urine and further signs of compartment syndrome if this diagnosis has not already been made. Although some of the laboratory values could be similar in cases of myocardial infarction or malignant hyperthermia, there are no other signs and symptoms to suggest these diagnoses. Hemorrhage may be the initial cause of compartment syndrome but is not the direct cause of the muscle necrosis. (Edwards S: Acute compartment syndrome, *Emerg Nurse* 12[3]:32-38, 2004; Quinn D, Schick L, editors: *ASPAN's perianesthesia nursing core curriculum: preoperative, Phase I and Phase II PACU nursing*, Philadelphia, 2004, Saunders.)

6.44. Correct Answer: **c**
A patient with diabetes may have neurovascular damage that could result in a lessened ability to recognize the early signs and symptoms of compartment syndrome as well as preexisting kidney disease. Although the other co-morbid conditions could eventually be of concern, a patient with diabetes might make early diagnosis difficult. (Edwards S: Acute compartment syndrome, *Emerg Nurse* 12[3]:32-38, 2004.)

6.45. Correct Answer: **a**
Patients with facial trauma who are having airway difficulties need to have interventions that will not cause further injury. Insertion of a nasal airway or nasal endotracheal tube has the potential to do more harm than good. If a patient could not be ventilated and progressed further to respiratory distress, oral intubation, depending on the injury and patient condition, is generally safer. Suctioning excess secretions and inserting an oral airway is the primary and safest way to intervene with this patient unless massive oral trauma would contraindicate any type of invasive airway intervention. In some cases, maxillofacial trauma is severe enough to warrant creation of a tracheostomy. (McQuillan KA et al: *Trauma nursing: from resuscitation through rehabilitation*, ed 3, Philadelphia, 2002, Saunders.)

6.46. Correct Answer: **a**
The timing of extubation can facilitate clearing of secretions and ideally prevent aspiration of oral secretions. If a patient is extubated with a cough or exhalation, his or her next respiratory activity will be inspiration. All oral contents or loose phlegm will then be inspired. By timing extubation to occur at the end of inspiration, the patient will probably cough or breathe out secretions. Having a patient "cough" the tube out can irritate

the airway and can potentially raise intrapulmonary pressures to dangerous levels. (Drain C, editor: *Perianesthesia nursing: a critical care approach*, ed 4, Philadelphia, 2003, Saunders; Quinn D, Schick L, editors: *ASPAN's perianesthesia nursing core curriculum: preoperative, Phase I and Phase II PACU nursing*, Philadelphia, 2004, Saunders.)

6.47. Correct Answer: **d**
Patients with an ICD sometimes require external defibrillation. In these cases, CPR should not be stopped while the ICD fires. The defibrillation pads or paddles should not be placed directly over the ICD because that may damage the implant and impair shock delivery. (Quinn D, Schick L, editors: *ASPAN's perianesthesia nursing core curriculum: preoperative, Phase I and Phase II PACU nursing*, Philadelphia, 2004, Saunders; Fetzer SJ: The patient with an implantable cardioverter defibrillator, *J PeriAnesthes Nurs* 18[6]:398-405, 2003.)

6.48. Correct Answer: **d**
A patient who has bradycardia accompanied by signs and symptoms such as hypotension and shortness of breath is experiencing an unsafe dysrhythmia requiring immediate intervention. Treating the bradycardia is a primary concern, but interventions for hypotension should also be initiated. These interventions include assessment for bleeding, increase in IV fluids, increase or initiation of supplemental oxygen, and potentially vasopressors and anticholinergics. (Cowling GE et al: Hypotension in the PACU: an algorithmic approach, *J PeriAnesthes Nurs* 17[3]:159-163, 2002; Drain C, editor: *Perianesthesia nursing:*

a critical care approach, ed 4, Philadelphia, 2003, Saunders.)

6.49. Correct Answer: **d**
In the case of symptomatic bradycardia, it is important to prepare/administer atropine and prepare to pace immediately. Support with vasopressors such as phenylephrine and ephedrine is also indicated. Dopamine, which will increase cardiac output and cause vasoconstriction, is generally indicated when atropine is not effective. Because pacing is part of the answer, some type of sedation, such as a mixture of fentanyl and midazolam, would be indicated. Amrinone is not generally indicated for treatment of symptomatic bradycardia. (American Heart Association: Part 6—Advanced cardiovascular life support: Section 7—Algorithm approach to ACLS emergencies, *Circulation* 102[90001]:136-165, 2000; Drain C, editor: *Perianesthesia nursing: a critical care approach*, ed 4, Philadelphia, 2003, Saunders; Quinn D, Schick L, editors: *ASPAN's perianesthesia nursing core curriculum: preoperative, Phase I and Phase II PACU nursing*, Philadelphia, 2004, Saunders.)

6.50. Correct Answer: **b**
During transcutaneous pacing, the nurse must monitor the ECG to troubleshoot any potential problems. Although all of the interventions listed with the problems are correct, failure to capture is the issue noted and can usually be remedied by simply increasing milliamp output on the device used until consistent capture is achieved. (Quinn D, Schick L, editors: *ASPAN's perianesthesia nursing core curriculum: preoperative, Phase I and Phase II PACU nursing*, Philadelphia, 2004, Saunders.)

SET 2

6.51.	a		**6.76.**	b
6.52.	c		**6.77.**	b
6.53.	b		**6.78.**	b
6.54.	d		**6.79.**	d
6.55.	d		**6.80.**	a
6.56.	d		**6.81.**	c
6.57.	b		**6.82.**	a
6.58.	a		**6.83.**	d
6.59.	c		**6.84.**	a
6.60.	d		**6.85.**	c
6.61.	b		**6.86.**	b
6.62.	a		**6.87.**	c
6.63.	c		**6.88.**	d
6.64.	b		**6.89.**	b
6.65.	a		**6.90.**	c
6.66.	b		**6.91.**	a
6.67.	c		**6.92.**	d
6.68.	b		**6.93.**	b
6.69.	b		**6.94.**	d
6.70.	d		**6.95.**	b
6.71.	c		**6.96.**	b
6.72.	c		**6.97.**	b
6.73.	c		**6.98.**	c
6.74.	a		**6.99.**	d
6.75.	b		**6.100.**	a

SET 2

6.51. Correct Answer: **a**
Tachycardia and tachypnea in the presence of rapidly rising expired carbon dioxide levels in a patient with a clenched jaw or any muscular rigidity should immediately cause the nurse to suspect malignant hyperthermia. Rises in body temperature can be a late sign. (Malignant Hyperthermia Association of the United States (MHAUS): Malignant hyperthermia: professional information center. Website: www.mhaus.org/index.cfm/fuseaction/Content.Display/PagePK/ProfessionalInfoCenter.cfm. Accessed October 21, 2005; Wedel DJ: Malignant hyperthermia. In Faust R, editor: *Anesthesiology review,* ed 3, New York, 2002, Churchill Livingstone.)

6.52. Correct Answer: **c**
It is an expected side effect for patients to occasionally experience tremors, headache, tachycardia, or nervousness during or after receiving inhaled albuterol. Neither discontinuing the medication nor warming the patient is indicated in this situation. Racemic epinephrine is generally indicated for patients with upper airway obstruction. (National Institutes of Health Medline Plus: *Bronchodilators, adrenergic.* Website: www.nlm.nih.gov/medlineplus/druginfo/uspdi/202095.html. Accessed December 21, 2005.)

6.53. Correct Answer: **b**
Post-extubation laryngeal edema is more common in children younger than 4 years and is a major reason why younger children are generally admitted at this age after adenotonsillectomy. The symptoms presented are classic for this condition. Other symptoms include use of accessory muscles, retractions, dysphonia, difficulty swallowing, tachypnea, and tachycardia. Asthma would generally present in this fashion and is easily ruled out by auscultation. Aspiration of gastric contents, a rare complication, would more likely present with wheezing and rhonchi and not with upper airway symptoms. (Lucier MM et al: Extubation of pediatric patients by PACU nurses, *J PeriAnesth Nurs* 18[2]:91-95, 2003; Quinn D, Schick L, editors: *ASPAN's perianesthesia nursing core curriculum: preoperative, Phase I and Phase II PACU nursing,* Philadelphia, 2004, Saunders; Ross AT, Kazahaya K, Tom LWC: Revisiting outpatient tonsillectomy in young children, *Otolaryngol Head Neck Surg* 128[3]:326-331, 2003.)

6.54. Correct Answer: **d**
Humidified oxygen, racemic epinephrine, reintubation, and dexamethasone all may be considered depending on the severity and accompanying vital signs. A nasal airway is contraindicated in this scenario, and a close-fitting mask will not help solve the problem and may actually make the patient more anxious. It is also important to prevent the event in the first place by avoiding intubation altogether, especially in children with an upper respiratory infection. (Lucier MM et al: Extubation of pediatric patients by PACU nurses, *J PeriAnesth Nurs* 18[2]:91-95, 2003; Quinn D, Schick L, editors: *ASPAN's perianesthesia nursing core curriculum: preoperative, Phase I and Phase II*

PACU nursing, Philadelphia, 2004, Saunders.)

6.55.

Correct Answer: **d**
A patient with a difficult airway requires careful assessment, evaluation, and preparation when the time comes for extubation. Although a normal extubation with close supervision is ideal, having the necessary emergency airway items and the skills to handle complications is still necessary. A Venturi mask, though helpful to deliver oxygen, would not be a priority item if there were difficulties after getting the patient extubated. An airway exchange catheter can allow for "extubation over a wire" allowing for easy reintubation and emergent ventilatory support if needed. A laryngeal mask airway (LMA) will sometimes be placed after endotracheal tube extubation to continue airway support but by less invasive means. A fiberoptic scope allows for pre-extubation visualization and a guided extubation if deemed safe as well as ports for medication administration. (Miller KA et al: Postoperative tracheal extubation, *Anesth Analg* 80[1]:149-172, 1995; Mort TC: Extubating the difficult airway: formulating the management strategy—use of accessory airway devices and alternative techniques may be key, *J Crit Illn* 18[5]:210-217, 2003.)

6.56.

Correct Answer: **d**
Malignant hyperthermia is characterized by rhabdomyolysis, or muscle breakdown and necrosis. As myoglobin from destroyed muscle cells is released into the bloodstream, it can lead to renal failure from tubular obstruction and ischemia. The nursing interventions specific to this aspect of malignant hyperthermia would probably include administration of mannitol and infusion of chilled IV fluids. Hypercalcemia and acidosis are common findings in patients with malignant hyperthermia and contribute to further patient deterioration. (Redmond MC: Malignant hyperthermia: perianesthesia recognition, treatment, and care, *J PeriAnesth Nurs* 16[4]:259-270, 2001; Quinn D, Schick L, editors: *ASPAN's perianesthesia nursing core curriculum preoperative, Phase I and Phase II PACU nursing*, Philadelphia, 2004, Saunders.)

6.57.

Correct Answer: **b**
There are multiple reversible causes of atrial fibrillation that should be investigated to guide therapy. The nurse is a vital part of this "detective work" and should be aware of the following that can lead to onset of atrial fibrillation: pericarditis, mitral valve disease, pulmonary embolism, sleep apnea or simple hypoxia, hyperthyroidism, high circulating catecholamines, alcohol/drug use, and multiple anti-dysrhythmic and anticholinergic drugs. Although sepsis can lead to dysrhythmia, it is not generally linked to atrial fibrillation. (Institute for Clinical Systems Improvement: *Atrial fibrillation*. Website: www.icsi.org/knowledge/detail.asp?catID=29&itemID=153. Accessed October 26, 2005; McNamara RL et al: Clinical guidelines: management of atrial fibrillation—review of the evidence for the role of pharmacologic therapy, electrical cardioversion, and echocardiography, *Ann Intern Med* 139[12]:1018-1033, 2003; Snow V et al: Clinical guidelines: management of newly detected atrial fibrillation, *Ann Intern Med* 139[12]:1009-1017,1032, 2003.)

6.58.

Correct Answer: **a**
Multiple studies on atrial fibrillation confirm the importance of anticoagulation for all patients with atrial fibrillation. Although therapeutic levels of anticoagulation are

not required for electrical cardioversion in the unstable patient with new onset atrial fibrillation, these patients generally will still receive anticoagulation of some sort during and/or after cardioversion. Transesophageal echocardiography has generally been indicated as a means of determining the risk for thromboembolic event in this patient population. Rate control is generally indicated as a priority for all patients with atrial fibrillation regardless of length of time in which the patient has been in the rhythm. (Institute for Clinical Systems Improvement: *Atrial fibrillation.* Website: www.icsi.org/knowledge/detail.asp?catID=29&itemID=153. Accessed October 26, 2005; Kellen JC: Implications for nursing care of patients with atrial fibrillation: lessons learned from the AFFIRM and RACE studies, *J Cardiovasc Nurs* 19[2]:128-137, 2004; McNamara RL et al: Clinical guidelines: management of atrial fibrillation—review of the evidence for the role of pharmacologic therapy, electrical cardioversion, and echocardiography, *Ann Intern Med* 139[12]:1018-1033,1032, 2003.)

6.59. Correct Answer: **c**
Patients with atrial fibrillation, whether it be chronic or new onset, have varying levels of signs and symptoms. Patients may complain of palpitations, dyspnea, fatigue, and chest pain. They may also feel malaise, exhibit confusion, or be completely asymptomatic. Loss of consciousness and/or seizure activity is generally not a classic sign of atrial fibrillation. (Institute for Clinical Systems Improvement: *Atrial fibrillation.* Website: www.icsi.org/knowledge/detail.asp?catID=29&itemID=153. Accessed October 26, 2005; Kellen JC: Implications for nursing care of patients with atrial fibrillation:

lessons learned from the AFFIRM and RACE studies, *J Cardiovasc Nurs* 19[2]:128-137, 2004.)

6.60. Correct Answer: **d**
A patient experiencing laryngospasm reflects a clinical emergency in which the vocal cords are partially or fully closed. Although it would be hard for the patient to breath, he or she would not be able to speak in the event of a true laryngospasm. The other items listed are more representative of bronchospasm. A patient experiencing laryngospasm may not be moving any air and therefore may not even experience stridor. In the event of partial laryngospasm, high-pitched stridor, tracheal tug, and patient anxiety/agitation are common. (Drain C, editor: *Perianesthesia nursing: a critical care approach*, ed 4, Philadelphia, 2003, Saunders; Quinn D, Schick L, editors: *ASPAN's perianesthesia nursing core curriculum: preoperative, Phase I and Phase II PACU nursing*, Philadelphia, 2004, Saunders.)

6.61. Correct Answer: **b**
Although pulmonary embolism or other cardiorespiratory event is implied here, the nurse should prioritize determination of the cause of the tachypnea, diaphoresis, and worsening oxygenation. Simply moving the patient on his or her side or giving breaths per Ambu bag will not necessarily assist in this process. Narrowing possible causes or intervention paths via chest X-ray and 12-lead ECG will help guide therapy. (Cardin T et al: Pulmonary embolism, *Crit Care Nurs Q* 27[4]:310-324, 2004; European Society of Cardiology: Guidelines on diagnosis and management of acute pulmonary embolism. Task Force on Pulmonary Embolism, *Eur Heart J* 21[16]:1301-1336, 2000; Quinn D, Schick L, editors: *ASPAN's perianesthesia nursing core curriculum: preoperative, Phase I and Phase II*

PACU nursing, Philadelphia, 2004, Saunders.)

6.62.

Correct Answer: **a**
The PACU nurse should immediately suspect inadequate reversal of muscle relaxant. Anxiolytics, especially those with amnesiac effect, can facilitate reduction of anxiety because the experience can be tremendously frightening for the patient. These drugs can also facilitate intubation, which may be necessary if airway support is insufficient to maintain adequate oxygenation. Phenobarbital or valium would be indicated if the patient were having a seizure. Narcotic and/or benzodiazepine overdose should not cause the symptoms seen in this patient. (Kervin MW: Residual neuromuscular blockade in the immediate postoperative period, *J PeriAnesth Nurs* 17[3]:152-158, 2002; Quinn D, Schick L, editors: *ASPAN's perianesthesia nursing core curriculum: preoperative, Phase I and Phase II PACU nursing*, Philadelphia, 2004, Saunders.)

6.63.

Correct Answer: **c**
Phenylephrine and ephedrine are both vasoconstrictors that are effective in treating patients with hypotension. Their effect is more venous than arterial. Phenylephrine can be administered in bolus doses (under close monitoring) or via continuous infusion depending on the care situation. Ephedrine cannot be administered indefinitely because its indirect action on norepinephrine receptor sites is limited by supply of intermediary chemical messengers. (Golembiewski JA: Vasopressors used in the critical care setting, *J PeriAnesth Nurs* 18[6]:414-416, 2003.)

6.64.

Correct Answer: **b**
Although all the answers listed are important measures of extubation readiness and determinants of neuromuscular function, the most important indicator identified in the literature is a sustained head lift. Other factors to consider include the surgical procedure that occurred, the patient's respiratory effort, and oxygenation status. (Kervin MW: Residual neuromuscular blockade in the immediate postoperative period, *J PeriAnesth Nurs* 17[3]:152-158, 2002; Miller KA et al: Postoperative tracheal extubation, *Anesth Analg* 80[1]:149-172, 1995; Quinn D, Schick L, editors: *ASPAN's perianesthesia nursing core curriculum: preoperative, Phase I and Phase II PACU nursing*, Philadelphia, 2004, Saunders.)

6.65.

Correct Answer: **a**
All these patients require special care and attention during the extubation course. Any patient undergoing neurosurgery, however, must be carefully observed because of potential for increases in intracranial pressure (ICP) that may occur with prolonged intubation or with coughing while intubated. Increased ICP as a result of inappropriate or poor extubation technique can lead to cerebral herniation and/or cerebral ischemia and edema that can be life threatening. A patient who has experienced high blood loss should not be at greater risk for complications from delayed endotracheal tube extubation. The patient who has undergone a LeFort I generally should be wide awake and able to handle his or her secretions before extubation. A patient who has had a dehisced wound could be at risk for pain or re-damaging suture lines if he or she is coughing against the endotracheal tube. (Miller KA et al: Postoperative tracheal extubation, *Anesth Analg* 80[1]:149-172, 1995; Mirski MA et al: Sedation for the critically ill neurologic patient,

Crit Care Med 23[12]:2038-2053, 1995.)

6.66. Correct Answer: **b**
A care priority in the patient after carotid endarterectomy surgery is to manage tight control of the blood pressure. Hypertension can threaten stability of the repaired vessels leading to hemorrhage and/or stroke. Nausea and vomiting can cause transient or sustained rises in blood pressure that should be promptly managed in this patient population. Tighter control of blood pressure in light of poorly controlled nausea and vomiting may eventually require a vasoactive drip. (Golembiewski JA, O'Brien D: A systematic approach to the management of postoperative nausea and vomiting, *J PeriAnesth Nurs* 17[6]:364-376, 2002; Jordan P et al: Decreasing process variation in the care of carotid endarterec-tomy patients, *Top Health Inf Manage* 22[2]:24-34, 2001; Nelson TP: Postoperative nausea and vomiting: understanding the enigma, *J PeriAnesth Nurs* 17[3]:178-189, 2002.)

6.67. Correct Answer: **c**
This patient may require immediate evacuation of a hematoma. Deviation of the trachea can threaten a patient's ability to breathe normally and should prompt immediate calls to the surgical and anesthesia teams. Crepitus can occur after this procedure and is generally self-resolving and benign if stable. (Drain C, editor: *Perianesthesia nursing: a critical care approach*, ed 4, Philadelphia, 2003, Saunders.)

6.68. Correct Answer: **b**
Review of the ACLS algorithms frequently points us back to looking for a cause for whatever rhythm might be occurring. This scenario hints at pulseless electrical activity as a result of massive blood loss

from the chest tube. A chest tube may allow for rapid blood loss if an artery was nicked during the surgical procedure. Urine output or lower extremity pulses are neither the quickest nor the most effective means of finding a cause and guiding intervention. Events such as pulmonary embolism or a massive MI may be a cause, as well as tension pneumothorax or cardiac tamponade, which might be discernible via auscultation of heart and lung sounds but might be secondary assessments. (American Heart Association: Part 6—Advanced cardiovascular life support: Section 7—Algorithm approach to ACLS emergencies, *Circulation* 102 [90001] :136-165, 2000.)

6.69. Correct Answer: **b**
The patient who has undergone a carotid endarterectomy requires a special set of focused assessments including a full neurologic assessment (motor and sensory functioning) and at a minimum should have the following cranial nerves assessed because these nerves could be injured during the surgical procedure: VII (facial), IX (glossopharyngeal), X (vagus), XI (spinal accessory), XII (hypoglossal). Blood pressure is a priority in preventing stress on delicate vascular surgical sites. (Fowler SB, Cococa R, Keller I: Patient care following carotid endarterectomy, *Medsurg Nurs* 8[1]:47-52, 1999; Kallenbach AM, Rosenblum J: Carotid endarterectomy: creating the pathway to 1-day stay, *Crit Care Nurse* 20[4]:23-26, 28-29, 31-36, 2000.)

6.70. Correct Answer: **d**
Age alone is not highly predictive of an MI after a surgical procedure, especially since no co-morbid conditions that would worsen with age are listed. Although the surgical procedure may put the patient at risk if bleeding was extensive, this

is not the case in the scenario. Patients who have had an MI at least 3 years in the past with no recurring cardiac problems have an MI risk that is equal to that of the general population. The main risk factor in this scenario is the fact that he is hypothermic. (Quinn D, Schick L, editors: *ASPAN's perianesthesia nursing core curriculum: preoperative, Phase I and Phase II PACU nursing*, Philadelphia, 2004, Saunders; Devereaux PJ et al: Perioperative cardiac events in patients undergoing noncardiac surgery: a review of the magnitude of the problem, the pathophysiology of the events and methods to estimate and communicate risk, *CMAJ* 173[6]:627-634, 2005; Drain C, editor: *Perianesthesia nursing: a critical care approach*, ed 4, Philadelphia, 2003, Saunders.)

6.71. Correct Answer: **c**
ST elevation or depression, depending on the location of the infarct, would be expected on review of a patient's 12-lead ECG. Elevated CK-MB and troponins are expected as a result of muscle breakdown. Pericardial friction rub, diaphoresis, cool and clammy skin, and/or S3/S4 heart sounds would be possible findings upon physical examination of the patient. Generally, because of the body's stress response, hyperglycemia, not hypoglycemia, would occur. (Quinn D, Schick L, editors: *ASPAN's perianesthesia nursing core curriculum: preoperative, Phase I and Phase II PACU nursing*, Philadelphia, 2004, Saunders; McCance KL, Huether SE: *Pathophysiology: the biologic basis for disease in adults and children*, ed 4, St. Louis, 2002, Mosby.)

6.72. Correct Answer: **c**
The American College of Cardiology/American Heart Association (ACC/AHA) guidelines for patients presenting with acute myocardial infarction make it easy for nurses and physicians to plan and be ready for this emergent situation. **M**orphine as an analgesic, **o**xygen therapy, **n**itrates to dilate coronary arteries, and **a**spirin complete the useful "MONA" acronym. The patient in this scenario was also hypothermic. Shivering can lead to further oxygen demand and stress on the heart. Fibrinolytics are an essential part of the reperfusion process. Intubation is neither warranted in this situation nor an implicit part of the ACC/AHA guidelines. (Connor EL et al: Detrimental effects of hypothermia: a systems analysis, *J PeriAnesth Nurs* 15[3]:151-155, 2000; Roettig ML et al: Emergency management of acute coronary syndromes, *J Emerg Nurs* 26[6 Pt 2]:1-42, 2000.)

6.73. Correct Answer: **c**
Urine output of 30 mL or less for 2 consecutive hours is a concern. Considering that these patients generally have poor vasculature to start (related to the most common cause of aneurysm, which is vascular disease), pulses obtainable only by Doppler are not uncommon but should be monitored closely. A CVP/RA reading of 3 mmHg would be indicative of a normovolemic patient. These patients generally require a great deal of fluid so this value also should be closely monitored. Poor pain control is a concern because it can lead to release of vasoconstriction hormones in the body (epinephrine, norepinephrine), which can alter coagulation processes and tissue perfusion. (Bryant C et al: Abdominal aortic aneurysm repair: a look at the first 24 hours, *J PeriAnesth Nurs* 17[3]:164-169, 2002; Drain C, editor: *Perianesthesia nursing: a critical care*

approach, ed 4, Philadelphia, 2003, Saunders.)

6.74. Correct Answer: **a**

Inflating the balloon on the end of the distal port is how a pulmonary artery wedge pressure might be measured. In general, this is **not** a part of obtaining a cardiac output reading. Aspirating the contents of the proximal port is important so that whatever is infusing in that port is not bolused into the patient. Iced or room temperature injectate is normally used for this procedure. Usually three to five injections are standard to ensure consistent results. (Gawlinski A: Protocols for practice: measuring cardiac output—intermittent bolus thermodilution method, *Crit Care Nurse* 20[2]:118-120, 122-124, 2000; Quinn D, Schick L, editors: *ASPAN's perianesthesia nursing core curriculum: preoperative, Phase I and Phase II PACU nursing*, Philadelphia, 2004, Saunders.)

6.75. Correct Answer: **b**

Dampened and abnormal waveforms after "shooting" a cardiac output require the nurse to troubleshoot for the cause. Much like any type of invasive line, an intact system is essential. Loose connections, air bubbles, and kinking can alter the readings, as can patient positioning. A flush solution at 300 mmHg must be maintained. Verifying that other parts of the central line, such as the balloon on the distal port, are not altering readings can be helpful in problem solving. Additionally, since patient positioning can affect results, patients should be repositioned onto their side as a part of troubleshooting. (Gawlinski A: Protocols for practice: measuring cardiac output—intermittent bolus thermodilution method, *Crit Care Nurse* 20[2]:118-120, 122-124, 2000; Quinn D, Schick L, editors: *ASPAN's perianesthesia nursing*

core curriculum: preoperative, Phase I and Phase II PACU nursing, Philadelphia, 2004, Saunders.)

6.76. Correct Answer: **b**

An ejection fraction (EF) of less than 40% (normal is 60%-75%) is indicative of some type of ventricular failure and/or congestive heart failure. NSAIDs can interfere with the important effect that ACE inhibitors have in this patient population and may lead to fluid overload. A low EF can cause an increasing mix of oxygenated and unoxygenated blood, which can affect oxygenation. A patient with shortness of breath, crackles, and/or S3/S4 heart sounds is most likely fluid overloaded and/or in the midst of an exacerbation of his or her CHF and should be treated accordingly. A cough is a known side effect of ACE inhibitors, but it should not be accompanied by shortness of breath. (Gilmore JC: Heart failure and treatment: part I, *J PeriAnesth Nurs* 18[2]:83-90, 2003; Gilmore JC: Heart failure and treatment: part II. Perianesthesia management, *J PeriAnesth Nurs* 18[4]:242-246, 2003; McCance KL, Huether SE: *Pathophysiology: the biologic basis for disease in adults and children*, ed 4, St. Louis, 2002, Mosby.)

6.77. Correct Answer: **b**

Cricothyrotomy is generally considered only as a last resort or when other means of ventilation have been exhausted. A Combitube may be an effective means of securing a difficult airway if respiratory distress would occur in this patient. A large-bore oral airway could make matters worse and would not help much in this scenario. A fiberoptic bronchoscope can be an excellent tool for facilitating safe extubation in the patient with a known difficult airway. (Mort TC: Extubating the difficult airway: formulating the management strategy—use of accessory airway devices and alternative techniques may be key, *J Crit Illn* 18[5]:210-217, 2003; Ovassapian A: Management of the difficult airway, *Curr Rev PeriAnesth Nurs* 24[18]:211-216, 2002; Quinn D, Schick L, editors: *ASPAN's perianesthesia nursing core curriculum: preoperative, Phase I and Phase II PACU nursing*, Philadelphia, 2004, Saunders.)

6.78. Correct Answer: **b**
Hyperventilation has been indicated as a short-term means of decreasing intracranial pressure by allowing for hypocarbia, which causes cerebral vasoconstriction. Generally, acid-base imbalances are treated through other modalities. Blood pressure is generally tightly controlled pharmacologically in these types of patients as a means of maintaining mean arterial pressure and cerebral perfusion pressures within safe parameters. (LeJeune GM et al: Nursing assessment and management of patients with head injuries, *Dimens Crit Care Nurs* 21[6]:226-231, 2002; Letvak S et al: Postanesthesia care of the patient suffering from traumatic brain injury, *J PeriAnesth Nurs* 18[6]:380-385, 406-413, 2003; McQuillan KA et al: *Trauma nursing: from resuscitation through rehabilitation*, ed 3, Philadelphia, 2002, Saunders; Nolan S: Traumatic brain injury: a review, *Crit Care Nurs Q* 28[2]:188-194, 2005; Quinn D, Schick L, editors: *ASPAN's perianesthesia nursing core curriculum: preoperative, Phase I and Phase II PACU nursing*, Philadelphia, 2004, Saunders.)

6.79. Correct Answer: **d**
Patients with traumatic brain injury require intensive neurologic and cardiopulmonary management and assessment. Thorough neurologic evaluation should include pupil checks, cranial nerve assessment, Glasgow Coma Scale scoring, and potentially an external ICP/CPP monitoring device. Sedation may be necessary both as a means of keeping ICP low and of promoting hemodynamic stability. Frequent suctioning can cause elevations in ICP and should be done sparingly. (LeJeune GM et al: Nursing assessment and management of patients with head injuries, *Dimens Crit Care Nurs* 21[6]:226-231, 2002; Letvak S et al: Postanesthesia care of the patient suffering from traumatic brain injury, *J PeriAnesth Nurs* 18[6]:380-385,406-413, 2003; McQuillan KA et al: *Trauma nursing: from resuscitation through rehabilitation*, ed 3, Philadelphia, 2002, Saunders; Nolan S: Traumatic brain injury: a review, *Crit Care Nurs Q* 28[2]:188-194, 2005; Quinn D, Schick L, editors: *ASPAN's perianesthesia nursing core curriculum: preoperative, Phase I and Phase II PACU nursing*, Philadelphia, 2004, Saunders.)

6.80. Correct Answer: **a**
Cerebral perfusion pressure (CPP) is an important variable in the care of a patient with traumatic brain injury and a patient with head injury and in neurosurgical patients. It is calculated by subtracting the mean arterial pressure (MAP) from the intracranial pressure (ICP). A normal CPP is 70 to 100 mmHg. Elevating CPP has no proven benefits and can actually be harmful to the patient. Measurement of CPP and ICP requires an invasive device. (LeJeune GM et al: Nursing assessment and management of patients with head injuries, *Dimens Crit Care Nurs* 21[6]:226-231, 2002; Letvak S et al: Postanesthesia care of the patient suffering from traumatic brain injury, *J PeriAnesth Nurs* 18[6]:380-385, 406-413, 2003;

McQuillan KA et al: *Trauma nursing: from resuscitation through rehabilitation*, ed 3, Philadelphia, 2002, Saunders; Nolan S: Traumatic brain injury: a review, *Crit Care Nurs Q* 28[2]:188-194, 2005; Quinn D, Schick L, editors: *ASPAN's perianesthesia nursing core curriculum: preoperative, Phase I and Phase II PACU nursing*, Philadelphia, 2004, Saunders.)

6.81. Correct Answer: **c**
The changes seen in the vital signs are called *Cushing's Triad* and are a classic sign of increasing intracranial pressure that needs to be treated immediately. The Cushing's Triad includes hypertension, irregular respirations and bradycardia. Narcotics are contraindicated because they can blunt awareness and prevent accurate neurologic checks. Turning the patient may agitate his condition further and is not indicated as a treatment for increasing ICP. Hyperventilation can blow off CO_2, causing hypocarbia and cerebral vasoconstriction that may reduce ICP. Raising the head of the bed can lead to further elevation of ICP and should be avoided in this situation. (Cook N: Respiratory care in spinal cord injury with associated traumatic brain injury: bridging the gap in critical care nursing interventions, *Intensive Crit Care Nurs* 19[3]:143-153, 2003; LeJeune GM et al: Nursing assessment and management of patients with head injuries, *Dimens Crit Care Nurs* 21[6]:226-231, 2002; Letvak S et al: Postanesthesia care of the patient suffering from traumatic brain injury, *J PeriAnesth Nurs* 18[6]: 380-385, 406-413, 2003; McQuillan KA et al: *Trauma nursing: from resuscitation through rehabilitation*, ed 3, Philadelphia, 2002, Saunders; Nolan S: Traumatic brain injury: a review, *Crit Care Nurs Q* 28[2]:188-194, 2005; Quinn D, Schick L,

editors: *ASPAN's perianesthesia nursing core curriculum: preoperative, Phase I and Phase II PACU nursing*, Philadelphia, 2004, Saunders.)

6.82. Correct Answer: **a**
A patient who is being treated for atelectasis can benefit greatly from either positive end-expiratory pressure (PEEP) and/or continuous positive airway pressure (CPAP). Generally, CPAP is reserved for patients who are breathing spontaneously. Increasing the FiO_2 will not improve atelectasis but will increase the percent of oxygen being delivered. A tidal volume of 800 mL is generally far too high for prolonged periods and should be based on the patient's weight (usually 6-8 mL/kg, which would be 600-800 mL in this patient). The I:E ratio for a normal person is 1:2. A long inspiratory time such as a ratio of 4:1 could lead to lung damage and altered cardiovascular functioning. (Drain C, editor: *Perianesthesia nursing: a critical care approach*, ed 4, Philadelphia, 2003, Saunders; Quinn D, Schick L, editors: *ASPAN's perianesthesia nursing core curriculum: preoperative, Phase I and Phase II PACU nursing*, Philadelphia, 2004, Saunders; Spritzer CJ: Unraveling the mysteries of mechanical ventilation: a helpful step-by-step guide, *J Emerg Nurs* 29[1]:29-36, 87-92, 2003.)

6.83. Correct Answer: **d**
There can be multiple causes for a high-pressure alarm, many of which require immediate nursing assessment and intervention. In this scenario, the patient might be biting on the tube or fighting the ventilator-administered breaths or the tube could have migrated or the patient could be coughing. Bronchospasm, pneumothorax, and other respiratory conditions may

also cause this alarm. Tubing air leaks and apnea usually cause low-pressure alarms (though kinked tubing can cause a high-pressure alarm). Lowering the pressure support setting would not solve the root of the problem. Placing a bite block would be the best answer in this scenario. (Drain C, editor: *Perianesthesia nursing: a critical care approach*, ed 4, Philadelphia, 2003, Saunders; Quinn D, Schick L, editors: *ASPAN's perianesthesia nursing core curriculum: preoperative, Phase I and Phase II PACU nursing*, Philadelphia, 2004, Saunders; Spritzer CJ: Unraveling the mysteries of mechanical ventilation: a helpful step-by-step guide, *J Emerg Nurs* 29[1]:29-36, 87-92, 2003.)

6.84. Correct Answer: **a**
A sustained head lift for longer than 5 seconds, tongue protrusion for longer than 5 seconds, and tidal volumes of 5 mL/kg are all excellent indicators of adequate reversal of neuromuscular blockade. Also included in this list are a strong cough, strong hand squeeze for longer than 5 seconds, as well as meeting other similar criteria of extubation readiness. Train-of-four measurement with peripheral nerve stimulator showing four strong twitches (which still could indicate 70% blockade of acetylcholine receptors) would be the acceptable level at which residual neuromuscular blockage might be ruled out as a cause of the problem in this scenario. (Drain C, editor: *Perianesthesia nursing: a critical care approach*, ed 4, Philadelphia, 2003, Saunders; Kervin MW: Residual neuromuscular blockade in the immediate postoperative period, *J PeriAnesth Nurs* 17[3]:152-158, 2002; Quinn D, Schick L, editors: *ASPAN's perianesthesia nursing core curriculum: preoperative, Phase I and Phase II*

PACU nursing, Philadelphia, 2004, Saunders.)

6.85. Correct Answer: **c**
The PACU nurse should know that this patient is at risk for aspiration because of an inability to handle his or her own secretions, dysphagia, and impaired cough. The patient would be too weak to pull out the tube or cause his or her own extubation or to cough heavily enough on the tube to cause pulmonary edema. Cor pulmonale would generally not be associated with this condition. The nurse would closely monitor the patient, be aggressive with suctioning, elevate the head of the bed, and provide anti-emetics or anxiolytics if prescribed and appropriate. (Drain C, editor: *Perianesthesia nursing: a critical care approach*, ed 4, Philadelphia, 2003, Saunders; Kervin MW: Residual neuromuscular blockade in the immediate postoperative period, *J PeriAnesth Nurs* 17[3]:152-158, 2002; Quinn D, Schick L, editors: *ASPAN's perianesthesia nursing core curriculum: preoperative, Phase I and Phase II PACU nursing*, Philadelphia, 2004, Saunders.)

6.86. Correct Answer: **b**
Recent research places emphasis on control of the source of sepsis as a primary means of reducing mortality. Antibiotic administration is a high enough priority that it is recommended that it occurs within the first hour of identification of severe sepsis. It is recommended that a central line is placed within the first 6 hours of diagnosis. Placement of the arterial line and placement of a urinary catheter might be more efficiently accomplished in the OR setting and are lower priorities than the antibiotics. (Dellinger RP et al: Surviving Sepsis Campaign guidelines for management of severe sepsis and septic shock, *Crit Care Med*

32[3]:858-873, 2004; Kleinpell RM: Working out the complexities of severe sepsis, *Nurse Pract* 30[4]:43-44, 46-48, 2005.)

6.87. Correct Answer: **c**
Steroids, especially in high doses, are contraindicated in sepsis if shock is not present. Sepsis alone is not indication enough for steroids, and they may actually do more harm than benefit. Light sedation would probably be insufficient to promote hemodynamic stability, ventilator synchrony, and greater tolerance of the stress and care required in this situation. Recent research has indicated that intermittent "wake-ups" can promote positive outcomes in ventilated patients requiring heavy sedation. Deep vein thrombus has been consistently identified as a concern in patients facing sepsis, not only because of prolonged bedrest and immobility but also because of coagulopathies that can occur. High-pressure ventilation has been linked to lung trauma and should be avoided. (Dellinger RP et al: Surviving Sepsis Campaign guidelines for management of severe sepsis and septic shock, *Crit Care Med* 32[3]:858-873, 2004; Noble KA: Inflammation II: sepsis, *J PeriAnesth Nurs* 20[2]:135-140, 2005; Schweickert WD et al: Daily interruption of sedative infusions and complications of critical illness in mechanically ventilated patients, *Crit Care Med* 32[6]:1272-1276, 2004; Wheeler AP et al: Treating patients with severe sepsis, *N Engl J Med* 340[3]:207-214, 1999.)

6.88. Correct Answer: **d**
A patient who is hypovolemic may be at risk for tachycardia and life-threatening dysrhythmias when a dopamine infusion is running or initiated. At high doses, there is increasing demand on the heart, as well as myocardial oxygen consumption. Treating hypovolemia and careful observation of the patient's vital signs and ECG become even more important. If dopamine infiltrates, it is tremendously caustic to the subcutaneous tissue and must be recognized and treated immediately. Dopamine is generally run centrally for this reason. (Dellinger RP et al: Surviving Sepsis Campaign guidelines for management of severe sepsis and septic shock, *Crit Care Med* 32[3]:858-873, 2004; Quinn D, Schick L, editors: *ASPAN's perianesthesia nursing core curriculum: preoperative, Phase I and Phase II PACU nursing*, Philadelphia, 2004, Saunders; Wheeler AP et al: Treating patients with severe sepsis, *N Engl J Med* 340[3]:207-214, 1999.)

6.89. Correct Answer: **b**
ARDS appears frequently with sepsis. It is important to consider the full clinical picture and to treat whatever acid-base imbalance that is accompanying the ARDS. There are multiple treatments and considerations when this is the case. Permissive hypercapnia is sometimes used as a means of reducing the risk of lung damage, and altered hemodynamics is often considered but only when it will not cause further harm to the patient as it would in the case of metabolic acidosis. To correct metabolic acidosis, sodium bicarbonate and insulin are frequently administered. Plasmapheresis is not indicated in this scenario. (Dellinger RP et al: Surviving Sepsis Campaign guidelines for management of severe sepsis and septic shock, *Crit Care Med* 32[3]:858-873, 2004; Kane C et al: Adult respiratory distress syndrome, *Crit Care Nurs Q* 27[4]: 325-335, 2004; Kleinpell RM: Working out the complexities of severe sepsis, *Nurse Pract* 30[4]: 43-44, 46-48, 2005; Wheeler AP et al: Treating patients with severe

sepsis, *N Engl J Med* 340[3]:207-214, 1999.)

6.90. Correct Answer: **c**
Patients who take nitroglycerin for a long period may see a tolerance develop that can alter therapy and efficacy. Nitrates actually have both a vasodilatory and antithrombic/antiplatelet effect, not a vasoconstrictive effect. Side effects include bradycardia, hypotension, and headaches. (National Institutes of Medicine Medline Plus: *Nitrates.* Website: www.nlm.nih.gov/medline-plus/druginfo/uspdi/202411.html. Accessed November 14, 2005; Quinn D, Schick L, editors: *ASPAN's perianesthesia nursing core curriculum: preoperative, Phase I and Phase II PACU nursing*, Philadelphia, 2004, Saunders.)

6.91. Correct Answer: **a**
It is important to consider that during inspiration, a patient's intrathoracic pressure is less than atmospheric pressure. If the cap is off of a central line, air will be pulled down into the catheter and result in an air embolism. By clamping the line and/or having the patient bear down, this potentially life-threatening complication can be avoided. When working with any central lines, all entry points and connections should be treated as sterile to prevent infection and sepsis. KVO fluids are not required as long as flushing protocols are followed and tunneled lines with Dacron or other internal cuffs do not require a dressing. (Dougherty L: Reducing the risk of complications in IV therapy, *Nurs Stand* 12[5]:40-42, 1997; Intravenous Nurses Society: Infusion nursing standards of practice, *J Intraven Nurs* [23]:6S, 2000; Masoorli S: Managing complications of central venous access devices, *Nursing* 27[8]:59-64, 1997.)

6.92. Correct Answer: **d**
In this scenario, the nurse should suspect that the patient might be experiencing an episode of autonomic dysreflexia. Bowel distention and "scope" procedures can put a patient with a spinal cord injury at risk for this complication postoperatively. Other signs and symptoms of autonomic dysreflexia include profuse sweating, pallor, stroke, seizures, cardiac arrest, headache, and severe acute hypertension. Raising the head of the bed, loosening restrictive closing, and administering oxygen will help with both the hypoxia associated with seizures and the dysreflexia episode. Epinephrine is not indicated here and may actually worsen the situation because of its sympathetic effects. (Quinn D, Schick L, editors: *ASPAN's perianesthesia nursing core curriculum: preoperative, Phase I and Phase II PACU nursing*, Philadelphia, 2004, Saunders; Blackmer J: Rehabilitation medicine: 1. Autonomic dysreflexia, *CMAJ* 169[9]: 931-935, 2003.)

6.93. Correct Answer: **b**
Nitroprusside provides rapid and titratable management of hypertension via reduction in both preload and afterload. Nitroprusside's metabolites can cause toxicity in patients only after prolonged use but not after just a few hours. Although antihypertensives are important, a complete bowel and bladder assessment may determine the actual cause of the dysreflexia in the first place. Nitroprusside does not generally cause altered sensorium nor is it associated with refractory hypertension unless the infusion is abruptly stopped. (Quinn D, Schick L, editors: *ASPAN's perianesthesia nursing core curriculum: preoperative, Phase I and Phase II PACU nursing*, Philadelphia, 2004, Saunders;

Blackmer J: Rehabilitation medicine: 1. Autonomic dysreflexia, *CMAJ* 169[9]:931-935, 2003.)

6.94. Correct Answer: **d**
Both CPAP and BiPAP deliver PEEP to a patient. BiPAP confers the added benefit of also providing pressure support and timed breaths. These added features make BiPAP the noninvasive equivalent to having a patient on a ventilator. BiPAP is often considered for patients who are not tolerating CPAP (CPAP delivers a constant pressure rather than reacting to the pressure changes of inhalation and exhalation). (Cross AM et al: Non-invasive ventilation in acute respiratory failure: a randomized comparison of continuous positive airway pressure and bi-level positive airway pressure, *Emerg Med J* 20[6]:531-534, 2003; Vanpee D et al: Effects of nasal pressure support on ventilation and inspiratory work in normocapnic and hypercapnic patients with stable COPD, *Chest* 122[1]:75-83, 2002.)

6.95. Correct Answer: **b**
Third-degree AV block is considered a lethal rhythm that presents in patients who have a history of cardiac disease or who are taking cardiac medications (digoxin, calcium channel blockers, beta blockers, and/or amiodarone). The patient may be dizzy or have a syncopal episode and the patient can quickly become hemodynamically unstable. On the ECG, the nurse should verify that there is no correlation between the P waves and the QRS cycles that are driven by an escape rhythm. Transcutaneous pacing and eventual placement of a permanent pacemaker are the mainstays of therapy for this rhythm and the main way to return the patient to a stable state. Atropine is usually not administered or administered cautiously until a myocardial infarction is first ruled out. (American Heart Association: Part 6—Advanced cardiovascular life support: Section 7—Algorithm approach to ACLS emergencies, *Circulation* 102[90001]:136-165, 2000; Paul S: ECGs and pacemakers: understanding advanced concepts in atrioventricular block, *Crit Care Nurse* 21[1]:56-68, 2001.)

6.96. Correct Answer: **b**
The nurse should not take blood pressures, give injections, or place IVs in the arm with an arteriovenous (AV) fistula, nor should he or she wrap dressings circumferentially around that arm. Verification of a bruit through both auscultation and palpation is an important part of the basic assessment of the fistula. (Quinn D, Schick L, editors: *ASPAN's perianesthesia nursing core curriculum: preoperative, Phase I and Phase II PACU nursing*, Philadelphia, 2004, Saunders; Ignatavius DD et al: *Medical-surgical nursing: critical thinking for collaborative care*, ed 4, Philadelphia, 2002, Saunders.)

6.97. Correct Answer: **b**
ACE inhibitors disrupt a vital step in the renin-angiotensin pathway. Renin, an enzyme, breaks apart angiotensinogen to form angiotensin I. Angiotensin I is converted to angiotensin II, a vasoconstrictive agent, by the angiotensin-converting enzyme (ACE). When this process is blocked, blood pressure will drop through dilation of vessels in the absence of angiotensin II. The improved survival rates in patient with hypertension and congestive heart failure and the endothelial and inflammatory mediator effects of these drugs are proving them to be valuable clinical tools. (Dzau VJ et al: A symposium: the relevance of tissue angiotensin-converting enzyme—manifestations in mechanistic and endpoint data, *Am J Cardiol* 88(9A):120-120L, 2001; McCance

KL, Huether SE: *Pathophysiology: the biologic basis for disease in adults and children*, ed 4, St. Louis, 2002, Mosby; Quinn D, Schick L, editors: *ASPAN's perianesthesia nursing core curriculum: preoperative, Phase I and Phase II PACU nursing*, Philadelphia, 2004, Saunders.)

6.98. Correct Answer: **c**
A decline in renal function pointing to renal failure can be the result of multiple factors that may be exacerbated by the surgical procedure or its complications. High blood loss is one way in which renal perfusion may be altered. Administering Lasix may exacerbate low fluid volumes and is generally recommended in this situation only if there is elevated potassium and/or congestive heart failure. Because potassium levels may already be elevated, determining serum potassium first would be important. Contrast dye and NSAIDs could further harm the kidneys and should be avoided. Requesting for cancellation or delay of the CT (which is a non-emergent test) and consulting about whether the contrast dye is safe is the best option. Renal-dose dopamine has been shown to be ineffective in decreasing renal dysfunction or associated mortality. (Agodoa L: Acute renal failure in the PACU, *J PeriAnesth Nurs* 17[6]:377-383, 2002; Agrawal M et al: Acute renal failure, *Am Fam Physician* 61(7):2077-2088, 2000; Friedrich JO et al: Meta-analysis: low-dose dopamine increases urine output but does not prevent renal dysfunction or death, *Ann Intern Med* 142[7]:510-524, 2005.)

6.99. Correct Answer: **d**
Endovascular procedures continue to increase in frequency and often present patients with a shorter-stay remedy to severe medical problems. Care of endovascular sites and sheaths requires basic assessments

of pulses, vital signs, and monitoring for complications. Complications include hematoma, pseudoaneurysm, AV fistula, retroperitoneal hematoma, and arterial occlusion. Neuropathy, pain at the insertion site with activity, change in thigh girth, altered vital signs, and changes in pulses should signal to the nurse that one of these complications may be occurring. Flushing the sheath would not determine the cause or act as an intervention. (Davis C et al: Vascular complications of coronary interventions, *Heart Lung* 26[2]:118-127, 1997; Hall SW: Home study program: endovascular repair of abdominal aortic aneurysms, *AORN J* 77[3]:630-642, 645-648, 2003.)

6.100. Correct Answer: **a**
Patients who have a sheath in place are generally required to lie flat or to be on extended bedrest to allow the site to heal. Neurologic/neurovascular checks are essential because of both the neurologic and neurovascular aspects of this procedure. Application of TED stockings and a sequential compression device are standard postoperative orders, and there is no contraindication in this case. Many of these patients, if hemodynamically stable, will not require intensive care and will generally not need the arterial lines. (Davis C et al: Vascular complications of coronary interventions, *Heart Lung* 26[2]:118-127, 1997; Hall SW: Home study program: endovascular repair of abdominal aortic aneurysms, *AORN J* 77[3]:630-642,645-648, 2003; Ignatavius DD et al: *Medical-surgical nursing: critical thinking for collaborative care*, ed 4, Philadelphia, 2002, Saunders; Quinn D, Schick L, editors: *ASPAN's perianesthesia nursing core curriculum: preoperative, Phase I and Phase II PACU nursing*, Philadelphia, 2004, Saunders.)

SET 3

	ANSWER KEY		

6.101.	c	**6.126.**	a
6.102.	a	**6.127.**	b
6.103.	d	**6.128.**	a
6.104.	a	**6.129.**	c
6.105.	c	**6.130.**	d
6.106.	d	**6.131.**	d
6.107.	c	**6.132.**	b
6.108.	d	**6.133.**	a
6.109.	b	**6.134.**	a
6.110.	d	**6.135.**	c
6.111.	a	**6.136.**	b
6.112.	d	**6.137.**	d
6.113.	c	**6.138.**	d
6.114.	d	**6.139.**	a
6.115.	c	**6.140.**	c
6.116.	a	**6.141.**	c
6.117.	b	**6.142.**	b
6.118.	a	**6.143.**	d
6.119.	d	**6.144.**	c
6.120.	c	**6.145.**	b
6.121.	c	**6.146.**	a
6.122.	b	**6.147.**	c
6.123.	c	**6.148.**	a
6.124.	a	**6.149.**	b
6.125.	c	**6.150.**	b

SET 3

6.101. Correct Answer: **c**

DVT is a common but preventable postoperative complication that manifests with pain, swelling, edema, or with no symptoms at all. Virchow's Triad explains the three main categories of risk factors (venotrauma, venous stasis, and hypercoagulability). The four risk factors specific to this patient include obesity, orthopedic procedure, surgery longer than 45 minutes, and a history of DVT. Other risk factors include smoking, age, malignancy, oral contraceptives, peripheral vascular disease, and dehydration to name a few. (Aquila AM: Deep venous thrombosis, *J Cardiovasc Nurs* 15[4]:25-44, 2001; Day MW: Recognizing and managing DVT: deep vein thrombosis, *Nursing* 33[5]:36-42, 2003; Quinn D, Schick L, editors: *ASPAN's perianesthesia nursing core curriculum: preoperative, Phase I and Phase II PACU nursing*, Philadelphia, 2004, Saunders.)

6.102. Correct Answer: **a**

The mainstay treatment for DVT is anticoagulation. Although there is debate about how long a patient should be on bedrest with a known DVT, generally, patients are not asked to ambulate immediately. Massaging the site of a DVT is contraindicated, and, generally, application of heat and leg elevation are recommended. The nurse may also administer analgesics and closely monitor PT/INR values once anticoagulation therapy has been initiated. (Aquila AM: Deep venous thrombosis, *J Cardiovasc Nurs* 15[4]:25-44, 2001; Day MW: Recognizing and managing DVT: deep vein thrombosis, *Nursing* 33[5]:36-42, 2003; Quinn D, Schick L, editors:

ASPAN's perianesthesia nursing core curriculum: preoperative, Phase I and Phase II PACU nursing, Philadelphia, 2004, Saunders.)

6.103. Correct Answer: **d**

In this scenario, the patient appears to be fluid overloaded, which is being exacerbated by the multiple blood transfusions. Although suctioning the patient might be a temporary fix, it will not treat the underlying problem. A chest X-ray will help determine the cause and elucidate the extent, but again, does not treat the patient's immediate symptoms. The blood infusion probably should be stopped, the IV site kept KVO with normal saline, and supportive measures initiated. Answer **d** is the best choice because it treats the immediate issues and includes an intervention that may eliminate one of the causes of the pulmonary edema. (Drain C, editor: *Perianesthesia nursing: a critical care approach*, ed 4, Philadelphia, 2003, Saunders; Quinn D, Schick L, editors: *ASPAN's perianesthesia nursing core curriculum: preoperative, Phase I and Phase II PACU nursing*, Philadelphia, 2004, Saunders.)

6.104. Correct Answer: **a**

The patient is dealing with ventilation and not oxygenation issues. The respiratory acidosis is probably a result of inadequate respiratory rate, which could be easily resolved by increasing it. The ABGs reveal that the patient's FiO_2 does not need to be adjusted, and a tidal volume of 6 to 8 mL/kg is recommended and would also not need to be adjusted in this scenario. Increasing PEEP is unnecessary, and if it were, it is recommended that it be increased by 2- to 3-cm intervals with close monitoring for hemodynamic effect. (Drain C, editor: *Perianesthesia nursing: a critical care approach*, ed 4, Philadelphia, 2003, Saunders; Quinn D, Schick L, editors: *ASPAN's perianesthesia nursing core curriculum: preoperative, Phase I and Phase II PACU nursing*, Philadelphia, 2004, Saunders; Spritzer CJ: Unraveling the mysteries of mechanical ventilation: a helpful step-by-step guide, *J Emerg Nurs* 29[1]:29-36, 87-92, 2003.)

6.105.   Correct Answer: **c**
Knowledge of lung anatomy explains many postoperative pulmonary complications. The right bronchus is larger and has less of an angle toward the lung and therefore is the more common site of aspiration, receives greater ventilation, and is commonly where an endotracheal tube may end up if it is placed too far into the trachea. (Quinn D, Schick L, editors: *ASPAN's perianesthesia nursing core curriculum: preoperative, Phase I and Phase II PACU nursing*, Philadelphia, 2004, Saunders; National Institutes of Health Medline Plus: *Bronchial anatomy*. Website: www.vh.org/adult/provider/radiology/LungAnatomy/BronchAnatomy/BronchAnat.html. Accessed December 1, 2005.)

6.106.   Correct Answer: **d**
After free-flap reconstruction, a white to light-gray coloration of the flap site is normal in the immediate postoperative period as long as this coloration does not persist. Low continuous suction is the norm for these patients, which can be accomplished with a Jackson-Pratt drain. Subcutaneous heparin or other anticoagulants can help prevent occlusion of the vasculature of the flap. A patient who is hypothermic is generally vasoconstricted, which puts him or her at risk for a lack of perfusion to the new flap. A patient with this body temperature would require immediate intervention. (Black SB et al: Repair and care of chest wall defects, *Plast Surg Nurs* 21[1]:13-21, 2001; Drain C, editor: *Perianesthesia nursing: a critical care approach*, ed 4, Philadelphia, 2003, Saunders; Haskins N: Intensive nursing care of patients with a microvascular free flap after maxillofacial surgery, *Intensive Crit Care Nurs* 14[5]:225-230, 1998; Quinn D, Schick L, editors: *ASPAN's perianesthesia nursing core curriculum: preoperative, Phase I and Phase II PACU nursing*, Philadelphia, 2004, Saunders.)

6.107.   Correct Answer: **c**
It is important to keep tension to a minimum on the wound bed and surgical site. It is also important that positioning limit pressure on the wound bed as well. Patients should not rest on their operative side, and if a patient absolutely cannot tolerate a supine position, special beds or bed coverings may be needed to avoid altering perfusion to the flap. Adjusting the head of bed and administering ordered analgesics are the best options. (Black SB et al: Repair and care of chest wall defects, *Plast Surg Nurs* 21[1]:13-21, 2001; Drain C, editor: *Perianesthesia nursing: a critical care approach*, ed 4, Philadelphia, 2003, Saunders; Haskins N: Intensive nursing care of patients with a microvascular free flap after maxillofacial surgery, *Intensive Crit Care Nurs* 14[5]:225-230, 1998; Quinn D, Schick L, editors: *ASPAN's perianesthesia nursing core curriculum: preoperative, Phase I and Phase II PACU nursing*, Philadelphia, 2004, Saunders.)

6.108. Correct Answer: **d**
The two main complications that can threaten the viability of flap tissue relate to arterial insufficiency and venous congestion. The speed of capillary refill can differentiate these two conditions as can the color of the skin at the flap site. Generally, arterial insufficiency will result in capillary refill longer than 3 seconds and a flap that becomes increasingly pale. Venous congestion will result in rapid capillary refill and a flap site that is purple or blue and may ooze dark blood. A warm flap with pulses that can be heard by Doppler is a normal finding. (Black SB et al: Repair and care of chest wall defects, *Plast Surg Nurs* 21[1]:13-21, 2001; Drain C, editor: *Perianesthesia nursing: a critical care approach*, ed 4, Philadelphia, 2003, Saunders; Haskins N: Intensive nursing care of patients with a microvascular free flap after maxillofacial surgery, *Intensive Crit Care Nurs* 14[5]:225-230, 1998; Quinn D, Schick L, editors: *ASPAN's perianesthesia nursing core curriculum: preoperative, Phase I and Phase II PACU nursing*, Philadelphia, 2004, Saunders.)

6.109. Correct Answer: **b**
Chest tube placement is important for drainage of air and fluid from the thoracic cavity. Because air rises, placement of the chest tube higher up will remove air. The removal of fluid or blood requires placement of a chest tube between the sixth and eighth intercostal space. Mediastinal chest tubes are generally placed for postoperative drainage after open heart surgery. (Drain C, editor: *Perianesthesia nursing: a critical care approach*, ed 4, Philadelphia, 2003, Saunders; Goss JF: Complexities of blunt chest trauma: prehospital assessment and management of rib fractures, flail chest, pulmonary contusions, pneumothorax, hemothorax, traumatic asphyxia & diaphragmatic rupture, *JEMS* 29[11]:44-46, 48-57, 2004.)

6.110. Correct Answer: **d**
Commercially available chest tube drainage systems generally have three sections, chambers, or columns. A collection chamber allows for collection of actual fluid that comes from the chest cavity for recording and sometimes for re-infusion. A water seal chamber is the one-way pressurizing seal that allows air out but not in. Bubbling in the water seal chamber indicates an air leak somewhere from the patient through to the device. Tidaling, or the up-and-down movement of the fluid in the water seal chamber, is an expected finding that correlates with respiration. The final chamber is the suction chamber that creates a "pull" or negative pressure that works to remove air and fluid. Bubbling in this chamber is created by "wall suction," which helps maintain the negative pressure. Wall suction does not directly pull air or fluid. (Quinn D, Schick L, editors: *ASPAN's perianesthesia nursing core curriculum: preoperative, Phase I and Phase II PACU nursing*, Philadelphia, 2004, Saunders; Drain C, editor: *Perianesthesia nursing: a critical care approach*, ed 4, Philadelphia, 2003, Saunders.)

6.111. Correct Answer: **a**
An *endoleak* is defined as a continued flow of blood into the original aneurysm sack despite repair. Unfortunately, this complication is frequently asymptomatic and is usually diagnosed via serial CT scans. Often they spontaneously repair, and the only intervention is close observation. Occasionally re-operation via open or endovascular route may be required. Neither fluid

resuscitation, pressure to the femoral sites, nor nitroglycerin are indicated in this scenario. (Anderson LA: Abdominal aortic aneurysm, *J Cardiovasc Nurs* 15[4]:1-14, 2001; Latessa V: Endovascular stent-graft repair of descending thoracic aortic aneurysms: the nursing implications for care, *J Vasc Nurs* 20[3]:86-95, 2002.)

6.112. Correct Answer: **d**
Lidocaine has been shown to decrease the cough reflex and decrease intracranial pressure. There are mixed reports of its cardio-protective effect during induction. It is not known to protect the patient against aspiration or pulmonary edema. (Butler J: Lidocaine premedication before rapid sequence induction in head injuries, *Emerg Med J* 19[6]:554, 2002; Frakes MA: Rapid sequence induction medications: an update, *J Emerg Nurs* 29[6]:533-540, 587-594, 2003; Pousman R: Rapid sequence induction for prehospital providers, *Internet Journal of Advanced Nursing Practice* 3[2]:17, 1999.)

6.113. Correct Answer: **c**
Rapid sequence induction (RSI) (or intubation) is commonly performed in patients who might be at risk for aspiration. RSI is the simultaneous delivery of sedative and paralytic agent with preoxygenation and careful, but quick, intubation. A patient who may be extremely difficult to intubate is not considered a good candidate for RSI. (Frakes MA: Rapid sequence induction medications: an update, *J Emerg Nurs* 29[6]:533-540,587-594, 2003; Pousman R: Rapid sequence induction for prehospital providers, *Internet Journal of Advanced Nursing Practice* 3[2]:17, 1999.)

6.114. Correct Answer: **d**
The key ingredients for success and reduction of complications in a rapid sequence induction (RSI) (or intubation) includes the appropriate pharmacologic mix. Preoxygenation is followed by the administration of some of type of amnesic/hypnotic (etomidate) administered simultaneously with a paralytic agent (succinylcholine). (Frakes MA: Rapid sequence induction medications: an update, *J Emerg Nurs* 29[6]:533-540, 587-594, 2003; Pousman R: Rapid sequence induction for prehospital providers, *Internet Journal of Advanced Nursing Practice* 3[2]:17, 1999.)

6.115. Correct Answer: **c**
Immediately after a seizure, the patient may have excessive oral secretions and/or vomit in the mouth. Although a CT scan is frequently done for a patient with seizures after a craniotomy, the immediate priority of care is airway assessment and management. Bite blocks or placement of anything in the mouth when a patient is having a seizure is generally not recommended, since it may further obstruct the airway or cause unnecessary trauma. Although patients may have a desaturation episode during the seizure, it is not an indication for reintubation unless the patient continues to be unable to manage his or her airway independently or oversedation occurs from treatment with antiseizure/sedatives used to treat an ongoing seizure. (Ignatavicius DD et al: *Medical-surgical nursing: critical thinking for collaborative care*, ed 4, Philadelphia, 2002, Saunders; Peña CG: Seizure, *Am J Nurs* 103[11]:73,75,77-78, 2003.)

6.116. Correct Answer: **a**
Calcium ions are essential for transmission of nerve impulses, bone growth, muscle contraction, and multiple other physiologic processes. For patients with poor

cardiac function, calcium has a positive inotropic effect (increases myocardial contractility). (Drain C, editor: *Perianesthesia nursing: a critical care approach*, ed 4, Philadelphia, 2003, Saunders; Wilson BA, Shannon MT, Stang CL: *Nurse's drug guide 2006*, Upper Saddle River, NJ, 2006, Prentice Hall.)

6.117. Correct Answer: **b**
One co-morbidity that perianesthesia nurses are faced with includes any variety of cardiac valvular dysfunction including mitral valve stenosis or regurgitation. The key issues to consider in this patient population include high rates of atrial fibrillation, pulmonary hypertension, "backing up" of blood into the pulmonary vasculature, high-pitched murmur on auscultation, and a need for close hemodynamic monitoring and fluid management. (Quinn D, Schick L, editors: *ASPAN's perianesthesia nursing core curriculum: preoperative, Phase I and Phase II PACU nursing*, Philadelphia, 2004, Saunders; Segal BL: Valvular heart disease, part 1: Diagnosis and surgical management of aortic valve disease in older adults, *Geriatrics* 58[9]:31-36, 2003; Segal BL: Valvular heart disease, part 2: Mitral valve disease in older adults, *Geriatrics* 58[10]:26-32, 2003.)

6.118. Correct Answer: **a**
Lasix is an important part of the medical regimen because it reduces fluid retention and overload, which could be exacerbated by a fluid bolus. Generally, these patients are to be extubated rapidly with early ambulation to promote respiratory functioning and limit high pressures in the lungs. Anticoagulants are an essential part of preventing and reducing the risk of the variety of thromboembolic events that can occur with this condition but would

not necessarily be given to this patient if he did not have a previous stroke or atrial fibrillation. (Quinn D, Schick L, editors: *ASPAN's perianesthesia nursing core curriculum: preoperative, Phase I and Phase II PACU nursing*, Philadelphia, 2004, Saunders; Salem DN et al: Antithrombotic therapy in valvular heart disease—native and prosthetic: the seventh ACCP conference on antithrombotic and thrombolytic therapy, *Chest* 126[3]:457S-482S, 2004; Segal BL: Valvular heart disease, part 1: Diagnosis and surgical management of aortic valve disease in older adults, *Geriatrics* 58[9]:31-36, 2003. Segal BL: Valvular heart disease, part 2: Mitral valve disease in older adults, *Geriatrics* 58[10]:26-32, 2003.

6.119. Correct Answer: **d**
The patient has multiple risk factors for cerebral emboli and stroke including gender (male), age older than 55 years, atrial fibrillation, and mitral valve regurgitation. (National Guidelines Clearing house: *Diagnosis and initial treatment of ischemic stroke*. Website: www.guideline.gov/summary/summary.aspx?doc_id=6497&nbr =004070&string=CVA. Accessed January 15, 2006; Quinn D, Schick L, editors: *ASPAN's perianesthesia nursing core curriculum: preoperative, Phase I and Phase II PACU nursing*, Philadelphia, 2004, Saunders.)

6.120. Correct Answer: **c**
Patients experiencing a stroke require emergency medical interventions that should include high-flow oxygen to maintain adequate cerebral oxygenation. Having the head of the bed at 30° helps promote venous return. Frequent neurologic evaluations (every 15-30 minutes) are essential to diagnosis and ongoing patient evaluation. Treatment of thermic and

glycemic imbalances and diagnostic tests including blood work, CT, ECG and potential tPA administration would also be considered. Management of a patient's blood pressure has remained somewhat controversial because aggressive treatment may affect the body's ability to perfuse the ischemic area of the brain. Literature on the topic has suggested that treatment needs to occur with blood pressure higher than 185/110 mmHg. (Adams HP, Jr et al: Guidelines for the early management of patients with ischemic stroke: a scientific statement from the stroke council of the American Stroke Association, *Stroke* 34[4]:1056-1083, 2003; National Guidelines Clearing house: *Diagnosis and initial treatment of ischemic stroke.* Website: www.guideline.gov/summary/summary.aspx?doc_id=6497&nbr=004070&string=CVA. Accessed January 15, 2006; Quinn D, Schick L, editors: *ASPAN's perianesthesia nursing core curriculum: preoperative, Phase I and Phase II PACU nursing*, Philadelphia, 2004, Saunders.)

6.121. Correct Answer: **c**
After an ischemic event, the kidneys may be inadequately perfused and display clear signs of damage and dysfunction including urine output less than 0.5 mL/kg/hour and renal-sensitive laboratory tests that are outside normal parameters (BUN, creatinine). Tracking and reviewing the patient's blood pressure and MAP can help determine how long the kidneys may have been underperfused and to what extent the damage may be. MAP should have been consistently greater than 60 to 75 mmHg to promote adequate perfusion. In this scenario, a bedside bladder ultrasound would be minimally helpful in determining function and damage. (Quinn D, Schick L, editors: *ASPAN's perianesthesia*

nursing core curriculum: preoperative, Phase I and Phase II PACU nursing, Philadelphia, 2004, Saunders.)

6.122. Correct Answer: **b**
Although it is essential to aggressively treat infection if it is the cause of renal failure, the ischemic event is the identified cause. Vancomycin can be extremely nephrotoxic and may not be appropriate in this situation. Dialysis is appropriate for treatment in some circumstances but would not be the first thing the nurse could do to help treat and prevent further worsening of renal function. Renal-dose dopamine infusions continue to be shown in current research to not have renal protective effects as once thought. Ensuring adequate volume would be essential in this scenario, and both albumin and isotonic saline are excellent choices to achieve this. (Agodoa L: Acute renal failure in the PACU, *J PeriAnesth Nurs* 17[6]:377-383, 2002; Friedrich JO et al: Meta-analysis: low-dose dopamine increases urine output but does not prevent renal dysfunction or death, *Ann Intern Med* 142[7]:510-524, 2005; Lameire N et al: Acute renal failure, *Lancet* 365[9457]:417-430, 2005.)

6.123. Correct Answer: **c**
Patients with pelvic and long bone fractures are at high risk for mortality and fat emboli that can manifest as respiratory distress or ARDS. The patient in this situation needs immediate respiratory assistance. Care of the patient with a fat embolus often requires careful ventilator support and adjustment and aggressive hydration and extensive cardiopulmonary support. Although all the options are appropriate and may occur during the course of care, being prepared for imminent intubation is essential.

(Hussain A: A fatal fat embolism, *Internet Journal of Anesthesiology* 8[2]:18, 2004; Quinn D, Schick L, editors: *ASPAN's perianesthesia nursing core curriculum: preoperative, Phase I and Phase II PACU nursing*, Philadelphia, 2004, Saunders; Rose DD, Rowen DW: AANA journal course 1: update for nurse anesthetists: Perioperative considerations in major orthopedic trauma: pelvic and long bone fractures, *AANA J* 70[2]:131-137, 2002.)

6.124. Correct Answer: **a**
Unfortunately, little can be done to prevent fat embolus. Primary prevention involves stabilization of fractured extremities and oxygen administration. Corticosteroids are sometimes used for treatment, but their use is controversial. The statin family of drugs is not indicated as part of treatment. Close monitoring of oxygen saturations and the ECG are a part of diagnosing and monitoring for, rather than preventing, fat emboli. (Hussain A: A fatal fat embolism, *Internet Journal of Anesthesiology* 8[2]:18, 2004; Quinn D, Schick L, editors: *ASPAN's perianesthesia nursing core curriculum: preoperative, Phase I and Phase II PACU nursing*, Philadelphia, 2004, Saunders; Rose DD, Rowen DW: AANA journal course 1: update for nurse anesthetists: Perioperative considerations in major orthopedic trauma: pelvic and long bone fractures, *AANA J* 70[2]:131-137, 2002.)

6.125. Correct Answer: **c**
After an extensive back surgery in the prone position, all the concerns and assessments listed are common. The biggest concern would be the neck and face swelling because this may also translate to swelling of tissues in the airway as well. Extubation of this patient may

allow those tissues to close off and compromise the patient's airway. (Quinn D, Schick L, editors: *ASPAN's perianesthesia nursing core curriculum: preoperative, Phase I and Phase II PACU nursing*, Philadelphia, 2004, Saunders.)

6.126. Correct Answer: **a**
Hypothermia and vascular surgery patients are a dangerous combination in that a patient's body temperature and physiologic processes can hamper perfusion and healing. Hypertension is more commonly seen with shivering and hypothermia. Both difficulty with palpating peripheral pulses and slow capillary refill may be expected with this type of patient, it is not related to hypothermia. Depending on the extent of hypothermia, patients may range in level of consciousness from somnolent to anxious. (Connor EL et al: Detrimental effects of hypothermia: a systems analysis, *J PeriAnesth Nurs* 15[3]:151-155, 2000; Quinn D, Schick L, editors: *ASPAN's perianesthesia nursing core curriculum: preoperative, Phase I and Phase II PACU nursing*, Philadelphia, 2004, Saunders.)

6.127. Correct Answer: **b**
Essential to understanding any aspect of cardiovascular care is basic knowledge of the vascular system and the affect of disease on it. Low fluid volumes actually decrease peripheral vascular resistance. Baroreceptors do in fact decline in function with age, altering a patient's ability to self-regulate blood pressure changes. Age, smoking, diabetes, hypertension, and a host of other factors alter vessel wall elasticity and compliance, which directly alters blood pressure and general cardiovascular functioning. (McCance KL, Huether SE: *Pathophysiology: the*

biologic basis for disease in adults and children, ed 4, St. Louis, 2002, Mosby; Quinn D, Schick L, editors: *ASPAN's perianesthesia nursing core curriculum: preoperative, Phase I and Phase II PACU nursing*, Philadelphia, 2004, Saunders.)

6.128. Correct Answer: **a**
The difficulty for the nurse and the medical team is simultaneously locating the source of the bleed while managing the sequelae. A retroperitoneal bleed would manifest with back pain and potentially ecchymosis and would need to be visualized and palpated to rule it out. Abdominal bleeds may be indicated by rigidity, tenderness, and ecchymosis. Deep breathing, anxiolytics, bowel sounds, nor laboratory results will not help the medical team locate the source of the bleed. (Ernits M et al: A retroperitoneal bleed induced by enoxaparin therapy, *Am Surg* 71[5]:430-433, 2005; Ignatavius DD et al: *Medical-surgical nursing: critical thinking for collaborative care*, ed 4, Philadelphia, 2002, Saunders.)

6.129. Correct Answer: **c**
Hyperthyroidism and hypovolemia will generally cause tachycardia, whereas stimulation of baroreceptors will cause bradycardia. Reversal agents such as atropine and glycopyrrolate generally cause tachycardia that is relatively benign and short-lived in healthy patients. (Quinn D, Schick L, editors: *ASPAN's perianesthesia nursing core curriculum: preoperative, Phase I and Phase II PACU nursing*, Philadelphia, 2004, Saunders; Wilson BA, Shannon MT, Stang CL: *Nurse's drug guide 2006*, Upper Saddle River, NJ, 2006, Prentice Hall.)

6.130. Correct Answer: **d**
Although bronchoscopy is a simple procedure that is usually done under light sedation and on an outpatient basis, there can be potentially dangerous concerns that the PACU nurse must be knowledgeable of and prepared for. Laryngospasm and bronchospasm are of the greatest concern, but pneumothorax, aspiration, and even anatomic perforation can also occur. Nurses should be concerned by the presence of frank bleeding. Atrial ectopy and heavy nonproductive coughing are common and generally benign. Numbness of the mouth and difficulty swallowing are generally associated with the local lidocaine or analgesic used to numb the throat pre-procedure. Fever is particularly concerning because it is generally indicative of an infection. (Belli M: Critical care extra: Bronchoscopy, *Am J Nurs* 99[7]:24AA-BB,24, 1999; National Institutes of Health Medline Plus: *Bronchoscopy*. Website: www.nlm.nih.gov/medlineplus/ency/article/003857.htm. Accessed December 21, 2005; Quinn D, Schick L, editors: *ASPAN's perianesthesia nursing core curriculum: preoperative, Phase I and Phase II PACU nursing*, Philadelphia, 2004, Saunders.)

6.131. Correct Answer: **d**
The risk for pneumothorax exists for both procedures, whereas subcutaneous emphysema is more common with mediastinoscopy because entrance is gained through the chest as opposed to through the trachea. Although biopsies can be taken for both, mediastinoscopy is more commonly done as a means of getting tissue from lymph nodes. Both procedures call for some sedation to promote comfort and tolerance of the procedure for the patient. (National Institutes of Health Medline Plus: *Mediastinoscopy*. Website: www.nlm.nih.gov/medlineplus/ency/article/003864.htm. Accessed

December 21, 2005; Quinn D, Schick L, editors: *ASPAN's perianesthesia nursing core curriculum: preoperative, Phase I and Phase II PACU nursing*, Philadelphia, 2004, Saunders.)

6.132. Correct Answer: **b**
Lung volume reduction surgery can help the patient by removing diseased or poorly functioning lung material. Full to near-full expansion of remaining and/or healthy lung tissue is normal, and there should be limited reduction in lung sounds even on the operative side. Because of the positioning during thoracoscopy (lateral decubitus), there is potential for some short-term neuromuscular effects such as paresthesias on the side where the arm was elevated. Atelectasis is also very common because of this positioning. An end-tidal CO_2 level of 50 mmHg is high but not life threatening and can generally be corrected with a stir-up regimen. A minimal chest tube air leak is also common until postoperative day 3. (Quinn D, Schick L, editors: *ASPAN's perianesthesia nursing core curriculum: preoperative, Phase I and Phase II PACU nursing*, Philadelphia, 2004, Saunders.)

6.133. Correct Answer: **a**
In all these scenarios, beta blockers should be used cautiously. A patient with Raynaud's probably already has peripheral vascular problems and may have further exacerbation with administration of beta blockers. Diabetic patients need to be carefully watched for hypoglycemia as a result of administration of this drug. Because the diabetic patient had a minor procedure under light sedation, he or she may be more able to notice hypoglycemia. Patients with asthma can be put at risk for worsening bronchospasm from beta blockers. Concomitant administration of beta blockers

and calcium channel blockers can cause severe hypotension. (National Institutes of Health Medline Plus: *Beta-adrenergic blocking agents*. Website: www.nlm.nih.gov/medlineplus/druginfo/uspdi/202087.html. Accessed December 21, 2005; Nunnelee JD et al: Assessment and nursing management of hypertension in the perioperative period, *J PeriAnesth Nurs* 15[3]:163-168, 2000; Quinn D, Schick L, editors: *ASPAN's perianesthesia nursing core curriculum: preoperative, Phase I and Phase II PACU nursing*, Philadelphia, 2004, Saunders; Walker JR: Antihypertensive agents, *J PeriAnesth Nurs* 14[5]:278-283, 1999.)

6.134. Correct Answer: **a**
The basics of care for children with congenital heart defects of any type include ensuring that air filters are in all IV tubing because any air can cause a stroke. Frequently these children have mixing of oxygenated and unoxygenated blood and by all appearances are cyanotic and hypoxemic with symptoms such as tachypnea, clubbing of the fingers, and low oxygen saturations. Heat lamps and external warming devices are important in the care of any infant because of the infant's large body surface area and poor thermoregulation ability. (Quinn D, Schick L, editors: *ASPAN's perianesthesia nursing core curriculum: preoperative, Phase I and Phase II PACU nursing*, Philadelphia, 2004, Saunders; Suddaby EC: Contemporary thinking for congenital heart disease, *Pediatr Nurs* 27[3]: 233-238, 253-254, 270, 2001.)

6.135. Correct Answer: **c**
Although ECG monitoring is frequently the standard of care for all patients in the postanesthesia environment, there are certain patient populations for which ECG

monitoring is not as essential; these include, for example, patients at very low risk for cardiac dysrhythmias (ASA I patients) who have undergone uncomplicated surgical procedures and patients for whom monitoring is almost impossible, such as extremely agitated patients. A situation in which the patient may be at risk for QT prolongation should prompt the nurse to advocate for/initiate ECG monitoring (e.g., the drugs listed that put a patient at risk for QT prolongation). (ASPAN: Resource 4 in *2006-2008 Standards of perianesthesia nursing practice,* Cherry Hill, NJ, 2006, ASPAN; Drew BJ et al: AHA scientific statement: practice standards for electrocardiographic monitoring in hospital settings, *J Cardiovasc Nurs* 20[2]:76-106, 2005.)

6.136. Correct Answer: **b**
A wide range of medications have been implicated as causative agents of a prolonged QT interval. Although the severity of their effects varies, they come from every class of drug ranging from antiemetics and antipsychotics to antibiotics and antidysrhythmics. Although QT interval more than 0.5 second does not always lead to torsades, it is frequently a precursor. (Drew BJ et al: AHA scientific statement: practice standards for electrocardiographic monitoring in hospital settings, *J Cardiovasc Nurs* 20[2]:76-106, 2005; Reilly JG et al: QTc-interval abnormalities and psychotropic drug therapy in psychiatric patients, *Lancet* 355[9209]:1048-1052, 2000.)

6.137. Correct Answer: **d**
It is important to select the correct size nasopharyngeal airway to minimize trauma, optimize airway patency, and reduce obstruction. The distal tip should not touch the epiglottis, and the length should be

approximated by holding the tube up to the naris and measuring it back to the earlobe. (Quinn D, Schick L, editors: *ASPAN's perianesthesia nursing core curriculum: preoperative, Phase I and Phase II PACU nursing,* Philadelphia, 2004, Saunders.)

6.138. Correct Answer: **d**
Lubricant, vasoconstrictive agents, local anesthetics, and the pointing of the bevel in a posterior and medial direction can all reduce the risk for trauma and bleeding and make insertion easier. Choosing the correct size is also essential, and ensuring that the patient is not overly awake or agitated assists in smooth insertion. (Drain C, editor: *Perianesthesia nursing: a critical care approach,* ed 4, Philadelphia, 2003, Saunders; McQuillan KA et al: *Trauma nursing: from resuscitation through rehabilitation,* ed 3, Philadelphia, 2002, Saunders; Quinn D, Schick L, editors: *ASPAN's perianesthesia nursing core curriculum: preoperative, Phase I and Phase II PACU nursing,* Philadelphia, 2004, Saunders.)

6.139. Correct Answer: **a**
Bundle branch blocks reflect a mismatch of the signaling and depolarization of the ventricles of the heart, which is the main reason the "bunny ears" of a prolonged QRS cycle are seen on ECG. They can both be asymptomatic and benign, but a left bundle branch block always indicates past ischemia, hypertension, or other cardiac disease and is thus the more concerning block. (Geiter HB, Jr: Understanding bundle-branch blocks: go beyond left and right to recognize the ECG clues for these ventricular conduction problems, *Nursing* 33[4]:321-322, 324-326, 2003; Jain AC et al: Etiologies of left bundle branch block and

correlations with hemodynamic and angiographic findings, *Am J Cardiol* 91[11]:1375-1378, 2003.)

6.140. Correct Answer: **c**
The mainstay treatment for low oxygen saturation and the inevitable atelectasis is coughing and deep breathing. The physiologic reasoning for these exercises entails high inspiratory volumes, which promotes loosening and clearing of airway secretions, redistribution of lung surfactant, and recruitment of deflated alveoli with the intent of promoting oxygenation. (McCance KL, Huether SE: *Pathophysiology: the biologic basis for disease in adults and children*, ed 4, St. Louis, 2002, Mosby.)

6.141. Correct Answer: **c**
Poor planning for cardiac or respiratory arrest in the obese patient can result in disaster. Having appropriate physiologic monitoring is an important start, since most blood pressure cuffs will fit poorly on a patient's arm whether it be because of excess tissue or the conical shape of the arm. Frequently, arterial lines will be placed in these patients even if the procedure does not dictate a need for them to allow for close hemodynamic monitoring. Airway management adjuncts such as CPAP and BiPAP are a must considering the high rates of both diagnosed and undiagnosed obstructive sleep apnea in the obese population. Unless the patient has a cardiac condition requiring a higher voltage rate for defibrillation, standard defibrillators should work just as well in this cohort. (Davidson JE et al: Critical care of the morbidly obese, *Crit Care Nurs Q* 26[2]: 105-118, 2003; Hurst S et al: Bariatric implications of critical care nursing, *Dimens Crit Care Nurs* 23[2]:76-83, 2004; Quinn D, Schick L, editors: *ASPAN's perianesthesia nursing core curriculum:*

preoperative, Phase I and Phase II PACU nursing, Philadelphia, 2004, Saunders.)

6.142. Correct Answer: **b**
Although there is some controversy regarding the advantages of colloids versus crystalloids, an important study investigating mortality related to fluid resuscitation using albumin and normal saline showed no differences. Usually rates can run as fast as pump technologies and infusion sites can handle but, generally, only in relatively healthy populations whose lungs and cardiovascular system can handle the fluid. There is still risk in healthy patients of pulmonary problems and fluid overload if liberal fluid is given with poor monitoring of patient outcomes. In small quantities (usually not more than one or two units), artificial colloids can be helpful with fluid resuscitation, but they can also have negative side effects such as coagulation problems even when given in these doses. (Drain C, editor: *Perianesthesia nursing: a critical care approach*, ed 4, Philadelphia, 2003, Saunders; Kelley DM: Hypovolemic shock: an overview, *Crit Care Nurs Q* 28[1]:2-21, 2005; SAFE (Saline versus Albumin Fluid Evaluation) Study Investigators: A comparison of albumin and saline for fluid resuscitation in the intensive care unit, *N Engl J Med* 350[22]:2247-2256, 2004; Vincent J et al: Fluid resuscitation in severe sepsis and septic shock: an evidence-based review, *Crit Care Med* 32[11]:S451-S454, 2004.)

6.143. Correct Answer: **d**
Cheyne-Stokes respirations are characterized by a pattern of rising rate and depth that descends to apnea with repetition of the rising and falling with an apneic endpoint. The breathing pattern is commonly seen in brain-injured patients

with increasing intracranial pressure, bilateral cerebral hemispheric damage, or injury to the midbrain or pons. The pattern can also be seen in stroke victims, patients with heart failure, and obstructive sleep apnea. It may also be seen as a normal assessment finding for children or after ascents to high altitudes. (Drain C, editor: *Perianesthesia nursing: a critical care approach*, ed 4, Philadelphia, 2003, Saunders; Nopmaneejumrus-lers C et al: Cheyne-stokes respiration in stroke: relationship to hypocapnia and occult cardiac dysfunction, *Am J Respir Crit Care Med* 171[9]:1048-1052, 2005; Spieker ED et al: Sleep-disordered breathing in patients with heart failure: pathophysiology, assessment, and management, *J Am Acad Nurse Pract* 15[11]:487-493, 2003.)

6.144. Correct Answer: **c**
A patient with a large amount of secretions may not be a good candidate for CPAP because of poor fit and tolerance. Drugs that block acetylcholine generally cause dry mouth, which might negate this concern. For a patient who has just undergone an upper airway procedure, CPAP is generally contraindicated because it may injure the patient and damage surgical sites. A patient's face shape and presence of facial hair may alter fit of the mask, lowering its efficacy. A tight seal is essential to optimal functioning. (Liesching T et al: Acute applications of noninvasive positive pressure ventilation, *Chest* 124[2]:699-713, 2003.)

6.145. Correct Answer: **b**
Pneumothorax is a common complication after thoracotomy and is generally treated only if lung field deflation is greater than 20% or if the patient is symptomatic. Although hypoxia may occur,

support with supplemental oxygen will assist the patient until re-expansion occurs. (Quinn D, Schick L, editors: *ASPAN's perianesthesia nursing core curriculum: preoperative, Phase I and Phase II PACU nursing*, Philadelphia, 2004, Saunders.)

6.146. Correct Answer: **a**
Pulmonary function tests such as vital capacity measurement can determine a great deal about lung function and the severity of trauma or the disease process. Multiple vital capacity measurements describe different or combined phases of the respiratory cycle. Comparison of normal values and the patient's results can help determine severity of disease or effectiveness of treatment. The amount of air left in the lungs after exhalation is called *physiologic dead space*. The other options described in the question are not directly measured with vital capacity. (McCance KL, Huether SE: *Pathophysiology: the biologic basis for disease in adults and children*, ed 4, St. Louis, 2002, Mosby; Smith AD et al: Diagnosing asthma: comparisons between exhaled nitric oxide measurements and conventional tests, *Am J Respir Crit Care Med* 169[4]:473-478, 2004.)

6.147. Correct Answer: **c**
Most pacemakers have the ability to pace, sense, and respond to the atria and/or the ventricles in a variety of different ways. The first letter of the description of the settings always corresponds to the chamber being paced, and the second letter corresponds to the chamber being sensed (V = ventricle; A = atrium; D = both; O = none). The third letter relates to the mode of response and reflects the pacemaker's ability to sense intrinsic rhythm or pace over the heart's activity. In this case, the "I" refers to a setting where the pacemaker will not fire

over a set level of intrinsic beats. A "T" would refer to a timed delivery of an electrical impulse, a "D" would indicate a setting of atrial triggering and ventricle inhibition (O = none). (Quinn D, Schick L, editors: *ASPAN's perianesthesia nursing core curriculum: preoperative, Phase I and Phase II PACU nursing*, Philadelphia, 2004, Saunders; Van Orden Wallace C: Dual-chamber pacemakers in the management of severe heart failure, *Crit Care Nurse* 18[2]:57-67, 1998.)

6.148. Correct Answer: **a**
Although these beats have some similarities, they look quite different on an ECG monitor or strip largely because of the differences in the QRS complex. In the case of ventricular tachycardia, the QRS complex will be wide (0.14-0.16 seconds) and it will appear normal for PSVT (0.10 seconds or less). Both can have rates ranging from 140+, and the P waves, though absent with ventricular tachycardia, may be hidden in the T waves in PSVT. The patient may be hemodynamically unstable and may exhibit anxiety with either rhythm. (Huff J: *ECG workout: exercises in arrhythmia interpretation*, ed 5, Philadelphia, 2006, Lippincott Williams & Wilkins; Quinn D, Schick L, editors: *ASPAN's perianesthesia nursing core curriculum: preoperative, Phase I and Phase II PACU nursing*, Philadelphia, 2004, Saunders.)

6.149. Correct Answer: **b**
The nurse should immediately recognize this as ventricular fibrillation

and at least be prepared to administer electrical therapy. Adenosine will not help in this scenario and is indicated for PSVT and not for ventricular tachycardia or fibrillation. Waiting to call for a 12-lead ECG or ABGs could further endanger the patient. A precordial thump is not indicated in the current ACLS algorithms. (American Heart Asso-ciation: Part 6—Advanced cardiovascular life support: Section 7—Algorithm approach to ACLS emergencies, *Circulation* 102[90001]:136-165, 2000; Quinn D, Schick L, editors: *ASPAN's perianesthesia nursing core curriculum: preoperative, Phase I and Phase II PACU nursing*, Philadelphia, 2004, Saunders.)

6.150. Correct Answer: **b**
Administration of adenosine slows and interrupts conduction through the AV and SA nodes in the heart with the purpose of restoring sinus rhythm during paroxysmal supraventricular tachycardia. Frequently, a short "pause" or bradycardia will result that often makes the patient feel like his or her heart has stopped. This medication is given only through the IV, and headache is not a listed side effect. Burning at the IV site, flushing, chest pain, and dyspnea are listed side effects. (Quinn D, Schick L, editors: *ASPAN's perianesthesia nursing core curriculum: preoperative, Phase I and Phase II PACU nursing*, Philadelphia, 2004, Saunders; Wilson BA, Shannon MT, Stang CL: *Nurse's drug guide 2006*, Upper Saddle River, NJ, 2006, Prentice Hall.)

Chapter 7

Physiologic Balance

Scenarios and items in this section focus on issues of *physiologic balance* of the body's internal *chemical* (acid-base, oxygen, and electrolyte), *fluid, coagulation, endocrine*, and *thermal* environment. These concepts are considered together because each:

- Has defined ''balance'' parameters (normal values)

- Causes measurable outcomes related to deficit (hypo) or excess (hyper)
- Produces pharmacokinetic and pharmacodynamic effects related to anesthetics and medications
- Suggests nursing process responses to restore balance

ESSENTIAL CORE CONCEPTS	AFFILIATED CORE CURRICULUM CHAPTERS
Nursing Process	
Assessment	**Chapters 3, 35, 56**
Planning and Implementation	**Chapters 3, 4, 57**
Evaluation	
Chemical and Electrolyte Balance	
Acid-Base Concepts	**Chapters 25, 31**
Acidosis	
Respiratory	
Metabolic	
Alkalosis	
Respiratory	
Metabolic	
Compensation, Mixed Imbalances	
Buffers	
Renal	
Respiratory	
Interpreting Arterial Blood Gases (ABGs)	
Oxygenation	**Chapter 25**
Hypoventilation	
Hypoxemia	
Oxygen Delivery Systems	**Chapter 31**
Toxicity	
Restoring Balance	

Electrolyte Stability   **Chapter 24**

Concentration
Anions
Cations
Deficits and Excesses
Causes
Symptoms
Nursing Assessment and Intervention
Principles
Diffusion
Restoring Balance

Fluid Balance   **Chapter 24**

Composition: Extracellular, Intracellular
Distribution and Volumes
Fluid Regulation: Loss, Gain, and Balance
Causes
Compartment Shifts
Symptoms
Principles and Concepts
Hydrostatic Pressure
Osmosis
Osmolality
Tonicity (iso-, hypo-, and hyper-)
Volume Replacement
Colloid
Crystalloid
Restoring Balance

Hematologic Balance   **Chapter 34**

Blood Components
Structure and function
Antigens and Antibodies: ABO, Rh, and Immunity
Platelets and Thrombin: Hemostasis and Clots
Red Cells: Anemias, Hemolysis, and Sickling
White Cells: Leukemias

Order and Disorder
Characteristics and Symptoms
Blood Loss
Coagulation Cascade
Disseminated Intravascular Coagulation (DIC)
Normal Values
Restoring Balance
Transfusion Therapy
Blood Components
Hemolysis, Allergy, and Anaphylaxis
Infection Transmission (Hepatitis)

Set 1

7.1. Aldosterone release does all the following *except:*
a. promotes reabsorption of potassium and excretion of sodium.
b. increases circulating blood volume.
c. prevents acidosis.
d. increases reabsorption of sodium and excretion of potassium.

7.2. Which of the following factors places the patient most at risk for acidosis?
a. A $PaCO_2$ of 46 mmHg on O_2 at 6 L/min
b. A temperature of 35.4° C (95.7° F) with shivering
c. A 5-year history of smoking
d. An HCO_3 level of 23 mEq/L

7.3. After a bilateral adrenalectomy because of metastatic cancer, a cortisone titration was administered during general anesthesia and is continued in the PACU to:
a. promote catecholamine level stability.
b. prevent hemorrhagic shock.
c. prevent hypernatremia.
d. vasoconstrict the renal blood vessels.

7.4. The most common blood transfusion risk is:
a. acquisition of hepatitis.
b. exposure to bacterial contaminates.
c. ABO/Rh incompatibility reaction.
d. transfusion-related acute lung injury.

7.5. While caring for an adrenalectomy patient, the PACU nurse can anticipate:
a. polyuria related to intraoperative manipulation of the kidneys.
b. positioning the patient on the non-operative side.
c. vigilant cardiac assessment for signs of shock.
d. collecting serum electrolytes every 6 hours postoperatively.

7.6. Which of the following statements about electrolytes is *not* true?
a. Electrolytes dissociate in solution to form ions.
b. Composition of electrolytes in each compartment varies.
c. Electrical balance of cations is greater than anions.
d. The major ions found in extracellular fluid are chloride and sodium.

7.7. The perianesthesia nurse observes that a patient with cirrhosis and an actively bleeding gastric ulcer received 5 units of packed red blood cells (RBCs) during a partial gastrectomy, vagotomy, and pyloroplasty. A unit of whole blood infuses now, and bleeding has abated. This patient has an increased potential for which of the following?
a. Hypoglycemia related to banked packed cells
b. Hyperkalemia related to respiratory alkalosis
c. Hypocalcemia related to citrate preservative
d. Hyponatremia related to hemodilution

7.8. One type of surgery that may include planned perioperative hypothermia includes:
a. vascular procedures.
b. neurosurgical procedures.
c. eye procedures.
d. orthopedic procedures.

7.9. Blood type O negative is considered the "universal donor" because it carries:
a. no antigens.
b. no antibodies.
c. antigens to blood types A, B, and O.
d. antibodies for type O.

7.10 The approximate percentage of total body weight (TBW) contained in a child's extracellular fluid (ECF) is:
a. 66%.

b. 70%.

c. 75%.

d. 81%.

7.11 A preoperative complete blood count (CBC) is:

a. a requirement for Medicare patients ages 65 years and older.

b. an effective screening tool for undiagnosed coagulopathies.

c. recommended before any surgical case requiring endotracheal intubation.

d. indicated on a selective basis related to patient history and surgical procedure.

NOTE: Consider items 7.12-7.14 together.

7.12 A male patient is recovering from general anesthesia in the Phase 1 PACU after a 3-hour partial gastrectomy. Arterial blood gases (ABGs) ordered by the surgeon, collected 30 minutes after PACU admission, showed pH = 7.28; PaO_2 = 80 mmHg; $PaCO_2$ = 67 mmHg; HCO_3 = 26 mEq/L. These results indicate:

a. uncompensated metabolic acidosis.

b. partially compensated respiratory acidosis.

c. simultaneous respiratory and metabolic acidosis.

d. uncompensated respiratory acidosis.

7.13 Based on the ABG results, the nurse can anticipate the patient demonstrating all the following *except:*

a. tachycardia.

b. opioid deprivation.

c. mental confusion.

d. slow, shallow breathing.

7.14 After ensuring the patient has a patent airway with an adequate oxygen device in place, the next *most immediate* nursing action is to:

a. report the ABG results to the surgeon.

b. call for a ventilator.

c. initiate a stir-up regimen.

d. check the intubation equipment.

7.15 The primary goal of transfusing packed RBCs is to:

a. maintain hemoglobin level of 10 g/dL.

b. increase circulating oxygen-carrying capacity.

c. replace diminishing clotting factors.

d. stimulate production of clotting factors.

7.16 The nurse caring for a postoperative type 1 diabetic patient who received epidural anesthesia is aware that:

a. gastroparesis increases intestinal mobility in type 1 diabetics.

b. peripheral neuropathy will not affect bladder function.

c. pain assessment is uncompromised by physiologic changes.

d. urinary catheterization is guardedly performed in the absence of spontaneous voiding before discharge.

7.17 After the infusion of 1 unit of packed RBCs, the postanesthesia nurse would expect a post-transfusion hemoglobin and hematocrit (Hgb & Hct) to show an increase of:

a. 0.5 g Hgb and 1.5% Hct.

b. 1 g Hgb and 3% Hct.

c. 1.5 g Hgb and 5% Hct.

d. 2 g Hgb and 10% Hct.

7.18 The preanesthesia nurse admits a type 1 diabetic patient to a preoperative unit on the morning of elective surgery. The patient was seen in the facility's preanesthesia education and testing unit. While reviewing the medical record, the admitting nurse is *most likely* to find documentation on which of the following:

a. ECG results, serum electrolyte and cholesterol levels, hemoglobin A_{1C} level

b. Serum blood urea nitrogen (BUN) and creatinine results, urine ketone and acetone levels, serum blood sugar

c. Instructions for the patient to hold all insulin on the day of surgery, electrocardiogram (ECG) results, and serum electrolyte and blood glucose results

d. Hemoglobin A_{1C} level, urine ketone and acetone levels, serum blood sugar

7.19 Thyroid storm can occur up to 18 hours postoperatively and is characterized by:
  a. decreased respirations, atrial flutter, and convulsions.
  b. sweating, dehydration, and tachycardia.
  c. hypotension followed by hypertension and hyperthermia.
  d. agitation, atrial fibrillation, and pulmonary system collapse.

7.20 The specific indication for fresh frozen plasma (FFP) is to:
  a. expand circulating volume.
  b. replace acute blood loss.
  c. correct coagulation deficiencies.
  d. treat thrombocytopenia.

7.21 Body temperature is regulated in which part of the brain?
  a. Pons
  b. Hypothalamus
  c. Medulla
  d. Hypophysis

During a lumbar decompression and fusion of vertebrae L2 to S1, a female patient's estimated blood loss was 800 mL. Her Hgb in PACU is 7.2 g/dL, and the surgeon orders an infusion of 2 units of autologous blood. The blood bank technician informs the PACU nurse that the patient has "cold agglutinins."

7.22 Safe infusion of autologous blood requires:
  a. a 22-gauge, intermediate-length catheter.
  b. concurrent infusion with 5% dextrose in water.
  c. blood pressure assessment after infusing 150 mL.
  d. replacement of blood filter after the second unit.

SET 2

7.23 Red blood cell production is:
a. inhibited by the spleen.
b. stimulated by the kidney.
c. initiated by plasma proteins.
d. controlled by hepatic enzymes.

7.24 A female patient is having a hypophysectomy procedure under general anesthesia because of a diagnosed tumor. This tumor resulted in a decreased hormone secretion from the involved gland. The nurse can expect all the following *except:*
a. intolerance to hyperthermia.
b. decreased heart rate.
c. less anesthetic medications required.
d. intolerance to hypothermia.

7.25 The operative approach commonly used for a hypophysectomy procedure is:
a. temporal craniotomy.
b. transsphenoidal resection via a posterior palate incision.
c. occipital craniotomy.
d. transsphenoidal resection in front of the hard palate.

7.26 Old red blood cells are normally:
a. removed by the spleen.
b. excreted in bile.
c. absorbed by the liver.
d. broken down in the small intestine.

7.27 Which of the following statements regarding pulse oximetry is *true?*
a. Readings in the 80% to 100% range are considered an accurate comparison to ABGs.
b. Readings are less reliable in anemic patients and children.
c. Ambient light at the sensor site can alter readings.
d. Cardiac dysrhythmias do not affect readings.

7.28 A type 2 male diabetic has a history of successful blood sugar management by careful adherence to a diabetic exchange diet, regular brisk walks for exercise, and daily oral metformin doses. The patient arrives in the PACU with a blood glucose level of 251 mg/dL. The nurse understands that this elevation is *most likely* related to:
a. hemoconcentration.
b. an increase in adrenal cortisol secretion.
c. anesthetic inhibition of pancreatic enzyme production.
d. intraoperative hydration with 1000 mL of 5% dextrose solution in water.

7.29 The *primary* role of parathormone is to:
a. retain serum phosphorus.
b. regulate calcium concentration.
c. metabolize vitamin D.
d. stimulate calcitonin production.

7.30 Sickle cell disease is the result of:
a. bone marrow suppression.
b. an autoimmune disease.
c. endocrine insufficiency.
d. an inherited genetic trait.

7.31 A 23-year-old male with a history of sickle cell disease is scheduled for an open reduction of a fractured ankle. Among the interventions to reduce this patient's risk of an acute sickle cell crisis is:
a. spinal anesthesia for preemptive pain management.
b. intraoperative vasodilators to promote microcirculation.
c. fluid administration to prevent dehydration.
d. induced hypothermia to minimize blood loss.

7.32 Respiratory alkalosis may be caused by:
a. tumors of the medulla and brainstem.
b. pain, decreased carbonic acid levels, and anxiety.
c. appropriate mechanical ventilation.
d. pregnancy and surgical manipulation of the brainstem.

7.33 A patient on long-term steroid therapy experiences suppressed cortisone production. The incapacity to generate endogenous adrenocorticoids can:
a. cause an exaggerated response to surgical stressors.
b. necessitate postoperative administration of dexamethasone.
c. require postoperative administration of parenteral hydrocortisone.
d. require decreased steroid replacement doses in the preoperative period.

7.34 Hypertonic intravenous (IV) solutions:
a. cause water to move from the cell to the serum.
b. have an osmolality less than 340 mOsm/L.
c. are more concentrated in the intracellular fluid.
d. are infrequently used for ambulatory surgical procedures.

7.35 In the immediate postoperative period, the hemoglobin and hematocrit values of a stable 47-year-old male after elective total knee replacement are Hgb 11 g/dL and Hct 35%. Reported blood loss was 200 mL; IV fluids given were 2600 mL of lactated Ringer's. The postanesthesia nurse recognizes that the patient's Hgb and Hct:
a. are within normal ranges.
b. must be reported as crisis values.
c. may be a result of hemodilution.
d. indicate the need for colloid volume expansion.

7.36 During emergency treatment of abdominal hemorrhage, rapidly infusing 4 units of packed red blood cells through a blood warmer:
a. eliminates the potential for cell hemolysis.

b. increases the likelihood of serum hypokalemia.
c. reduces the risk of allergic reaction.
d. promotes peripheral vasodilation for comfort.

7.37 The drug of choice in the treatment of malignant hyperthermia (MH) is:
a. succinylcholine.
b. etomidate.
c. dantrolene.
d. diazepam.

7.38 During an inflammatory response, leukocytes function within the:
a. bone marrow.
b. endothelium.
c. capillary bed.
d. interstitial space.

7.39 Polycythemia may be a response to all the following *except:*
a. high altitude.
b. vitamin B_{12} deficiency.
c. acute infection.
d. leukemia.

7.40 Endocrine changes that occur in the elderly patient population result in which of the following?
a. The greatest decline in pancreatic function between ages 70 and 80 years
b. Decreased vitamin A absorption
c. A higher plasma concentration of antidiuretic hormone
d. Decreased ability to metabolize glucose

7.41 Serum calcium deficiency is of concern when administering muscle relaxants because hypocalcemia:
a. promotes repolarization of depolarizing neuromuscular blocking agents.
b. potentiates nondepolarizing neuromuscular blocking agents.
c. potentiates neuromuscular transmission.
d. increases the amount of acetylcholine release.

7.42 The most common diagnosis of leukemia is:
a. adults with acute myelocytic leukemia.

208

b. children with acute lymphocytic leukemia.

c. adults with chronic myelocytic leukemia.

d. children with chronic lymphocytic leukemia.

7.43 A 62-year-old female patient arrives in the preoperative unit at 8 AM for an exploratory bowel procedure. She reports completing the bowel prep as instructed with excellent results and maintaining NPO status for 8 hours; she states that she is feeling "exceptionally weak" today. Potential causes for the reported weakness include all *except:*
a. hypercalcemia related to fasting.
b. dehydration.
c. poor sleep from preoperative anxiety and the stress response.
d. hypokalemia related to electrolyte depletion from the bowel prep.

7.44 Clinical symptoms of Addisonian crisis include all the following *except:*
a. hypertension.
b. azotemia.
c. flaccid muscles in the extremities.
d. nausea and vomiting.

7.45 A male patient is admitted for repair of an incarcerated hernia. He has been on warfarin (Coumadin) since having a mitral valve replacement 2 years ago and took his usual dose 16 hours before admission. The admitting perianesthesia nurse recognizes that:
a. surgery must be postponed for 24 hours.
b. infusion of platelets may be therapeutic.
c. administration of vitamin K may be indicated.
d. the partial thromboplastin time (PTT) level will suggest appropriate perioperative management.

7.46 The drug of choice to administer in the PACU if Addisonian crisis is suspected would be:
a. hydrocortisone.
b. potassium sulfate.

c. sodium chloride.
d. dexamethasone.

7.47 Which of the following statements *best* describes properties of a nonrebreathing O_2 mask?
a. It requires a flow rate of 10 to 15 L/min of O_2.
b. The leaflet valves at both exhalation ports should close.
c. The O_2 delivery level can exceed 80%.
d. There is no risk of suffocation when using this device.

7.48 A diabetic patient exhibits symptoms of tachypnea, polyuria, tachycardia, hyperkalemia, and hypotension. The perianesthesia nurse recognizes these symptoms as consistent with:
a. insulin overdose.
b. diabetic acidosis.
c. lactic acidosis.
d. a blood sugar below 70 mg/dL.

7.49 The most important preoperative considerations for a patient after a total thyroidectomy procedure include all the following *except:*
a. management of cardiovascular requirements.
b. patient education regarding postoperative positioning of head and neck.
c. administration of antithyroid medications.
d. management of hyperthermia.

7.50 A female patient arrives in the PACU with a reaction from general anesthesia. She has a neck dressing with a Jackson-Pratt drain in place. The PACU nurse will:
a. apply a low-humidity oxygen facemask.
b. position the patient in high-Fowler position.
c. assess the patient's ability to swallow.
d. anticipate overproduction from tear ducts.

7.51 Under normal conditions, predominately mature blood cells are circulating in the blood. Which of the following statements is *true* about circulating immature blood cells?

a. Increased immature neutrophils are found in response to overwhelming infection.
b. Healthy bone marrow does not release immature blood cells.
c. Elevated counts of reticulocytes are a sign of coagulopathy.
d. Immature RBCs are a hallmark of pernicious anemia.

SET 3

ITEMS 7.52–7.70

7.52 A patient admitted to PACU after a femoral-tibial bypass graft is to receive a dose of protamine sulfate. The perianesthesia nurse knows that the drug is to be administered "slowly" and prepares to give 60 mg IV push in:
a. no less than 5 minutes.
b. no less than 10 minutes.
c. no less than 15 minutes.
d. divided doses of 10 mg every 5 minutes.

7.53 A 2-month-old infant's primary compensatory response to hypothermia is:
a. muscle fasciculation.
b. crying and agitation.
c. increased metabolism.
d. peripheral vasoconstriction.

7.54 Heparin is an anticoagulant that:
a. in high doses dissolves established clots.
b. cannot be effectively reversed.
c. disrupts platelet production.
d. inhibits circulating coagulation factors.

7.55 Based on the third-space concept and documentation of adequate replacement of intraoperative fluid losses, important information for the PACU nurse to include in the transfer-of-care report is the:
a. potential for fluid overload as third-space fluid shifts back to the extracellular fluid (ECF) compartment.
b. postoperative hemoglobin and hematocrit values.
c. most recent electrolyte panel results.
d. number of available units of reserved blood products.

7.56 A shift to the right in the oxyhemoglobin curve for a hyperthermic, acidotic patient indicates that:
a. there is less circulating hydrogen ions in the blood.

b. oxygen loading of the hemoglobin is decreased.
c. a lower pH increased hemoglobin saturation.
d. pH compensation will decrease oxygen saturation.

7.57 Which of the following statements is **true** regarding anesthesia concerns in patients undergoing transplantation of the pancreas?
a. Serum potassium levels remain fairly constant when glucose levels are well controlled.
b. Immunosuppressive agents are administered before graft reperfusion is facilitated.
c. Risk of aspiration is lower in this patient population.
d. End-stage renal disease patients receive succinylcholine for muscular maintenance blockade.

7.58 Low-molecular-weight heparin is:
a. an alternate to warfarin for prevention of deep vein thrombosis.
b. contraindicated within 24 hours of total joint replacement.
c. the oral delivery form of heparin.
d. used in weight-based heparin protocols.

7.59 On arrival to the PACU a patient has a temperature of 36° C (96.8° F). The perianesthesia nurse would institute the following interventions **except:**
a. increase ambient temperature.
b. assess temperature on admission and before discharge.
c. initiate active warming measures.
d. apply passive insulation.

7.60 To assess for erythrocyte sickling, the PACU nurse observes the patient for which of the following?
a. Bleeding from the site used for intraoperative epidural anesthesia

b. Abdominal pain and neurovascular changes in extremities
c. Muscle fasciculations and decreased consciousness
d. Unrelenting postoperative nausea and vomiting

7.61 After removal of the parathyroid glands, the PACU nurse can anticipate all of the following *except*:
a. rapid administration of calcium chloride to treat tetany.
b. laryngeal spasm.
c. a positive Chvostek's sign.
d. dysrhythmias.

7.62 Peripheral chemoreceptors are *best* described as:
a. the carotid and aortic bodies are located at the proximal end of the carotid artery.
b. peripheral chemoreceptors are made of highly vascular tissue and glomerular cells.
c. the carotid bodies are more physiologically important than the aortic bodies.
d. the aortic bodies respond to pH.

7.63 The anesthetist reports that no nondepolarizing muscle relaxants were administered during surgery. During assessment of a postanesthesia patient, the nurse notes flaccid paralysis that mimics nondepolarizing muscular blockade. Which of the following conditions can these signs be attributed?
a. Hypocalcemia
b. Hypercalcemia
c. Hypermagnesia
d. Hypernatremia

7.64 In 1999 The Joint Commission (formerly JCAHO) (TJC) issued a Sentinel Event alert on "Blood Transfusion Errors: Preventing Future Occurrences." Suggested strategies for reducing transfusion risks include all the following *except:*
a. educating staff on transfusion-related procedures.
b. limiting dependence on computer support.

c. changing the process of patient identification and blood verification procedures.
d. prohibiting simultaneous cross matching of multiple patients by the same technologist.

7.65 After the administration of 4 units of subcutaneous regular insulin for a serum glucose of 319 mg/dL, the nurse anticipates that the peak effect of this insulin dose is expected within:
a. ½ to 1 hour.
b. 1 to 2 hours.
c. 1 to 3 hours.
d. 2 to 4 hours.

7.66 While assessing perianesthesia risk in an elderly patient, the preanesthesia nurse obtains information about preexisting diseases and reviews laboratory results. Regarding laboratory analysis for an elderly patient, the nurse understands all of the following to be true *except:*
a. serum sodium levels may be elevated because of decreased antidiuretic hormone output.
b. glucose levels may be affected.
c. potassium levels can be lower because of diuretic medication use.
d. low hemoglobin levels are fairly common.

7.67 Leukocytosis is:
a. a normal response to inflammation.
b. an indication of bone marrow suppression.
c. a process to remove leukocytes from blood.
d. the maturation process of white blood cells.

NOTE: Consider items 7.68-7.69 together.

7.68 Arterial blood gas values of pH = 7.22, $PaCO_2 = 49$ mmHg, $PaO_2 = 89$ mmHg, and $HCO_3 = 14$ mEq/L are indicative of:
a. mixed and uncompensated metabolic and respiratory acidosis.
b. simultaneous and partially corrected respiratory and metabolic acidosis.

c. partially compensated metabolic acidosis with respiratory alkalosis.

d. mixed and uncompensated respiratory alkalosis with metabolic acidosis.

7.69 The nurse can anticipate all the following measures to treat these blood gases *except:*

a. administration of sodium bicarbonate.

b. increase in supplemental oxygen levels.

c. laboratory analysis of electrolytes.

d. increased emphasis on deep breathing.

7.70 The preservatives in blood products:

a. provide a 60-day "shelf life" for donated blood.

b. maintain the hematocrit of packed RBCs between 36% and 45%.

c. have the potential to cause electrolyte imbalance.

d. may prolong the bleeding time of the recipient.

SET 1

7.1	a
7.2	b
7.3	a
7.4	c
7.5	c
7.6	c
7.7	c
7.8	b
7.9	a
7.10.	c
7.11.	d

7.12.	d
7.13.	b
7.14.	c
7.15.	b
7.16.	d
7.17.	b
7.18.	a
7.19.	b
7.20.	c
7.21.	b
7.22.	d

SET 1

7.1. Correct Answer: **a**
Aldosterone, released from the adrenal cortex in response to decreased sodium or increased potassium levels, triggers the kidneys to reabsorb more sodium and excrete more potassium. The effect of this mineralocorticoid release is conservation of water and sodium, an increase in blood pressure, and prevention of acidosis. Adverse effects include a decrease in organ perfusion and systemic vasoconstriction. (Quinn D, Schick L, editors: *ASPAN's perianesthesia nursing core curriculum: preoperative, Phase I and Phase II PACU nursing*, Philadelphia, 2004, Saunders.)

7.2. Correct Answer: **b**
The healthy body will self-regulate to maintain normal acid-base parameters, although acid-base changes are common in the perianesthesia patient population. Many factors can impact chemical balance such as acute or chronic illness, anesthetic effects, and surgical fluid shifts. Perianesthesia nurses must recognize that acidosis is more likely to occur in the hypoxic and hypothermic patient. In this scenario, the patient with a low temperature and higher oxygen consumption caused by shivering is most at risk for acidosis. Active warming and supplemental oxygenation must be implemented. (Quinn D, Schick L, editors: *ASPAN's perianesthesia nursing core curriculum: preoperative, Phase I and Phase II PACU nursing*, Philadelphia, 2004, Saunders.)

7.3. Correct Answer: **a**
The adrenal glands are located on top of the kidneys and function as a secretory organ for catecholamines released during stress situations, making an adrenalectomy a potentially dangerous procedure. To maintain catecholamine levels and blood pressure levels, cortisone titrations are indicated when bilateral resection is performed. Discontinuation of the cortisone titration in the PACU triggers hypovolemia and hyponatremic shock. Specific postoperative dosing instructions should be provided by the anesthesia provider or the surgeon. (Drain C, editor: *Perianesthesia nursing: a critical care approach*, ed 4, Philadelphia, 2003, Saunders.)

7.4. Correct Answer: **c**
Among the noninfectious serious hazards of transfusions, ABO/Rh incompatibility is the most common cause of transfusion-related morbidity and mortality in the United States. Improved viral screening and donor selection have resulted in a significant decrease in blood transfusion transmission of disease. Transfusion-related acute lung injury (noncardiogenic pulmonary edema) ranks third (behind ABO incompatibility reactions and bacterial contamination) as a cause of transfusion injury. (Hoffman R: *Hematology: basic principles and practice*, ed 4, London, 2005, Churchill Livingstone; Hussain E, Kao E: Medication safety and transfusion errors in the ICU and beyond, *Crit Care Clin* 21[1]:91-110, 2005.)

7.5. Correct Answer: **c**
The PACU nurse must maintain a close watch on the cardiovascular status of the patient since shock and hemorrhage are the most

common complications after adrenalectomy. Removal of the adrenal glands and the subsequent decrease in serum catecholamines compounded by the effects of preoperative antihypertensive medications may produce profound hypotension. This could lead to circulatory shock that the body normally would compensate by releasing catecholamines from the adrenal glands. Hourly electrolyte levels and urine output should be assessed; output of less than 1 mL/kg/hr can indicate a shock state. Preferred positioning for a high abdominal incision is semi-Fowler or on the operative side to help prevent bleeding. (Drain C, editor: *Perianesthesia nursing: a critical care approach*, ed 4, Philadelphia, 2003, Saunders.)

7.6. Correct Answer: **c**
Although composition of electrolytes in each compartment varies, the numeric balance of cations and anions maintains electrical neutrality. Cations have a positive charge and include calcium, magnesium, potassium, and sodium. Anions carry a negative charge and include phosphate, sulphate, chloride, and bicarbonate. Electrolytes occupy a tiny proportion of body weight, yet they are essential to normal body function; therefore assessment of electrolyte levels in the perianesthesia care period based on clinical indication is extremely important. (Drain C, editor: *Perianesthesia nursing: a critical care approach*, ed 4, Philadelphia, 2003, Saunders.)

7.7. Correct Answer: **c**
Hypocalcemia may develop after large volumes of stored blood are rapidly infused. Citrate from the preservative citrate phosphate dextrose (CPD) used in banked blood binds to ionized calcium, thereby reducing circulating unbound calcium. Signs of hypocalcemia include neuromuscular irritability, such as muscle tremors, extremity paresthesias, tingling, or cramps, and cardiac dysrhythmias. A positive Chvostek's sign could also be present. To check for the Chvostek's sign tap around the facial nerve. If an abnormal spasm of the facial muscles occurs then the patient had a positive Chvostek's sign. Potassium shifts among body fluid compartments restore any possible transient hypokalemia related to transfusion. Hyperkalemia is associated with acidosis, not alkalosis. Coffland FI, Sheleton DM: Blood component replacement therapy, *Crit Care Nurs Clin North Am* 5[3]:543-556, 1993; Drain C, editor: *Perianesthesia nursing: a critical care approach*, ed 4, Philadelphia, 2003, Saunders.; Quinn D, Schick L, editors: *ASPAN's perianesthesia nursing core curriculum: preoperative, Phase I and Phase II PACU nursing*, Philadelphia, 2004, Saunders.)

7.8. Correct answer: **b**
Planned perioperative hypothermia is seen in neurosurgical procedures because it decreases both bleeding and intracranial pressure. Planned perioperative hypothermia is also beneficial with cardiac surgery, especially those procedures involving cardiopulmonary bypass since this decreases the oxygen requirements of myocardial cells and reduces metabolic demands. Intentionally-induced hypothermia also has been effective with the management of perinatal asphyxia, acute stroke, severe head injury and neurological outcome after a cardiac arrest. (Quinn D, Schick L, editors: *ASPAN's perianesthesia nursing core curriculum: preoperative, Phase I and Phase II PACU nursing*, Philadelphia, 2004, Saunders.)

7.9. Correct Answer: **a**
Antigens are proteins carried on the surface of RBCs and stimulate antibodies carried in blood serum. Because type O blood is free of antigens, it will not trigger a response from the antibodies carried in A, B or AB blood types. O negative blood is also free of the D antigen called the *Rh factor*. (Bryan S: Hemolytic transfusion reaction: safeguards for practice, *J PeriAnesth Nurs* 17[6]:399-403, 2002.)

7.10. Correct Answer: **c**
Seventy-five percent of TBW is contained in a child's ECF. ECF circulates outside of cells and includes the intravascular fluid within plasma, as well as interstitial fluid. Between 33%-40% of an adult's TBW is contained in their ECF. Anesthetic medications expand the ECF through dilation of vasculature. Consideration of fluid spacing in children and adults is important for management of fluid replacement infusions. (Quinn D, Schick L, editors: *ASPAN's perianesthesia nursing core curriculum: preoperative, Phase I and Phase II PACU nursing*, Philadelphia, 2004, Saunders.)

7.11. Correct Answer: **d**
Neither Medicare nor the American Society of Anesthesiologists has routine preoperative testing requirements. Each supports the use of the preoperative CBC when indicated by a patient's age, history, risks, and complexity of the surgical procedure. The CBC reports information about the components of blood and is not selective for coagulation disorders. (American Society of Anesthesiologists: *Statement on routine preoperative laboratory and diagnostic screening* (amended October 2003). Website: www.asahq.org/publicationsandservices/standards/28.pdf. Accessed

November 2, 2005; George-Gay B: Understanding the complete blood count with differential, *J PeriAnesth Nurs* 18[2]:96-117, 2003.)

7.12. Correct Answer: **d**
A $PaCO_2$ above the normal range is characteristic of acute respiratory acidosis, whereas all other causes of acidosis tend to be metabolic in nature. To determine respiratory system acidosis, assess for an acute rise in $PaCO_2$ with a corresponding decrease in pH and a normal HCO_3 level. (Drain C, editor: *Perianesthesia nursing: a critical care approach*, ed 4, Philadelphia, 2003, Saunders; Quinn D, Schick L, editors: *ASPAN's perianesthesia nursing core curriculum: preoperative, Phase I and Phase II PACU nursing*, Philadelphia, 2004, Saunders.)

7.13. Correct Answer: **b**
Causes of respiratory acidosis include neuromuscular blocking agents, general anesthesia, hypothermia, airway obstruction, constrictive dressings, increased intracranial pressure, restlessness and apprehension, and pain. A lack of opioid administration would not contribute to slow, shallow breathing found in respiratory acidosis. (Ireland D, editor: *Redi-Ref 2004: ambulatory/PACU/pediatric*, Cherry Hill, NJ, 2004, ASPAN.)

7.14. Correct Answer: **c**
Hypoventilation is the primary cause of acute respiratory acidosis. Although the other nursing actions listed are prudent, by initiating a stir-up regimen and instructing and reminding the patient to breathe deeply, the CO_2 level will decrease and the pH will become less acidic. (Quinn D, Schick L, editors: *ASPAN's perianesthesia nursing core curriculum*

preoperative, Phase I and Phase II PACU nursing, Philadelphia, 2004, Saunders.)

7.15. Correct Answer: **b**
The primary goal of transfusing packed RBCs is to improve oxygen transport to tissues. No specific hemoglobin level is used as the sole indicator for blood transfusion. Packed cells do not contain clotting factors or influence their production. (Drain C, editor: *Perianesthesia nursing: a critical care approach*, ed 4, Philadelphia, 2003, Saunders; Quinn D, Schick L, editors: *ASPAN's perianesthesia nursing core curriculum: preoperative, Phase I and Phase II PACU nursing*, Philadelphia, 2004, Saunders.)

7.16. Correct Answer: **d**
Spontaneous voiding is highly preferable to urinary catheterization in the type 1 diabetic population to avoid the risk of urinary tract infection. Autonomic neuropathy of the bladder can increase the incidence of anesthesia-related voiding difficulty. If urinary catheterization is required, this must be performed under strict aseptic technique. Gastroparesis is a reduced motility of the esophagus and intestines often found in type 1 diabetics. This condition causes pooling of gastric contents, thereby increasing the risk of aspiration in the perianesthesia period. Peripheral neuropathy decreases awareness of pressure and pain in a diabetic patient's extremities, which can complicate the assessment and reporting of postoperative pain. (Quinn D, Schick L, editors: *ASPAN's perianesthesia nursing core curriculum: preoperative, Phase I and Phase II PACU nursing*, Philadelphia, 2004, Saunders.)

7.17. Correct Answer: **b**
Hemoglobin and hematocrit levels are parallel. For each unit of packed RBCs, the expected rise in Hgb is 1 g and the Hct 3%. (George-Gay B: Understanding the complete blood count with differential, *J PeriAnesth Nurs* 18[2]: 96-117, 2003.)

7.18. Correct Answer: **a**
Usual preoperative management for the type 1 diabetic patient undergoing elective surgery includes a 12-lead ECG interpretation and cardiac history assessment; serum glucose and acetone analysis; BUN and serum creatinine analysis and assessment of urinary output; and instructions regarding insulin dosage on the day of surgery. The urine glucose concentration offers a late indicator of serum glucose level and is less desirable than a serum glucose evaluation. Although clinicians may differ on how to manage preoperative insulin dosages, the usual preoperative course of insulin management includes subcutaneous administration of half the daily dosage of intermediate-acting insulin on the morning of surgery for an early morning case or one third of the daily dosage of intermediate-acting insulin for a surgery scheduled later in the day. (Drain C, editor: *Perianesthesia nursing: a critical care approach*, ed 4, Philadelphia, 2003, Saunders; Ireland D, editor: *Redi-Ref 2004: ambulatory/PACU/pediatric*, Cherry Hill, NJ, 2004, ASPAN; Quinn D, Schick L, editors: *ASPAN's perianesthesia nursing core curriculum: preoperative, Phase I and Phase II PACU nursing*, Philadelphia, 2004, Saunders.)

7.19. Correct Answer: **b**
Thyroid storm, or thyrotoxic crisis, is caused by a rapid rise in

circulating thyroid hormone levels. The mortality rate when left untreated is about 70%. Symptoms of this crisis can be confused with those of malignant hyperthermia, and they include profuse sweating; tachycardia; hyperthermia; agitation, delirium, convulsions, psychosis, and coma; atrial fibrillation; tachypnea; congestive heart failure; and hypertension followed by hypotension. (Quinn D, Schick L, editors: *ASPAN's perianesthesia nursing core curriculum: preoperative, Phase I and Phase II PACU nursing*, Philadelphia, 2004, Saunders.)

7.20. Correct Answer: **c**
FFP contains all coagulation factors except platelets and is used specifically to correct coagulation abnormalities. Serum albumin, 5% or 25%, is a blood component used for acute volume expansion and management of hypovolemia. Fluid therapy with crystalloid solutions rather than blood components is initiated for acute blood loss. Thrombocytopenia is a reduction in platelets, and transfusion of platelet concentrates is a specific therapy. (Drain C, editor: *Perianesthesia nursing: a critical care approach*, ed 4, Philadelphia, 2003, Saunders; Quinn D, Schick L, editors: *ASPAN's perianesthesia nursing core curriculum: preoperative, Phase I and Phase II PACU nursing*, Philadelphia, 2004, Saunders.)

7.21. Correct Answer: **b**
Several autonomic controls, including thermoregulation, are based in the hypothalamus. Feedback relays between thermoreceptors in the hypothalamus and skin detect thermal variations and alter metabolism, blood vessel size, sweat production, and muscular movements (shivering) to balance heating and cooling. The medulla oblongata joins the spinal cord and pons to form the brainstem; motor and sensory relays and involuntary cardiopulmonary regulation occur here. The hypophysis refers to pituitary, glandular activity. (Hudak CM et al: *Critical care nursing: a holistic approach*, ed 6, Philadelphia, 1994, Lippincott; Stalheim-Smith A, Fitch GK: *Understanding human anatomy and physiology*, Belmont, Calif, 1993, Wadsworth.)

7.22. Correct Answer: **d**
There are no differences in policies between allogenic and autologous blood transfusions. Recommended transfusion practice includes replacing blood tubing and filter after every 2 units of cells. The filter of a blood administration set can clog. A large-gauge needle (16-18 gauge) and normal saline, never water, are used to prevent hemolysis. As the patient pre-donated their own blood, compatibility reactions are unlikely unless identification errors mismatch blood or patient. Monitor vital signs and temperature after the first 50 mL of each unit of blood has infused to detect blood reactions. Autologous blood is subject to the same administration requirements as any other banked blood as there remains a potential for clerical error during processing of the blood. Patients who have had seizures or have an active infection cannot donate autologous blood. (Drain C, editor: *Perianesthesia nursing: a critical care approach*, ed 4, Philadelphia, 2003, Saunders; Quinn D, Schick L, editors: *ASPAN's perianesthesia nursing core curriculum: preoperative, Phase I and Phase II PACU nursing*, Philadelphia, 2004, Saunders.)

SET 2

7.23.	b		**7.38.**	d
7.24.	a		**7.39.**	b
7.25.	d		**7.40.**	d
7.26.	a		**7.41.**	b
7.27.	c		**7.42.**	a
7.28.	b		**7.43.**	a
7.29.	b		**7.44.**	a
7.30.	d		**7.45.**	c
7.31.	c		**7.46.**	d
7.32.	d		**7.47.**	c
7.33.	c		**7.48.**	b
7.34.	a		**7.49.**	d
7.35.	c		**7.50.**	c
7.36.	d		**7.51.**	a
7.37.	c			

SET 2

RATIONALES AND REFERENCES

7.23. Correct Answer: **b**
The production of red blood cells is stimulated by low oxygen levels in peritubular cells of the kidney. In this process, a renal enzyme interacts with a plasma protein to form the hormone *erythropoietin*; the hormone then circulates to the bone marrow and stimulates production of red blood cells. (George-Gay B: Understanding the complete blood count with differential, *J PeriAnesth Nurs* 18[2]:96-117, 2003.)

7.24. Correct Answer: **a**
A hypophysectomy procedure involves the pituitary gland. Hyposecretion of the anterior pituitary gland decreases thyroid-stimulating hormone (TSH) and adrenocorticotropic hormone (ACTH). The physiologic results of hyposecretion of the involved pituitary hormones include bradycardia, intolerance to hypothermia, and decreased anesthetic agent requirements related to hypothyroidism. (Quinn D, Schick L, editors: *ASPAN's perianesthesia nursing core curriculum: preoperative, Phase I and Phase II PACU nursing*, Philadelphia, 2004, Saunders.)

7.25. Correct Answer: **d**
A common operative approach for a hypophysectomy procedure is either by using the transsphenoidal approach (making an incision in front of the hard palate inside the superior upper lip) or by performing a frontal craniotomy. This procedure is performed to treat primary pituitary disease and tumors and as a palliative treatment measure in prostate and breast cancer. (Quinn D, Schick L, editors: *ASPAN's perianesthesia nursing*

core curriculum: preoperative, Phase I and Phase II PACU nursing, Philadelphia, 2004, Saunders.)

7.26. Correct Answer: **a**
One of the spleen's functions is to disintegrate old or damaged RBCs. The process frees hemoglobin, which the liver converts into bilirubin; bilirubin is then taken up by liver cells and is eventually excreted in bile. (Drain C, editor: *Perianesthesia nursing: a critical care approach*, ed 4, Philadelphia, 2003, Saunders; Quinn D, Schick L, editors: *ASPAN's perianesthesia nursing core curriculum: preoperative, Phase I and Phase II PACU nursing*, Philadelphia, 2004, Saunders.)

7.27. Correct Answer: **c**
Pulse oximetry measures the ratio of oxygenated hemoglobin to total hemoglobin and expresses the ratio in a saturation percentage. This technology is now a standard monitoring tool in postanesthesia units. Motion at the sensor site, interference from electrical or light sources, hypotension and low perfusion of the arterial bed, significant dysrhythmias, and severe anemia can alter the accuracy of readings. Readings in the 70% to 100% range are considered an accurate comparison to arterial blood gases. (Burden N et al: *Ambulatory surgical nursing*, ed 2, Philadelphia, 2000, Saunders.)

7.28. Correct Answer: **b**
Surgery produces a physiologic stress response that promotes increased serum glucose levels resulting from secretion of epinephrine and cortisol. An elevated blood sugar results from the stress

response and resultant hormonal action. The perianesthesia goal is to maintain a serum glucose level of less than 200 mg/dL and to prevent hypoglycemia. Preoperative and intraoperative hydration with 1000 mL of 5% dextrose solution in water is recommended to prevent a hypoglycemic event, and use of the dextrose-based solution should cue the PACU nurse to be observant of postoperative serum glucose levels. (Drain C, editor: *Perianesthesia nursing: a critical care approach*, ed 4, Philadelphia, 2003, Saunders.)

7.29. Correct Answer: **b**
The parathyroid glands, located on the posterior aspect of the thyroid gland, release parathormone via a negative feedback process dependent on serum calcium concentration. Low calcium levels trigger parathormone release, whereas a high serum calcium concentration will suppress production. Other calcium regulatory mechanisms include magnesium, phosphorus, vitamin D, and calcitonin, but parathormone action serves as the principal regulator of serum calcium. (Drain C, editor: *Perianesthesia nursing: a critical care approach*, ed 4, Philadelphia, 2003, Saunders.)

7.30. Correct Answer: **d**
Bone marrow suppression, autoimmune disease, and endocrine insufficiency can all affect red blood cell production and cause anemia, but this patient's medical condition is caused by an inherited genetic trait. Sickled cells are subject to destruction in the circulatory system and have a life expectancy of 20 days or less (versus 120 days for normal red blood cells), resulting in chronic anemia. (Quinn D, Schick L, editors: *ASPAN's perianesthesia nursing core curriculum: preoperative, Phase I and Phase II*

PACU nursing, Philadelphia, 2004, Saunders.)

7.31. Correct Answer: **c**
Fluid administration to prevent dehydration and decrease viscosity of the blood is an appropriate intervention. Intraoperative management of a patient with sickle cell disease is aimed at preventing hypoxia or increased oxygen consumption because deoxygenation of red blood cells causes defective hemoglobin to distort the shape of affected red blood cells. The misshapen, or "sickled," cells loose their normal flexibility and become wedged in the capillary bed, occluding normal flow and increasing blood viscosity. The result is localized tissue hypoxia and possible tissue or organ infarct. Common sickling triggers are dehydration, stress, pain, cold, infection, hypoventilation, or acidosis. Because of the possibility of hypotension (another precipitating factor), spinal anesthesia and vasodilators should be avoided. Temperature monitoring and thermoregulation devices to maintain optimal body temperature between 36° and 37° C are preferred. (Drain C, editor: *Perianesthesia nursing: a critical care approach*, ed 4, Philadelphia, 2003, Saunders; Goss J: Blood disorders: sickle cell disease and leukemia—more similar than you may think, *JEMS* 28[10]:72-84, 2003.)

7.32. Correct Answer: **d**
Respiratory alkalosis occurs when there is hyperventilation of the alveoli with oversecretion of carbonic acid as the respiratory rate increases from a normal range. Clinical causes include pain, panic, anxiety, excessive mechanical ventilation, surgical manipulation of the brainstem, and tumors of the medulla and pons. This condition

is a normal finding in pregnant women. (Quinn D, Schick L, editors: *ASPAN's perianesthesia nursing core curriculum: preoperative, Phase I and Phase II PACU nursing*, Philadelphia, 2004, Saunders.)

7.33. Correct Answer: **c**

A patient on long-term steroid therapy experiences suppressed cortisone production and adrenocortical insufficiency. The incapacity to generate endogenous adrenocorticoids can cause a limited response to surgical stressors impacting heart rate and blood pressure regulatory ability. Patients on long-term steroid management should be given an increase in oral dosage the day before surgery, and an IV hydrocortisone phosphate infusion should be available during the intraoperative period and in the PACU to treat signs of acute adrenal insufficiency. Dexamethasone, an incomplete corticosteroid, is contraindicated because it is inadequate for replacement use. (Quinn D, Schick L, editors: *ASPAN's perianesthesia nursing core curriculum: preoperative, Phase I and Phase II PACU nursing*, Philadelphia, 2004, Saunders.)

7.34. Correct Answer: **a**

Hypertonic IV solutions cause water to move from the cell to the serum and have an osmolality higher than 340 mOsm/L. The movement of water to the serum assists in maintaining circulating blood volume. Hypertonic solutions are more concentrated in the extracellular fluid, and these solutions include D_5 in lactated Ringer's, D_5 in 0.5 normal saline, and D_{10} in water. (Quinn D, Schick L, editors: *ASPAN's perianesthesia nursing core curriculum: preoperative, Phase I and Phase II PACU nursing*, Philadelphia, 2004, Saunders.)

7.35. Correct Answer: **c**

Guidelines for men's normal ranges are Hgb, 14 to 18 g/dL; and Hct, 40% to 52%. The patient's hemoglobin and hematocrit are below normal ranges but not at crisis levels in an otherwise stable patient. The crystalloid volume to replace blood loss is usually 3 to 5 mL for each 1 mL of blood loss, and the amount of lactated Ringer's given to this patient may have caused a relative anemia secondary to hemodilution. Further volume expansion may not be indicated for this patient. (Drain C, editor: *Perianesthesia nursing: a critical care approach*, ed 4, Philadelphia, 2003, Saunders; Quinn D, Schick L, editors: *ASPAN's perianesthesia nursing core curriculum: preoperative, Phase I and Phase II PACU nursing*, Philadelphia, 2004, Saunders.)

7.36. Correct Answer: **d**

Using a blood warmer to quickly deliver multiple units of blood maintains body temperature, decreases vasoconstriction and acidosis, and may facilitate movement of potassium into cells. Rapid infusion of cold, stored red blood cells both vasoconstricts and promotes hypothermia. Blood must not be overheated because cells can hemolyze. Warming blood has no effect on occurrence of febrile reactions to blood. (Drain C, editor: *Perianesthesia nursing: a critical care approach*, ed 4, Philadelphia, 2003, Saunders; Litwack K: *Core curriculum for post anesthesia nursing practice*, ed 3, Philadelphia, 1995, Saunders.)

7.37. Correct answer: **c**

Dantrolene (dantrium) is the drug of choice in the treatment of MH. This drug is supplied in 20-mg vials and must be reconstituted with 60 ml of preservative-free sterile water and then shaken vigorously. The recommended dose of dantrolene is 2.5mg/kg body weight up to 10mg/kg. However if the crisis is not well controlled this dosage can be exceeded. (Quinn D, Schick L, editors: *ASPAN's perianesthesia nursing core curriculum: preoperative, Phase I and Phase II PACU nursing*, Philadelphia, 2004, Saunders)

7.38. Correct Answer: **d**
Leukocytes (white blood cells [WBCs]), are produced in bone marrow and carried in blood to the site of cell injury. Increased capillary permeability allows WBCs to pass into the interstitial spaces where they can phagocytize unwanted organisms and debris. (George-Gay B: Understanding the complete blood count with differential, *J PeriAnesth Nurs* 18[2]:96-117, 2003.)

7.39. Correct Answer: **b**
Polycythemia is an exaggeration of red blood cells, hemoglobin, hematocrit, or white blood cells. Causes may be normal adaptive responses, such as increased production of RBCs in people living at high altitudes or elevated WBCs in response to infection. Leukemia is a pathologic condition of excessive WBC proliferation. Vitamin B_{12} deficiency is a causative factor in pernicious anemia resulting in *lowered* amounts of RBCs. (Quinn D, Schick L, editors: *ASPAN's perianesthesia nursing core curriculum: preoperative, Phase I and Phase II PACU nursing*, Philadelphia, 2004, Saunders.)

7.40. Correct Answer: **d**
Endocrine changes in the elderly population result in reduced pancreatic function and glucose intolerance; decreased renin, aldosterone, and testosterone production; decreased absorption of vitamin D; and an increased plasma concentration of antidiuretic hormone. The elderly are more prone to develop type 2 diabetes mellitus and experience the greatest decline in pancreatic function between ages 60 and 70 years. (Quinn D, Schick L, editors: *ASPAN's perianesthesia nursing core curriculum: preoperative, Phase I and Phase II PACU nursing*, Philadelphia, 2004, Saunders.)

7.41. Correct Answer: **b**
Neuromuscular transmission involves impulse conduction along muscle fibers and the movement of acetylcholine, a chemical neurotransmitter, across the synaptic cleft. Acetylcholine is involved in the initiation of muscle contraction. Serum calcium deficiency is of concern when administering muscle relaxants because a calcium deficit prolongs effect of nondepolarizing neuromuscular blocking agents by decreasing acetylcholine release, and neuromuscular transmission is inhibited. Hypocalcemia also promotes depolarization, which acts to strengthen a depolarizing neuromuscular blocking agent. (Drain C, editor: *Perianesthesia nursing: a critical care approach*, ed 4, Philadelphia, 2003, Saunders.)

7.42. Correct Answer: **a**
Leukemia occurs in adults much more frequently than in children, and acute myelocytic leukemia (AML) is the most common adult form of the disease, accounting for 80% of adult leukemias. Acute lymphocytic leukemia (ALL) is the most common leukemia for children younger than 19 years, but the incidence of the disease is less than adult forms of leukemia. Both chronic myelocytic leukemia (CML) and chronic lymphocytic leukemia (CLL) are diseases that affect primarily adults and occur with increasing frequency after the age of 50 years. (The Leukemia &

Lymphoma Society: *Leukemia facts and statistics* (update August 2005). Website: www.leukemia-lymphoma.org/all_page?item_id=9346. Accessed November 2, 2005; Quinn D, Schick L, editors: *ASPAN's perianesthesia nursing core curriculum: preoperative, Phase I and Phase II PACU nursing*, Philadelphia, 2004, Saunders.)

7.43. Correct Answer: **a**
Hypercalcemia can result from a low PO_4 level, hyperparathyroidism, immobility, and malignancy. Healthy preoperative/pre-procedural patients are mildly dehydrated resulting from fasting and duration of NPO status, and the bowel preparation causes dehydration from fluid loss and hypokalemia related to electrolyte loss. Apprehension and stress with related cortisol release and a lack of sleep can contribute to feelings of physical weakness. (Quinn D, Schick L, editors: *ASPAN's perianesthesia nursing core curriculum: preoperative, Phase I and Phase II PACU nursing*, Philadelphia, 2004, Saunders.)

7.44. Correct Answer: **a**
Acute adrenal insufficiency, or Addisonian crisis, results from suppression of the adrenal axis. This situation is critical; therefore the PACU nurse must recognize clinical symptoms related to adrenal insufficiency in order to take rapid corrective action. Early clinical symptoms of Addisonian crisis include nausea and vomiting, hypotension, and muscular weakness. These early symptoms progress to hyperthermia, hypokalemia and hyponatremia, flaccid extremity muscles, azotemia, and shock. (Drain C, editor: *Perianesthesia nursing: a critical care approach*, ed 4, Philadelphia, 2003, Saunders.)

7.45. Correct Answer: **c**
Warfarin reduces the production of vitamin K–dependent coagulation factors resulting in anticoagulation. Administration of vitamin K is one intervention to restore the coagulation pathway, or in emergent situations, fresh frozen plasma can be given to replace inadequate clotting factors. Because warfarin's duration of effect is approximately 40 hours, postponement for 1 day would not reduce risks of intraoperative or postoperative bleeding. Warfarin does not influence platelet function, and infusion of platelets is not indicated. The INR/PT is the specific monitor for warfarin effects. The PTT monitors the effects of heparin. (Horton JD, Bushwick BM: Warfarin therapy: evolving strategies in anticoagulation, *Am Fam Physician* 59[3]:635-646, 1999; Quinn D, Schick L, editors: *ASPAN's perianesthesia nursing core curriculum: preoperative, Phase I and Phase II PACU nursing*, Philadelphia, 2004, Saunders.)

7.46. Correct Answer: **d**
When adrenal insufficiency signs and symptoms appear, the PACU nurse must immediately inform the physician responsible for the patient's care. A severely ill patient requires rapid treatment as substantiation of the Addisonian crisis diagnosis is being made. Intravenous dexamethasone is administered in a 2- to 4-mg dose via 5% dextrose in normal saline solution. Dexamethasone is the drug of choice because it provides necessary glucocorticoid coverage while not hindering diagnostic testing performed to confirm the diagnosis. (Drain C, editor: *Perianesthesia nursing: a critical care approach*, ed 4, Philadelphia, 2003, Saunders.)

7.47. Correct Answer: **c**

A nonrebreathing oxygen (O_2) mask can deliver an FiO_2 level higher than 80. For maximum effectiveness, the O_2 flow rate must be set at 15 L/min or higher. The leaflet valves should not close both exhalation ports because of the risk of suffocation. One exhalation port should remain open to allow for CO_2 escape. (Quinn D, Schick L, editors: *ASPAN's perianesthesia nursing core curriculum: preoperative, Phase I and Phase II PACU nursing*, Philadelphia, 2004, Saunders.)

7.48. Correct Answer: **b**

Diabetic acidosis in the postoperative diabetic patient can result from decreased insulin production and increased stress hormone production. Symptoms include elevated serum levels of potassium, acetone, and glucose; tachypnea, polyuria, tachycardia, and hypotension; an increase in serum osmolarity; elevated BUN, and a decrease in serum pH. Treatment includes fluid volume replacement and correction of the electrolyte balance. Insulin is administered to control serum glucose levels, and if the pH is acidic, bicarbonate may be administered to correct the pH level. (Quinn D, Schick L, editors: *ASPAN's perianesthesia nursing core curriculum: preoperative, Phase I and Phase II PACU nursing*, Philadelphia, 2004, Saunders.)

7.49. Correct Answer: **d**

In a hyperthyroid state, the patient's temperature may show an increase from normal because of the hypermetabolic condition. An elevated temperature presents the greatest concern during the perianesthesia period because of increased oxygen requirements, so intraoperative hyperthermia is aggressively treated. Routine preoperative thyroidectomy care focuses on control of hypertension and tachycardia encountered in a hyperdynamic cardiovascular state; preoperative patient education; creating a euthyroid state in the weeks before surgery through administration of antithyroid medications; and administering adequate sedation to counterbalance hyperactivity. (Quinn D, Schick L, editors: *ASPAN's perianesthesia nursing core curriculum: preoperative, Phase I and Phase II PACU nursing*, Philadelphia, 2004, Saunders.)

7.50. Correct Answer: **c**

Damage to the laryngeal nerve can impair the patient's ability to vocalize and swallow; therefore the nurse performs recurrent assessments of the ability to swallow and vocal quality in the postoperative period. Airway assessment for respiratory distress related to hematoma formation and postoperative edema of the glottis is critical. The reacted patient is positioned in semi-Fowler position with neck support, and oxygen is administered by aerosol or high-humidity face tent or mask. In the absence of tear production, artificial tears and lubricating ophthalmic ointment should be administered to protect exophthalmic eyes. (Quinn D, Schick L, editors: *ASPAN's perianesthesia nursing core curriculum: preoperative, Phase I and Phase II PACU nursing*, Philadelphia, 2004, Saunders.)

7.51. Correct Answer: **a**

Neutrophils are white blood cells that respond to acute bacterial infection. In the presence of overwhelming infection, stores of mature neutrophils are depleted and immature cells are released

226

from the bone marrow. Immature red blood cells are called *reticulocytes*; they are released from the bone marrow in large numbers in response to sudden RBC loss from hemorrhage or destruction and are not a measure of coagulation. Pernicious anemia, caused by insufficient vitamin B_{12}, is a condition of inadequate RBC *production*, not RBC *immaturity*. (George-Gay B: Understanding the complete blood count with differential, *J PeriAnesth Nurs* 18[2]:96-117, 2003; Quinn D, Schick L, editors: *ASPAN's perianesthesia nursing core curriculum: preoperative, Phase I and Phase II PACU nursing*, Philadelphia, 2004, Saunders.)

SET 3

ANSWER KEY

7.52.	c
7.53.	c
7.54.	d
7.55.	a
7.56.	b
7.57.	b
7.58.	a
7.59.	b
7.60.	b
7.61.	a

7.62.	c
7.63.	c
7.64.	b
7.65.	d
7.66.	a
7.67.	a
7.68.	a
7.69.	b
7.70.	c

SET 3

7.52. Correct Answer: **c**
The rate of administration for protamine sulfate should never exceed 50 mg in any 10-minute period. Too-rapid administration can cause anaphylaxis, bradycardia, dyspnea, flushing, sensation of warmth, or severe hypotension. Protamine is ordered to reverse effects of heparin, and dosage is related to the length of time elapsed since the heparin dose. Protamine doses are reduced by as much as one-half if 30 minutes has elapsed since the heparin was given. Giving the dose over ½ hour is not necessary and will not deliver the ordered dose in the optimal time frame. (Gahart BL, Nazareno AR: *Intravenous medications*, ed 21, St. Louis, 2005, Mosby.)

7.53. Correct Answer: **c**
The child's initial response to cold is increased norepinephrine production, which stimulates increased metabolism of brown fat, with lactic acid production. A child's insulating layer of subcutaneous fat is thinner and body surface area is greater than an adult's. Children tend to lose heat quickly because of a decreased body mass, an increased body surface area and the lack of insulating subcutaneous fat. Children will often exhibit mottling because of their immature temperature-regulating mechanism. Infants less than 6 months lack involuntary shivering mechanisms. (Burden N et al: *Ambulatory surgical nursing*, ed 2, Philadelphia, 2000, Saunders; Drain C, editor: *Perianesthesia nursing: a critical care approach*, ed 4, Philadelphia, 2003, Saunders; Quinn D, Schick L, editors: *ASPAN's perianesthesia nursing*

core curriculum: preoperative, Phase I and Phase II PACU nursing, Philadelphia, 2004, Saunders.)

7.54. Correct Answer: **d**
Heparin interrupts the *intrinsic* coagulation pathway (where factors to initiate clotting mechanism are found in the circulation) versus the *extrinsic* pathway (where clot formation is triggered by tissue injury). Heparin prolongs bleeding by reducing platelets' ability to stick together but has no influence on their production. Heparin does not dissolve well-established clots but may dissolve newer ones. Protamine sulfate is a heparin antagonist; each 1 mg of protamine neutralizes approximately 100 units of heparin. (Gahart BL, Nazareno AR: *Intravenous medications*, ed 21, St. Louis, 2005, Mosby; Quinn D, Schick L, editors: *ASPAN's perianesthesia nursing core curriculum: preoperative, Phase I and Phase II PACU nursing*, Philadelphia, 2004, Saunders.)

7.55. Correct Answer: **a**
Fluid accumulation into the third compartment is often referred to as "third spacing." Perioperative signs of hypovolemia reflect blood loss and third space fluid shifts, although the third space losses are hard to distinguish from blood loss. Although the other items are important to include in the transfer-of-care report, the risk of fluid overload is directly related to mobilization of third space fluid back into the ECF compartment or vascular space. (Drain C, editor: *Perianesthesia nursing: a critical care approach*, ed 4, Philadelphia, 2003, Saunders.)

7.56. Correct Answer: **b**
A shift to the right in the oxyhemoglobin curve means that oxygen loading of the hemoglobin is decreased. The oxygen-hemoglobin association portion of this curve is influenced by several factors, including temperature and pH. A temperature increase and the higher level of hydrogen ions associated with a decrease in pH alter the height and slope of the curve, thus shifting the curve to the right. This process leads to less loading or saturation of hemoglobin for an existing PaO_2 level. Increasing the patient's FiO_2 can help facilitate an improved hemoglobin saturation level, but this should be done only after arterial blood gases are drawn and analyzed. (Drain C, editor: *Perianesthesia nursing: a critical care approach*, ed 4, Philadelphia, 2003, Saunders.)

7.57. Correct Answer: **b**
Transplantation of the pancreas is currently the only treatment available for type 1 diabetics to attain a euglycemic condition. Anesthesia concerns in this patient population include rapid induction to prevent aspiration related to gastroparesis; use of atracurium for blockade maintenance in end-stage renal disease patients; induction with succinylcholine if the serum potassium level is within normal range; and vigilant control of serum potassium levels, which are prone to intraoperative variations despite good serum glucose control. Immunosuppressive agents are administered before graft reperfusion is facilitated to promote circulation of the agent before vascular circulation through the donor organ. (Quinn D, Schick L, editors: *ASPAN's perianesthesia nursing core curriculum: preoperative, Phase I and Phase II PACU nursing*, Philadelphia, 2004, Saunders.)

7.58. Correct Answer: **a**
Low-molecular-weight heparin is an anticoagulant/antithrombotic agent used in the prevention of deep vein thrombosis. It is administered subcutaneously and may be given the day of surgery (preoperatively as well as postoperatively). Weight-based heparin protocols are guidelines for determining the intravenous dose of continuous heparin infusions based on the weight of the patient. (Gahart BL, Nazareno AR: *Intravenous medications*, ed 21, St. Louis, 2005, Mosby; Hoffman R: *Hematology: basic principles and practice*, ed 4, London, 2005, Churchill Livingstone; Skidmore-Roth L: *Mosby's 2006 nursing drug reference*, St. Louis, 2006, Mosby.)

7.59. Correct Answer: **b**
This patient is defined as being hypothermic or having a temperature of less than 36° C. Patients who are hypothermic should have their temperature and comfort level assessed at least every 30 minutes until their temperature reaches 36° C (98.6° F), not just on admission and discharge. Interventions that the perianesthesia nurse should do include active warming measures (such as forced-air), apply passive insulation (warm cotton blankets, socks, head covering, reflective blankets, limited skin exposure), increase the ambient room temperature (minimum 68° to 75°), warm IV fluids, humidify and warm oxygen. Hypothermia has been associated with impaired wound healing, patient discomfort, untoward cardiac events, altered drug metabolism, coagulopathy, and increased medical costs. (Quinn D, Schick L, editors: *ASPAN's perianesthesia nursing core curriculum: preoperative, Phase I and Phase II PACU nursing*, Philadelphia, 2004, Saunders.)

7.60. Correct Answer: **b**
The patient is observed for signs of tissue ischemia and organ infarction because vascular occlusion often heralds crisis. Sickling obstructs vessels and produces severe ischemic pain or disrupts function of vital organs, especially the kidneys. Hypoventilation with hypoxemia and potential respiratory acidosis, thermal imbalance, and unrelieved pain, just the factors that prompt a sickle cell crisis, are highly possible during the immediate postanesthesia period. Sickle cell trait is a genetic trait of an estimated 10% of the African-American population and a factor to consider during preanesthesia assessment. (Burden N et al: *Ambulatory surgical nursing*, ed 2, Philadelphia, 2000, Saunders; Drain C, editor: *Perianesthesia nursing: a critical care approach*, ed 4, Philadelphia, 2003, Saunders.)

7.61. Correct Answer: **a**
Surgical removal of the parathyroid glands causes serum calcium levels to fall in the immediate postoperative period. Calcium uptake by bone can contribute to calcium depletion. Tetany results from acute hypocalcemia and decreased parathormone secretion. Symptoms of tetany include laryngeal spasm; positive Chvostek's sign observable by tapping the cheek over the facial nerve to educe muscle twitching; apprehension; a positive Trousseau's sign brought forth by impeded arm circulation from blood pressure cuff constriction resulting in carpopedal spasms; and tingling in the mouth, fingers, and toes. Treatment includes calcium chloride, administered slowly to prevent vein irritation, close observation of dysrhythmias, and vitamin D administration. (Quinn D, Schick L, editors: *ASPAN's perianesthesia nursing core curriculum:*

preoperative, Phase I and Phase II PACU nursing, Philadelphia, 2004, Saunders.)

7.62. Correct Answer: **c**
The carotid and aortic bodies are located at the arch of the aorta and the bifurcation of the common carotid arteries and are composed of highly vascular tissue and glomus cells. They are responsible for immediate ventilatory increase caused by lack of oxygen. The carotid bodies are more physiologically important because they respond, in order of the degree of importance, to decreased PaO_2, elevated PCO_2, and a decrease in pH. (Drain C, editor: *Perianesthesia nursing: a critical care approach*, ed 4, Philadelphia, 2003, Saunders.)

7.63. Correct Answer: **c**
An increased concentration of magnesium is dangerous because it results in flaccid paralysis that is similar to the effect of a nondepolarizing muscular blockade. Magnesium enters the nerve terminal and can decrease calcium volume or prevent calcium from entering, thus acting as a physiologic calcium blocker. This creates stabilization of the postsynaptic membrane. As acetylcholine release becomes more pronounced, a partial neuromuscular blockade occurs. Magnesium is known to boost the neuromuscular block produced by succinylcholine to a less significant degree. (Drain C, editor: *Perianesthesia nursing: a critical care approach*, ed 4, Philadelphia, 2003, Saunders.)

7.64. Correct Answer: **b**
TJC cites "human intervention" as a risk factor contributing to transfusion errors and recommends introducing a computerized verification step into the process of patient identification. TJC describes the

steps required for administration of blood products as a process "...that require(s) a higher level of consistency than is reasonably achievable by health care workers without computer support." Staff education and improved patient identification are suggested strategies for reducing risk. The prohibition of simultaneous cross matching of multiple patients by the same technologist is a specific action aimed at reducing error. (Joint Commission International Center for Patient Safety: *Sentinel Event alert issue 10: blood transfusion errors: preventing future occurrences*. Website: www.jcipatientsafety.org/14784/. Accessed June 20, 2007.)

7.65. Correct Answer: **d**
A patient's serum glucose should be monitored soon after arrival in the PACU because serum levels provide the most precise evidence of insulin requirements. Urine acetone and glucose levels reflect less current serum levels and may yield poor control of blood sugar levels. Regular insulin has an onset of action 30 minutes after administration, with peak action occurring between 2 and 4 hours. The duration of action is from 4 to 8 hours. (Quinn D, Schick L, editors: *ASPAN's perianesthesia nursing core curriculum: preoperative, Phase I and Phase II PACU nursing*, Philadelphia, 2004, Saunders.)

7.66. Correct Answer: **a**
Perianesthesia risk assessment in the elderly population should be based on known physiologic processes. The elderly experience increased plasma concentrations of antidiuretic hormone resulting in an inability to conserve sodium, leading to lower serum sodium levels, or hyponatremia. Assessment of glucose levels is important because serum blood sugar can be affected by a decline in pancreatic function, poor nutritional intake, and diabetic medication use. Non–potassium-sparing diuretic medications used in the treatment of hypertension and cardiac conditions may result in serum potassium losses, or hypokalemia. Anemia is a common finding in the elderly population, and they should be assessed preoperatively. (Quinn D, Schick L, editors: *ASPAN's perianesthesia nursing core curriculum: preoperative, Phase I and Phase II PACU nursing*, Philadelphia, 2004, Saunders.)

7.67. Correct Answer: **a**
Leukocytosis is an elevation in the white blood cell (WBC) count to greater than $11,000/mm^3$. It is part of the normal response to inflammation. Bone marrow suppression results in *leukopenia*, a decrease in the total WBC count to less than $4500/mm^3$. *Leukapheresis* is the process to remove WBCs from whole blood. (George-Gay B: Understanding the complete blood count with differential, *J PeriAnesth Nurs* 18[2]:96-117, 2003; *Taber's Cyclopedic Medical Dictionary*, ed 20, Philadelphia, 2005, FA Davis.)

7.68. Correct Answer: **a**
This patient's blood gas shows mixed and uncompensated metabolic and respiratory acidosis. Although the PaO_2 indicates adequate oxygenation, the pH of 7.22 and the elevated $PaCO_2$ of 49 mmHg reveal acidosis. The presence of a low HCO_3 (14 mEq/L) indicates metabolic acidosis. (Quinn D, Schick L, editors: *ASPAN's perianesthesia nursing core curriculum: preoperative, Phase I and Phase II PACU nursing*, Philadelphia, 2004, Saunders.)

7.69. Correct Answer: **b**
In acidosis, an abnormal increase of acids is within the body because of

increased hydrogen ions or loss of base or bicarbonate. Hypoventilation is a primary cause of respiratory acidosis. So the nurse instructs the patient to perform deep-breathing exercises without the need for an increase in supplemental oxygen levels because the PaO_2 level is within normal range at 89 mmHg. Causes of metabolic acidosis include diabetes, infection accompanied by high fever, diarrhea with loss of alkali, and hyperthyroidism; common treatment includes deep breathing, monitoring electrolytes, administering sodium bicarbonate, and administering insulin to control blood sugar as needed. (Burden N et al: *Ambulatory surgical nursing*, ed 2, Philadelphia, 2000, Saunders.)

7.70. Correct Answer: **c**
The preservative *citrate phosphate dextrose adenine* (CPD-A) functions as an anticoagulant by acting on calcium to interfere with the coagulation cascade. Although uncommon, after rapid transfusion of large volumes of citrated blood products, there is the potential for ionized calcium to bind with the citrate and cause a drop in circulating calcium levels. The shelf life of stored blood is 21 to 35 days. Packed cells are concentrated because of the removal of plasma, and the hematocrit is elevated to 70% to 80%, well above the normal range of 36% to 45% in circulating blood. The anticoagulant effect of CPD-A in packed cells does not affect the coagulation process of the recipient. (Hoffman R: *Hematology: basic principles and practice*, ed 4, London, 2005, Churchill Livingstone; Quinn D, Schick L, editors: *ASPAN's perianesthesia nursing core curriculum: preoperative, Phase I and Phase II PACU nursing*, Philadelphia, 2004, Saunders; *Dorland's Illustrated Medical Dictionary*, ed 30, Philadelphia, 2004, Saunders.).

Chapter 8

Neurologic, Neurovascular, and Musculoskeletal Systems

Scenarios and items in this section focus on perianesthesia concepts related to *intracranial* and *musculoskeletal* considerations of *neurologic function* and *orthopedics*. These concepts are considered together because:

- Vascular and nerve functions are intricately interrelated; altered nerve function often alters local blood flow
- Intracranial vascular alterations or tissue edema produces autoregulatory and compensatory shifts and may alter neurologic and musculoskeletal function
- Musculoskeletal procedures (both orthopedic and neurologic) share common patient management concepts, including methods to treat and monitor pain, concerns about blood loss and hemostasis, and circulation-promoting positions
- Postoperative nursing assessments involve monitoring neurovascular status and motor and sensory function after *both* orthopedic and spine-related surgical procedures

ESSENTIAL CORE CONCEPTS	AFFILIATED CORE CURRICULUM CHAPTERS
Nursing Process	**Chapters 3, 33, 40, 49**
Assessment	
Planning and Implementation	
Evaluation	
Intracranial Concerns	**Chapters 33, 40**
Anatomy: Structure and Function	
Blood-Brain Barrier	
Cerebrospinal Fluid	
Cranial Nerves	
Lobes and Ventricles	
Vessels and Spaces	
Physiology	
Intracranial Pressure Dynamics	
Autoregulation	
Herniation	
Hyperventilation	
Pharmacology	
Position, Ventilation, and Rest	
Neuronal Excitation	

Neuromuscular Junction: Transmitters
Pathology
Interventions and Anesthetic Consequences
Trauma, Tumors, Shunts, and Bleeding
Perianesthesia Specifics
Consciousness
Glasgow Coma Scale
Motor and Sensory Responses
Pupil Reaction
Reflexes and Vital Signs

Musculoskeletal: Spine and Orthopedics   **Chapters 33, 40, 49, 53**

Anatomy: Structure and Function   **Chapters 49, 53**
Ascending Tracts
Descending Tracts
Primary Extremity Nerves
Vertebrae, Disks, Bones, and Nerves
White Matter, Gray Matter, and Dura Mater
Physiologic Neurotransmission
Sympathetic: Adrenergic Response to
    Norepinephrine
Parasympathetic: Cholinergic Response to
    Acetylcholine
Neurologic and Vascular Concerns
Autonomic Hyperreflexia
Circulation: Capillary Refill, Temperature, and
    Color
Compartment Syndrome
Disks, Lesions, and Fractures
Edema, Embolism, and Ecchymosis
Innervation: Pain, Sensation, and Motor
    Control
Perianesthesia Specifics
Neurologic Function and Complications
Neurovascular Monitoring
Pain Management
Position and Comfort
Cardiorespiratory Risk Assessment

SET 1

ITEMS 8.1–8.40

8.1. To alter the course of malignant hyperthermia (MH), dantrolene sodium ***primarily:***
a. contracts vascular smooth muscle.
b. reverses cellular acidosis.
c. relaxes skeletal muscle.
d. augments hypothalamic temperature regulation.

8.2. A 48-year-old, nonsmoking, conversant, healthy woman sustained a pelvic fracture in a motor vehicle accident 28 hours ago. She has received morphine by patient-controlled analgesia (PCA), cefazolin, dexamethasone, and midazolam since hospital admission. The preanesthesia nurse considers the patient's potential for fat embolism, closely monitors her pulmonary status, and:
a. encourages active leg movement.
b. reports disorientation agitation.
c. releases traction 10 minutes each hour.
d. limits intravenous (IV) fluid volume.

8.3. The patient most likely to develop autonomic hyperreflexia had a/an:
a. 2-level anterior and posterior cervical fusion today.
b. anterior cord syndrome from incomplete T8 injury 3 days ago.
c. re-exploration after resection of lumbar tumor 2 weeks ago.
d. motor vehicle accident with cord transection at T2 5 months ago.

8.4. Documented post-craniotomy diabetes insipidus is treated with:
a. vasopressin and fluid replacement.
b. long-acting antihyperglycemics and bicarbonate.
c. 10% dextrose infusion and furosemide.
d. fluid restriction and hypertonic saline.

NOTE: Consider the scenario and items 8.5-8.6 together.

After 45 minutes in the PACU following her L4-5 decompression and fusion, a 64-year-old female patient is quickly responsive to touch and name call, oriented to her environment, dozes when undisturbed, and has three documented blood pressures of greater than 195/106 mmHg.

8.5. Of the following factors, the ***most likely*** contributor to the patient's blood pressure measures is:
a. moderate analgesia.
b. postspinal meningeal irritation.
c. evolving epidural hematoma.
d. preoperative hypertension.

8.6. Untreated hypertension increases the patient's potential to develop any of the following adverse outcomes ***except:***
a. release of blood vessel suture.
b. intrapulmonary rales.
c. myocardial hypoperfusion.
d. post-dural cerebral spinal fluid (CSF) leak.

8.7. Administering epinephrine to a patient who receives electroconvulsive therapy (ECT) 3 times weekly and regularly uses the antidepressant *amitriptyline* is ***most likely*** to result in:
a. unpredictable responses to ECT energy.
b. uncontrolled adrenergic stimulation.
c. profound vagal effect.
d. exaggerated agitation when wakening from ECT.

8.8. The incidence of post–dural puncture headache (PDPH) among ambulatory surgery patients is:
a. low; a small 27-gauge needle limits fluid leakage during local anesthetic injection.
b. high; patients must sit and stand early to prepare for discharge.
c. low; high-molecular-weight tetracaine injected through a 20-gauge needle seals any leak.

d. high; ambulatory surgery unit (ASU) patients should not receive large volumes of pre-hydrating fluid for vascular expansion.

8.9. After spinal anesthesia, a patient must meet the facility's discharge criteria and also should:
   a. repeat each postoperative instruction.
   b. urinate spontaneously.
   c. indicate pinprick sensation at S-2 dermatome.
   d. stand without orthostatic hypertension.

8.10. The patient with the least probable risk to develop an injury related to intraoperative positioning has:
   a. Crohn's disease, treated with a 4-hour proctocolectomy and continent ileostomy.
   b. arthritis, a 2-year-old left hip arthroplasty, and is a 64-year-old woman.
   c. non–insulin-dependent diabetes, is a 48-year-old man, and had a 50-minute surgery to revise an abdominal scar.
   d. a gastrostomy tube after gastric bypass surgery and weighs 88 kg at age 24 years.

8.11. Wide blood pressure variability after carotid endarterectomy most likely occurs because of intraoperative:
   a. fluid shifts and third spacing.
   b. vascular manipulation.
   c. intentional hypotensive technique.
   d. vagal nerve compression and trauma.

8.12. After craniotomy to remove an acoustic neuroma, the nurse asks the patient to clench his teeth to assess function of the:
   a. spinal accessory nerve.
   b. temporomaxillary nerve.
   c. glossopharyngeal nerve.
   d. trigeminal nerve.

8.13. The patient most likely to develop malignant hyperthermia crisis is a:
   a. 65-year-old woman with a fractured hip.
   b. 32-year-old man with Down syndrome.
   c. 15-year-old boy with muscular dystrophy.
   d. 6-month-old girl with cleft palate.

8.14. A 72-year-old man is admitted to Phase I PACU after repair of a right inguinal hernia with IV moderate sedation and analgesia with tissue infiltration of local anesthetic. Intraoperatively, the patient received 50 mcg of fentanyl and 2 mg of midazolam, both approximately 60 minutes ago. The patient is now restless and combative. A senior surgical resident orders 3 mg midazolam in the PACU. The PACU nurse's most appropriate response is to:
   a. tactfully consult with a second physician.
   b. evaluate causes for behavior and question the dose.
   c. ignore the order and restrain the patient.
   d. administer midazolam as ordered.

8.15. During patient assessment after spinal anesthesia, the PACU nurse considers the increased potential for both post–dural puncture headache (PDPH) and:
   a. hypotension.
   b. euphoria and diaphoresis.
   c. respiratory stimulation and alkalosis.
   d. tachycardia with vasoconstriction.

NOTE: Consider the scenario and items 8.16-8.17 together.

A female patient's myasthenia gravis is treated by her neurologist with pyridostigmine. The patient is in the PACU after an abdominal exploratory laparotomy and resection of a ruptured appendix.

8.16. While reviewing the surgeon's routine pre-printed postoperative orders, the PACU nurse questions the order for:
   a. hydrocortisone 100 mg.
   b. ketorolac 30 mg.
   c. gentamycin 80 mg.
   d. neostigmine 10 mg.

8.17. If the patient develops myasthenic crisis, the PACU nurse would expect to observe:

a. exophthalmos and hyperventilation.
b. mydriasis and dry mouth.
c. bradycardia and abdominal cramps.
d. ptosis and respiratory failure.

NOTE: Consider the scenario and items 8.18-8.19 together.

A male patient's intraoperative blood loss was 800 mL during a second right total knee replacement with spinal anesthetic. The patient received 2 units of packed red blood cells (RBCs) and 500 mL hetastarch during this surgery in addition to 2600 mL lactated Ringer's solution. In PACU, his hemoglobin is 10.3 g/dL, blood pressure rises to 194/96, central venous pressure (CVP) is 15 cm H_2O, heart rate is 96 bpm in normal sinus rhythm, he has an audible S3 heart sound, and the patient states he has "a pounding headache."

8.18. The patient's signs and symptoms are ***most probably*** related to acute:
a. intravascular hemolysis.
b. circulatory overload.
c. anxiety from spinal headache.
d. myocardial ischemia.

8.19. When assessing the patient, the PACU nurse considers that a hemolytic blood reaction usually produces symptoms of:
a. chills and chest or flank pain.
b. hypertension and dyspnea.
c. hypothermia and headache.
d. urticaria and hypotension.

NOTE: Consider items 8.20-8.21 together.

8.20. After exploration and excision of an intramedullary tumor and thoracic laminectomy, fusion, and instrumentation, an essential nursing aspect of the female patient's postoperative care is:
a. 100% immobility to "seat" instruments.
b. skeletal traction to prevent adhesions.
c. hypotension to minimize bleeding.
d. log rolling to ensure alignment.

NOTE: The scenario continues.

Thirty minutes later, the female patient reports new and sudden tingling in her left toes and severe back pain that does not decrease with pain medications. Neurologic assessment reveals decreased strength with both dorsiflexion and plantar flexion. Pedal and posterior tibial pulses are strong, and capillary refill is normal.

8.21. The female patient's symptoms probably result from:
a. intraspinal hematoma.
b. dural tear.
c. spinal muscle spasm.
d. nerve entrapment.

NOTE: Consider items 8.22-8.27 together.

8.22. A spinal anesthetic is planned for a male patient's knee arthrotomy and meniscus repair. The local anesthetic medication with longest duration of sensory anesthesia is:
a. 1% tetracaine in dextrose.
b. 10% procaine with meperidine.
c. 0.75% bupivacaine in saline.
d. 0.5% lidocaine with fentanyl.

8.23. An anesthesia provider may add epinephrine to a spinal anesthetic solution primarily to:
a. increase the anesthetic duration.
b. decrease duration of anesthetic effect.
c. increase vascular absorption of medication.
d. decrease potential for hypotension.

8.24. Achieving the desired level of dermatome blockade from the patient's spinal anesthetic is most determined by:
a. age and adding epinephrine to the solution.
b. body weight and extremity position.
c. anesthesiologist's experience and the needle size.
d. body position and density of anesthetic solution.

8.25. The patient is admitted to the PACU awake, alert, and slightly diaphoretic with pale color. Blood pressure is 84/52, heart rhythm sinus at a rate of 56 bpm, respiratory rate 20 breaths per minute, and oxygen saturation 98%. Preoperative blood pressure was 104/60,

with pulse 64 bpm. The patient denies pain and complains of nausea. The PACU nurse's intervention is directed toward minimizing:
a. potential for aspiration.
b. fluid volume deficit.
c. increased intrathoracic pressure.
d. local anesthetic movement in CSF.

8.26. Thirty minutes after PACU admission, the patient can raise his right knee from the bed. The nurse assesses his motor block at approximately derma- tome:
a. S1 to S2.
b. L2 to L3.
c. T12 to L1.
d. T4 to L5.

8.27. With a motor block at this level, the PACU nurse anticipates the patient's sensory block is:
a. higher than both sympathetic and motor block.
b. the same level as both motor and sym- pathetic block.
c. higher than motor but below sympa- thetic block.
d. equal to sympathetic block but below motor block.

8.28. Which of the following is the *best* indica- tor of neurologic change?
a. Change in level of consciousness
b. Pupillary changes
c. Motor changes
d. Vital sign changes

8.29. A 56-year-old man is scheduled for cra- niotomy to clip a leaking cerebral aneu- rysm. The patient is settled into the preanesthesia area for nursing observa- tion and to await the neurosurgeon's arrival. The preanesthesia nurse specifi- cally observes this patient for:
a. hyperventilation.
b. headache and neck stiffness.
c. tachycardia.
d. hypotension.

8.30. When applying a 100-mcg transdermal fentanyl patch to a patient with severe left calf injury, the nurse should:

a. pre-medicate the patient with 3 mL IV fentanyl.
b. rinse the skin with water.
c. shave chest hair.
d. scrub with povidone-iodine and apply patch below left knee.

NOTE: Consider the scenario and items 8.31- 8.40 together.

Forty minutes after evacuation of a left occipi- tal subdural hematoma, a male patient is drowsy but rouses when his name is called; the patient follows commands to move his extremi- ties, open his eyes, and deep breathe. Pupils are equal and pinpoint. A suction drain into the cranium is compressed and draining small amounts of red fluid.

8.31. The PACU nurse documents that this patient is:
a. disoriented.
b. stuporous.
c. lethargic.
d. awake.

8.32. Adverse influences on the patient's cur- rent level of consciousness could include any of the following factors *except:*
a. hypoxia.
b. hypocapnia.
c. hypoglycemia.
d. hypothermia.

NOTE: The scenario continues.

Twenty minutes later, the patient requires a louder voice and a stronger tap at his shoulder to arouse. The patient drifts to sleep immediately unless continuously stimu- lated. Pupils are equal, about 2 mm in size, and briskly reactive, and the patient slowly and weakly moves all extremities on command.

8.33. The PACU nurse's most appropriate intervention is to:
a. notify the neurosurgeon.
b. reassess the patient in 15 minutes.
c. administer naloxone 0.8 mg per protocol.
d. empty and recompress the patient's intracranial drain.

NOTE: The scenario continues.

The neurosurgeon requests dexamethasone 12 mg and frequent observation until he arrives in PACU. Within 20 minutes, the patient is considerably more difficult to rouse; eyes occasionally open to heavy touch, and the patient does not vocalize or move his right side when asked. His left arm moves fistlike toward his chest. The nurse applies the Glasgow Coma Scale to objectively grade the patient's neurologic function.

8.34. According to the Glasgow Coma Scale, this patient's motor response would best be described as:
   a. flaccid.
   b. decerebrate.
   c. localizing.
   d. abnormal flexion.

8.35. The bedside nurse most appropriately elicits a pain response by:
   a. twisting the nipple of the patient's left breast.
   b. applying nail bed pressure.
   c. applying pressure to the patient's left eye orbit.
   d. pinching the patient's right trapezius muscle vigorously.

NOTE: The scenario continues.

Further neurologic reassessments indicate that the patient consistently grimaces and flexes both arms and wrists toward his chest and extends his legs, pointing his toes downward and inward.

8.36. The nurse documents the patient's current response as:
   a. decerebrate rigidity.
   b. asynchronous reflex.
   c. decorticate posturing.
   d. withdrawal reaction.

8.37. With these clinical signs, the patient could imminently develop:
   a. transtentorial (central) herniation.
   b. cranial "blowout" with wound dehiscence.
   c. hydrocephalic shunting.
   d. compensatory cerebrospinal fluid displacement.

8.38. The PACU nurse anticipates that the patient's pupils would most likely dilate:
   a. equally.
   b. contralaterally.
   c. ipsilaterally.
   d. bilaterally.

NOTE: The scenario continues.

The anesthesiologist intubates the patient, and the neurosurgeon requests a mannitol infusion and a stat computed tomography (CT) scan.

8.39. In this situation, the patient's neurologic status is best protected when his:
   a. respiratory rate and depth are increased.
   b. airway is vigorously and regularly suctioned.
   c. body position is flat and supine.
   d. consciousness is continuously raised with stir-up regimen.

8.40. Dexamethasone was administered to the patient primarily to:
   a. support physiologic stress responses.
   b. reduce intracranial volume.
   c. increase blood flow to cerebral cells.
   d. decrease seizure threshold.

SET 2

NOTE: Consider items 8.41-8.42 together.

8.41. A patient received nitrous oxide with a total of 750 mcg of fentanyl in divided doses during a 2½-hour left thumb replantation because of a traumatic power saw injury. The PACU nurse most expects to observe fentanyl-induced:
a. dilated pupils and vomiting.
b. hypoventilation and pupillary constriction.
c. hypertension and hyperventilation.
d. bradycardia and emergence shivering.

8.42. Nursing care priorities for this patient focus on respiratory monitoring, neurovascular assessment, and providing:
a. ice to the inner midforearm to reduce posttrauma metabolic demand.
b. limited analgesia for quick detection of neurovascular changes.
c. a comfortable arm position that facilitates venous return.
d. fluid restriction to minimize extremity edema.

8.43. Awareness of sensory stimuli and degree of alertness occur through the:
a. limbic-pyramidal system.
b. reticular activating system.
c. corpus callosum system.
d. thalamic projection system.

8.44. Interrelationship between the cerebral hemispheres occurs through commissures of the:
a. corpus callosum.
b. longitudinal fissure.
c. lateral ventricle gyri.
d. central sulcus.

8.45. The most serious potential compromise to a diabetic surgical patient's recovery immediately after hip arthroplasty is:
a. absent responsiveness from unrecognized hypoglycemia.
b. infection from zealous glucose sampling.
c. hypercalcemia from citrated blood products.
d. altered intestinal flora from dual antibiotic therapy.

8.46. Mannitol's effectiveness occurs by:
a. hydrostatic pressure to increase renal excretion.
b. diffusion pressure to decrease electrolyte shifts.
c. oncotic pressure to increase solute removal.
d. osmotic pressure to decrease intracellular fluid.

8.47. Three hours ago during her 2-level lumbar diskectomy and fusion, a female patient's neurosurgeon injected a single epidural dose of preservative-free morphine 5 mg. Now in the PACU, the patient is drowsy, responds quickly to name call, and follows commands. When planning the patient's care, the PACU nurse reasons that any residual respiratory effects from this morphine sulfate (Duramorph) dose:
a. will not develop after only a single dose.
b. most likely will appear within 8 hours.
c. will require nalbuphine to treat opioid overdose.
d. probably occurred while the patient was intubated in the operating room (OR).

8.48. During the clonic phase of a seizure, the patient may elicit the following signs:
a. pupillary dilation, tachycardia, muscle spasm.
b. bladder incontinence, salivary frothing, jerking of the limbs.

c. loss of consciousness, apnea, generalized stiffness.

d. contracted throat muscles, hyperventilation, apnea.

8.49. Development of anisocoria in a 25-year-old man with a repair of a congenital arteriovenous malformation most likely reflects:
a. meningeal irritation.
b. undocumented cocaine use.
c. previous iridectomy.
d. temporal lobe displacement.

8.50. A 46-year-old healthy patient who is a smoker had a fusion of thoracic vertebrae T6 to T7 and T7 to T8 today. The most likely consequences related to his intraoperative position include any of the following *except:*
a. corneal abrasion.
b. impaired ear circulation.
c. sciatic nerve stretch.
d. skin redness at his ribs and iliac crest.

NOTE: Consider the scenario and items 8.51-8.54 together.

The anesthesiologist inserted an epidural catheter into the female patient's lumbar spine before her left total hip replacement. The anesthesiologist injected a total of 200 mcg fentanyl into the epidural catheter during surgery. Upon admission to PACU, the patient is awake and alert and denies pain. Blood pressure is 146/88, heart rate 86 bpm, and respiratory rate 16 breaths/min. Fifteen minutes later, the patient complains of moderate hip pain. The pharmacy is still preparing the fentanyl solution ordered by the anesthesiologist for continuous infusion.

8.51. In this situation, the PACU nurse's most appropriate intervention is to:
a. administer morphine sulfate 15 mg intramuscularly.
b. sedate the patient with midazolam for amnesia to pain.
c. inject fentanyl 150 mcg intravenously.
d. titrate IV morphine 2- to 3-mg doses to comfort.

8.52. The PACU nurse inspects the insertion site of the patient's epidural catheter and ensures that the epidural tubing is clearly labeled and has no injection ports to mistakenly inject any other medication. Before starting her epidural infusion, the nurse determines the catheter is located in the epidural space by:
a. aspirating less than 0.5 mL clear fluid.
b. ensuring 1 mL serosanguineous fluid flows from port.
c. observing 2 mL clear amber fluid drips from port.
d. injecting a 0.5-mL fentanyl test dose with ease.

8.53. Forty minutes later, the patient states less pain; fentanyl 1 mg, diluted in 100 mL normal saline, infuses epidurally at 8 mL/hr. While monitoring for the specific effects of epidurally injected fentanyl, the PACU nurse least expects to observe:
a. nausea with emesis.
b. respirations 8 breaths/min.
c. blood pressure 76/40.
d. strong left foot dorsiflexion.

8.54. During assessment for PACU discharge, the patient complains of "a lot of pain in my back where that tube is," indicating the epidural catheter, and mentions right leg weakness and heaviness. Assessment reveals diminished right dorsiflexion and plantar flexion, a change from the strong and equal leg activity noted upon PACU admission. The PACU nurse's most appropriate response is to:
a. transfer the patient to the orthopedic unit for frequent neurovascular assessment.
b. reassure the patient that symptoms are common and recede without consequence.
c. reposition the patient's leg and then increase the epidural infusion rate to decrease back spasm.
d. defer transfer from PACU for physician consultation and neurologic examination.

8.55. A healthy 22-year-old college student had surgery to repair his right shoulder rotator cuff. The patient received succinylcholine, fentanyl, and nitrous

oxide anesthesia. The patient is sedated and drowsy, breathes shallowly 14 times per minute, and has weak motor refl exes. A likely explanation for this situation is:
a. unusual narcotic and muscle relaxant overdose.
b. abnormal acetylcholine movement from the cell.
c. atypical pseudocholinesterase effect.
d. genetically inhibited glycopyrrolate response.

8.56. After a total hip replacement and general anesthesia, a patient is admitted to the PACU with an A-frame in place and is able to strongly dorsiflex and plantar flex her ankle. A loss of strength in the lower extremities is noted 30 minutes later. This loss of strength is most likely caused by which of the following?
a. The A-frame is causing pressure on the tibial and the peroneal nerves.
b. The A-frame is causing pressure resulting in decreased circulation.
c. Postoperative pain
d. Nerve damage from the surgery

NOTE: Consider the scenario and items 8.57-8.60 together.

The preanesthesia nurse observes a 57-year-old female patient who just received a brachial plexus block before repair of a wrist fracture. Lidocaine with epinephrine was injected by axillary approach. Before injection, the patient received midazolam 1 mg to decrease anxiety. Five minutes later, the patient mentions blurred vision and "not feeling right." Further assessment indicates tachycardia (heart rate 120 bpm) with palpitations, circumoral numbness, restlessness, dizziness, and tinnitus. Her current blood pressure is 160/72.

8.57. The perianesthesia nurse provides oxygen to the patient, informs the anesthesia provider of these symptoms, and:
a. prepares flumazenil to reverse midazolam.
b. encourages relaxation to decrease hyperventilation.
c. anticipates development of muscle tremors.

d. obtains labetalol to oppose adrenergic stimulation.

NOTE: The scenario continues.

The patient's symptoms abate. After observation by the preanesthesia nurse and family visitation, surgery proceeded uneventfully 2 hours later. Now, 6 hours after the brachial plexus block, the patient is alert, engaged in lively conversation with her daughter, tolerates food and fluids without nausea, and has urinated. Her vital signs have been stable since surgery. The patient requests to go home and receives approval from the anesthesiologist and surgeon.

8.58. To prepare for discharge, the perianesthesia nurse in Phase II ensures the patient has:
a. return of normal motor and sensory function in her hand.
b. strong train-of-four response to nerve stimulation.
c. adequate palmar circulation, assessed by Allen's test.
d. analgesic prescription and rapid capillary refill.

8.59. The patient learns to care for her plaster-casted arm by understanding the need for:
a. extremity elevation and resting the still-numbed arm against a table edge.
b. leaving the casted arm open to the air for 24 hours and applying ice.
c. preventing compression of the cast, which should be dry within 30 minutes.
d. controlling skin pruritus by spreading lotion under cast edge with a covered pen.

8.60. The patient is instructed to contact the orthopedic surgeon when any of the following occur *except:*
a. the right hand appears more purple than the left.
b. body temperature is 38.5° C at home.
c. the analgesic prescription slightly reduces her severe wrist pain for 2 hours.
d. she thinks her cast feels "warm" when discharged from Phase II.

8.61. The occipital lobe receives and interprets:
a. auditory data.

b. proprioception.

c. emotional events.

d. visual data.

8.62. After the patient's open reduction of a fracture to the left femoral neck, her spinal anesthetic continues to the T10 dermatome. Postoperative nursing considerations include:

a. promoting hip adduction and limiting flexion to 90 degrees.

b. assuring anatomic alignment and repositioning the patient only on her left side.

c. providing lateral leg supports and applying ice to the left hip.

d. inspecting sheets below hip for drainage and supporting the patient's legs behind the knees.

NOTE: Consider the scenario and items 8.63-8.66 together.

A female patient had a left lateral frontal lobotomy anterior to the central sulcus for placement of grids to map and control seizure activity. The patient opens her eyes, nods her head, and breathes well.

8.63. One primary assessment after surgery in the left frontal area is to identify this patient's ability to:

a. state her name.

b. hear music.

c. comprehend instructions.

d. focus on an object.

8.64. The patient's nurse is assessing function at:

a. Rolando's area.

b. Broca's area.

c. Brodmann's area.

d. Wernicke's area.

8.65. The patient's cranial nerve function is considered normal when neurologic assessment reveals ocular responses that are:

a. nystagmic and convergent.

b. consensual and equal.

c. constricted and exophthalmic.

d. conjugate and brisk.

8.66. The patient's upper arm function is best tested by asking her to:

a. sustain outstretched arms.

b. squeeze the nurse's hand.

c. adduct her shoulder.

d. hyperextend her hand and wrist.

8.67. Daily production of cerebrospinal fluid in adults is:

a. 100 mL.

b. 500 mL.

c. 1000 mL.

d. 2000 mL.

8.68. A patient with intracranial changes known as *Cushing's triad* has:

a. systolic increase, diastolic decrease, and bradycardia.

b. diastolic decrease, elevated glucose, and oliguria.

c. diastolic increase, decreased aldosterone, and polyuria.

d. systolic decrease, tachycardia, and hyperthermia.

8.69. Contralateral crossing of corticospinal tracts occurs at the:

a. brainstem.

b. dorsal horn.

c. cerebellum.

d. hippocampus.

NOTE: Consider the scenario and items 8.70-8.72 together.

A 12-year-old patient is in Phase I PACU after posterior fusion of L1 to L5 vertebrae and insertion of instrumentation to treat her scoliosis.

8.70. The nurse determines that the most important immediate nursing priority for the patient is:

a. mobilizing fluid volume with low-dose furosemide to relieve accumulated facial edema.

b. assisting the patient to use the bed trapeze for self-reposition and early mobility.

c. encouraging lung expansion while restoring fluid and oxygen-carrying deficits.

d. positioning her flat and nearly prone to drain secretions and relieve gastric distention.

8.71. Some of the patient's intraoperative blood loss was returned by an autotransfusion technique. Physiologic advantages of retransfusion include reduced potential for disease and:
  a. retained cell "freshness" for reinfusion 2 days later.
  b. immediate availability without need to filter small particles.
  c. normal potassium levels, preserved platelet number and function.
  d. risk of coagulopathy; processing reverses heparin and replaces thrombin.

8.72. To safely administer an autotransfusion of washed and processed blood cells from lost intraoperative blood, nursing responsibilities include the following *except* to:
  a. complete autotransfusion within 4 hours and flush tubing with saline.
  b. monitor temperature and infuse peripherally with morphine PCA.
  c. report abdominal cramping and circumoral tingling.
  d. observe for chills, hematuria, and increased wound drainage.

Set 3

Items 8.73–8.99

8.73. An interscalene block would **not** be used in which of the following types of surgery?
a. Total shoulder replacement
b. Reduction of a dislocated shoulder
c. Carpal tunnel release
d. Reduction of arm fracture

8.74. A patient who has received an interscalene block for shoulder surgery complains of numbness in his hand. The radial pulse is present and strong, and hand movement is intact. The perianesthesia nurse's immediate plan of care includes which of the following?
a. Inform the physician of the abnormal sensation.
b. Medicate for pain.
c. Reposition the arm.
d. Observe the patient and discharge to the receiving unit when stable.

NOTE: Consider the scenario and items 8.75-8.77 together.

After calibration of the subarachnoid monitoring system, the patient's intracranial pressure measures 18 mmHg.

8.75. Interventions to prevent further increases may include all the following **except**:
a. semi-Fowler's position with knees extended.
b. mechanical ventilation at 12 breaths per minute and 600 mL tidal volume.
c. nitroprusside infusion to increase cerebral blood flow.
d. immediate infusion of hyperosmotic solution.

8.76. Nursing responsibility with regard to invasively monitoring the patient's intracranial pressure includes:
a. administering scheduled steroid doses to suppress infection.

b. flushing the catheter system to ensure system patency.
c. reporting C waves promptly and calculating intracranial compliance.
d. recognizing plateau waves and identifying leaks at skull insertion site.

8.77. The Monro-Kellie hypothesis describes intracranial volume as a relationship among:
a. cerebral perfusion and mean arterial and systolic blood pressures.
b. oxygen and carbon dioxide partial pressures and cardiac index.
c. cerebrospinal fluid density, cerebral blood flow, and cellular oxygenation.
d. brain, cerebral blood, and cerebrospinal fluid volumes.

8.78. A cerebral perfusion pressure calculated at 43 mmHg probably represents:
a. inadequate brain blood flow.
b. compensated autoregulation.
c. normal cerebral circulation.
d. ischemia with active CSF loss.

NOTE: Consider the scenario and items 8.79-8.82 together.

A male patient is scheduled for a craniotomy to remove an infratentorial meningioma.

8.79. Characteristics of a meningioma that most increase the patient's potential for:
a. intraoperative hemorrhage.
b. malignancy-related death.
c. fluid volume excess.
d. postoperative hypertension.

8.80. Postoperatively the PACU nurse observes yellow-tinged drainage at the patient's posterior dressing. To confirm or refute a cerebrospinal fluid leak, the nurse most appropriately:
a. removes the dressing for incisional inspection.

b. lowers the ventriculostomy to observe flow increase.

c. determines the presence of glucose in drainage.

d. assesses the patient for position-related headache.

8.81. Immediate postsurgical complications after the patient's infratentorial surgery are most likely indicated by:

a. receptive aphasia.

b. serosanguineous nasal drainage.

c. altered respiratory pattern.

d. muscle paralysis.

8.82. Nursing intervention to best promote positive respiratory outcomes after the patient's infratentorial surgery includes:

a. mechanical ventilation with positive end-expiratory pressure (PEEP).

b. log-roll turns with neck support.

c. regular tracheobronchial suction.

d. achieving a functional Phase II block.

8.83. The PACU nurse is most concerned when, after left supratentorial craniotomy, the patient develops:

a. dilation of the right pupil.

b. weakness of the left arm.

c. inability to move the right leg.

d. nystagmus involving the left eye.

8.84. Nursing management of a patient with a ventriculostomy drain includes:

a. securing the system's "zero" point near the eye or by physician order.

b. ensuring system sterility and a minimum of 30 mL/hr drainage.

c. providing low, negative pressure suction to facilitate system patency.

d. complying with physician-specified volumes of fluid drainage.

NOTE: Consider the scenario and items 8.85-8.88 together.

The PACU nurse assesses a female patient's muscle strength after a right transthoracic diskectomy at T6 to T7. Comparative responses indicate the patient moves each arm without drift and resists the nurse's efforts to push them down or away. The patient easily lifts her left leg from the bed and has strong foot dorsiflexion and plantar flexion movements. The patient moves and lifts her right knee; the nurse moves the patient's right foot from the dorsiflexed position with little resistance.

8.85. Based on this assessment, the nurse documents muscle activity as:

a. equal bilaterally in arms and legs, with normal strength.

b. right leg moves with full range of motion against gravity and weakens to resistance.

c. left leg strong; right leg moves but with severe weakness against gravity.

d. arms have normal strength; legs move equally but with mild weakness to resistance.

NOTE: The scenario continues.

Thirty minutes later, the patient is much drowsier. The nurse sufficiently stimulates her and determines that she can still move her right leg but cannot lift it from the bed. Assessments of arm and left leg activity are unchanged.

8.86. The neurosurgeon requests an immediate CT scan and orders hourly doses of methylprednisolone, primarily to decrease:

a. autoimmune rejection of bone graft.

b. traumatic intraspinal edema.

c. intracranial pressure effects.

d. sepsis and future reherniation.

8.87. After this medication, the patient is at increased risk of developing infection, adrenal suppression, and:

a. gastric ulceration.

b. dehydration.

c. lethargy.

d. thromboembolism.

8.88. An important observation in the PACU related to the continuous infusion of sufentanil the patient received during surgery is:

a. relaxation of muscles, particularly in the chest.

b. altered consciousness and a staring, fixed gaze.

c. recurrent respiratory depression.

d. tachycardia and hypotension after large doses.

8.89. Neurologically, the term *nystagmus* describes:
  a. cerebellar dysfunction with uncoordinated, spastic extremity movements.
  b. coordinated eye movements away from the direction the head turns.
  c. parietal lobe disease with generalized skeletal muscle weakness.
  d. abnormally "jerky" eye movements that drift from a midline gaze.

8.90. The patient's leg deep tendon reflexes are described as "2+", which indicates:
  a. normal reflex responses.
  b. above-average responses in two of four limbs.
  c. suppression of reflexes.
  d. subnormal reactions and positive Babinski sign.

8.91. An autologous bone graft:
  a. substitutes for Luque rods during spinal fusion.
  b. transfers iliac bone to stabilize damaged bone.
  c. transplants bone acquired from an anonymous donor.
  d. requires high-dose steroids to prevent rejection.

8.92. After a male patient's total knee replacement, the nurse manages his pain, monitors for infection, and:
  a. provides high leg elevation, ice, and pillows behind the knee.
  b. checks regularly for accumulated drainage beneath the leg.
  c. limits leg movement to toe wiggling and foot flexion.
  d. informs the surgeon promptly that 180 mL red, clotty fluid collected in the wound drain.

8.93. Patients with greatest risk to develop compartment syndrome include all the following *except* a:
  a. 25-year-old muscular man with a warm cast 4 hours after repair of a left Pott's fracture.
  b. 48-year-old woman in lithotomy position for a 3-hour vaginal hysterectomy and pelvic floor repair.

  c. 65-year-old man with a sequential compression device 2 hours after a total hip replacement.
  d. 72-year-old obese woman with large left thigh hematoma 3 hours after removal of a femoral artery sheath.

8.94. An intramedullary rod and plates were inserted in a male patient's right leg to repair his tibia with three fractures. The patient is alert, has a long-leg cast propped high on three pillows, and describes severe, unrelenting leg pain after administration of 15 mg IV morphine sulfate. The nurse observes for drainage "hidden" beneath his cast and considers the patient's potential to develop compartment syndrome and then observes for altered capillary refill. Assessment for compartment syndrome includes all the following early signs *except:*
  a. burning sensation in extremity.
  b. diminishing dorsalis pedal pulse quality.
  c. muscle weakness against resistance.
  d. cyanotic toes and brisk "4+" tendon reflexes.

8.95. A contraindicated intervention in a patient with compartment syndrome is to:
  a. elevate the extremity.
  b. immobilize the extremity.
  c. bivalve the cast.
  d. monitor pressure with a catheter in the extremity.

8.96. Apneustic breathing, cluster breathing patterns, and central neurogenic hyperventilation are indicative of activity in the:
  a. cerebrum.
  b. cerebellum.
  c. brainstem.
  d. hypothalamus.

8.97. When using the Glasgow Coma Scale, a score of 3 or less is indicative of:
  a. a normal score.
  b. aphasia.
  c. dysphasia.
  d. coma.

NOTE: Consider the scenario and items 8.98-8.99 together.

A 76-year-old female with a history of hypertension, asthma, and renal dysfunction undergoes a right total knee replacement. The patient is breathing on her own with a respiratory rate of 28 and has minimal tracheal retraction. Blood pressure range during surgery was 180/90 to 110/56, and pulse ranged from 68 to 75. Arterial blood gases (ABGs) were within normal range during surgery, and no complications were noted upon extubation.

8.98. Which assessment would the perianesthesia nurse perform first, based on the patient's presentation?
a. Neurovascular assessment
b. Drainage tube assessment
c. Respiratory assessment
d. Surgical site assessment

NOTE: The scenario continues.

The patient received a respiratory treatment of albuterol. After the treatment was complete, the patient's lungs were clear, O_2 saturation was 97%, and respiratory rate was 20 and non-labored. The patient is complaining of pain, which is described as a "5" on a scale of 0 to 10.

8.99. Which of the following is contraindicated in an elderly patient with renal dysfunction?
a. Morphine
b. Dilaudid
c. Toradol
d. Demerol

SET 1

ANSWER KEY

8.1.	c		8.21.	a
8.2.	b		8.22.	c
8.3.	d		8.23.	a
8.4.	a		8.24.	d
8.5.	d		8.25.	b
8.6.	d		8.26.	b
8.7.	b		8.27.	c
8.8.	a		8.28.	a
8.9.	b		8.29.	b
8.10.	c		8.30.	b
8.11.	b		8.31.	c
8.12.	d		8.32.	b
8.13.	c		8.33.	a
8.14.	b		8.34.	d
8.15.	a		8.35.	b
8.16.	c		8.36.	c
8.17.	d		8.37.	a
8.18.	b		8.38.	c
8.19.	a		8.39.	a
8.20.	d		8.40.	b

SET 1

8.1. Correct Answer: **c**
Dantrolene sodium's direct effect on skeletal muscle suppresses release of intracellular calcium. Muscles relax, and rate of further contraction slows. In malignant hyperthermia, unsuppressed muscle contractions produce heat and increase body temperature up to $1°$ C ($1.8°$ F) each minute. Dantrolene does not alter contractile rate or strength of cardiac and smooth muscle. (Cole DJ, Schlunt M: *Adult perioperative anesthesia: the requisites in anesthesiology*, St. Louis, 2004, Mosby; Skidmore-Roth L: *Mosby's 2006 nursing drug reference*, St. Louis, 2006, Mosby; Quinn D, Schick L, editors: *ASPAN's perianesthesia nursing core curriculum: preoperative, Phase I and Phase II PACU nursing*, Philadelphia, 2004, Saunders; Roizen M, Fleisher L: *Essence of anesthesia practice*, ed 2, Philadelphia, 2002, Saunders.)

8.2. Correct Answer: **b**
Newly developing agitation, confusion, and disorientation in a trauma patient with orthopedic fractures should be reported and not ignored. Fat embolism is primarily a clinical diagnosis, and these symptoms of hypoxemia could indicate developing fat embolism syndrome, particularly within 24 to 72 hours after the fracture. Pelvic and long bone (femur) fractures are linked with high risk for fat embolism; the patient warrants a "high index of suspicion" and close observation. Some physicians believe early fracture stabilization and *generous* fluid infusion help reduce risk of fat embolism. *Limit*, not encourage, limb motion. Frequently assess sensorium, cardiopulmonary status, and relevant laboratory values, and provide adequate support to splint fractures. (Atlee JL: *Complications in anesthesia*, ed 2, Philadelphia, 2007, Saunders; Roizen M, Fleisher L: *Essence of anesthesia practice*, ed 2, Philadelphia, 2002, Saunders.)

8.3. Correct Answer: **d**
Patients most likely to develop autonomic hyperreflexia (or autonomic dysreflexia) had complete spinal cord transection, usually above T6, weeks, months, or years ago. Lesions below T6 rarely cause the syndrome. Evidence of autonomic hyperreflexia occurs after spinal shock from the initial injury has subsided. Spinal shock usually resolves within 10 days but may last longer. Patients with long-term spinal cord injury often are well aware of their own signs of impending autonomic hyperreflexia. (Atlee JL: *Complications in anesthesia*, ed 2, Philadelphia, 2007, Saunders; Cole DJ, Schlunt M: *Adult perioperative anesthesia: the requisites in anesthesiology*, St. Louis, 2004, Mosby; Drain C, editor: *Perianesthesia nursing: a critical care approach*, ed 4, Philadelphia, 2003, Saunders; Quinn D, Schick L, editors: *ASPAN's perianesthesia nursing core curriculum: preoperative, Phase I and Phase II PACU nursing*, Philadelphia, 2004, Saunders; Roizen M, Fleisher L: *Essence of anesthesia practice*, ed 2, Philadelphia, 2002, Saunders.)

8.4. Correct Answer: **a**
Diabetes insipidus (DI) is characterized by an impaired renal conservation of water, resulting in polyuria, low urine specific gravity, dehydration, and hypernatremia.

DI is a disorder of water imbalance resulting from a lack of production of or response to antidiuretic hormone (ADH); it is not a disease of glucose metabolism as is diabetes mellitus (DM). This patient is already hyperosmotic; giving additional glucose will only expound on this effect, with furosemide increasing the level of dehydration. The patient is already compromised with hypernatremia and needs fluid replacement, not restriction, as would be the treatment for the syndrome of inappropriate secretion of antidiuretic hormone (SIADH). DI is treated by replacing the posterior pituitary hormone (ADH) and fluid losses. ADH medications include vasopressin (Pitressin) and desmopressin (DDAVP), a synthetic ADH. DI represents ADH insufficiency and may transiently occur after intracranial trauma or pituitary removal (hypophysectomy). (Atlee JL: *Complications in anesthesia*, ed 2, Philadelphia, 2007, Saunders; Donohoe Dennison D: *Pass CCRN*, ed 2, St. Louis, 2000, Mosby; Papadakos PJ: *Critical care: the requisites in anesthesiology*, St. Louis, 2005, Mosby; Roizen M, Fleisher L: *Essence of anesthesia practice*, ed 2, Philadelphia, 2002, Saunders; Schumacher L, Chernecky CC: *Real world nursing survival guide: critical care and emergency nursing*, Philadelphia, 2005, Saunders.)

8.5. Correct Answer: **d**
History of preoperative hypertension, whether documented or undiagnosed, is a prime contributing factor to postoperative hypertension. Hypertension is defined as a blood pressure greater than 140/90 mmHg or 20% more than baseline blood pressure. Approximately 80% of postoperative hypertensive events occur within 30 minutes of surgery and resolve within 3 hours.

Postoperative hypertension may relate to increased catecholamine levels, cardiac output, or systemic vascular resistance. Unrelieved pain contributes to postoperative hypertension; providing analgesia may precede administration of antihypertensives in a patient with severe pain. Typically, hypertension abates as pain is managed and the patient relaxes; however, this patient remains hypertensive despite her drowsiness. Epidural hematomas typically develop insidiously, with back pain being present in fewer than half of patients. Bowel or bladder dysfunction, sensory changes, and/or motor weakness are more common presenting symptoms of this problem, after dissipation of the block. Moderate analgesia is the drug-induced depression of consciousness during which patients respond purposefully to commands. If this patient was under moderate analgesia, her anxiety level should be well controlled and not be contributing to her elevated BP. Post–spinal meningeal irritation would include nuchal rigidity, fever, headache, and photophobia, with the possibility of a positive Kernig sign. (Atlee JL: *Complications in anesthesia*, ed 2, Philadelphia, 2007, Saunders; Rathmell JP, Neal JM, Viscomi CM: *Regional anesthesia: the requisites in anesthesiology*, St. Louis, 2004, Mosby; Odom-Forren J, Watson DS: *Practical guide to moderate sedation/analgesia*, ed 2, St. Louis, 2005, Mosby; Morton PG et al: *Critical care nursing: a holistic approach*, ed 8, Philadelphia, 2005, Lippincott Williams & Wilkins; Papadakos PJ: *Critical care: the requisites in anesthesiology*, St. Louis, 2005, Mosby; Stoelting RK, Miller RD: *Basics of anesthesia*, ed 5, London, 2007, Churchill Livingstone; Woods A: Loosening the grip of hypertension, *Nursing* 34[12]:36-43, 2004.)

8.6. Correct Answer: **d**

In patients with preexisting cardiac damage, any increased systemic vascular resistance and cardiac output associated with hypertension can produce damaging myocardial ischemia. Treat pain, anxiety, hypoxia, hypercarbia, and fluid volume excess before initiating antihypertensive therapy. Infarction, dysrhythmias, congestive heart failure, cerebral hemorrhage, and bleeding or suture disruption at the surgical site are all possible consequences of untreated hypertension. (Cole DJ, Schlunt M: *Adult perioperative anesthesia: the requisites in anesthesiology*, St. Louis, 2004, Mosby; Fleisher LA: *Evidence-based practice of anesthesiology*, Philadelphia, 2004, Saunders; Quinn D, Schick L, editors: *ASPAN's perianesthesia nursing core curriculum: preoperative, Phase I and Phase II PACU nursing*, Philadelphia, 2004, Saunders.)

8.7. Correct Answer: **b**

The interaction of epinephrine and tricyclic antidepressants like amitriptyline (Elavil) or phenelzine (Nardil), a monoamine oxidase inhibitor, can produce severe hypertension and tachycardia. These medications potentiate norepinephrine (NE) and serotonin in the central nervous system (CNS) by blocking reuptake. Tricyclics have antihistamine, anticholinergic, and sedating effects so can interfere with atrioventricular (AV) conduction. Giving sympathomimetic medications such as epinephrine can release stored NE and produce unpredictable and exaggerated adrenergic responses. (Atlee JL: *Complications in anesthesia*, ed 2, Philadelphia, 2007, Saunders; Cole DJ, Schlunt M: *Adult perioperative anesthesia: the requisites in anesthesiology*, St. Louis, 2004, Mosby;

Roizen M, Fleisher L: *Essence of anesthesia practice*, ed 2, Philadelphia, 2002, Saunders.)

8.8. Correct Answer: **a**

Some clinicians believe the size of the needle used to puncture the dura is the most important determinant of whether post–dural puncture headache (PDPH) will occur. Very small (24- to 27-gauge) needles reduce potential for leakage of cerebrospinal fluid through the dural puncture. Specially designed needles split, not cut, fibers of the dura. With current anesthesia practice, the incidence of PDPH is low, typically 1% to 7% after spinal anesthetic. Tetracaine is a potent and long-duration agent that provides anesthesia for up to 150 minutes. Most ambulatory surgical procedures do not require that long of a duration of action, and it is rarely used in practice at this time. Because the vasculature is temporarily expanded because of the vasodilating effects of the spinal anesthesia, sufficient intravascular volume is necessary to maintain normotension. Often, healthy patients are hydrated with 500 mL or more of fluid before the start of spinal anesthesia to prevent hypotension. PDPH typically occurs 1 to 5 days postoperatively, well after the ASU patient is discharged. (Atlee JL: *Complications in anesthesia*, ed 2, Philadelphia, 2007, Saunders; Burden N et al: *Ambulatory surgical nursing*, ed 2, Philadelphia, 2000, Saunders; Drain C, editor: *Perianesthesia nursing: a critical care approach*, ed 4, Philadelphia, 2003, Saunders; Quinn D, Schick L, editors: *ASPAN's perianesthesia nursing core curriculum: preoperative, Phase I and Phase II PACU nursing*, Philadelphia, 2004, Saunders; Rathmell JP, Neal JM, Viscomi CM: *Regional anesthesia:*

the requisites in anesthesiology, St. Louis, 2004, Mosby.)

8.9. Correct Answer: **b**
Ability to control and empty the bladder and to stand without profound *hypo*tension indicates postspinal recovery of function of sacral nerves S3 to S5 and of sympathetic tone. Peripheral vasoconstriction and bladder control are the first functions to be blocked and the last to return. Return of movement and sensation (sympathetic block) after spinal anesthesia occurs in reverse from the order of loss. Requirements that a patient urinate before vary among facilities; this expectation is recommended for specific situations, including spinal and epidural blocks. Spinal anesthesia does not affect mentation; however, sedation and/or narcotics are normally given in conjunction with spinal analgesia. (ASPAN: *2006-2008 Standards of perianesthesia nursing practice,* Cherry Hill, NJ, 2006, ASPAN; Burden N et al: *Ambulatory surgical nursing,* ed 2, Philadelphia, 2000, Saunders.)

8.10. Correct Answer: **c**
Every patient has risk of nerve, soft tissue, and eye injury related to intraoperative position and anesthetic effects. Though this patient does have diabetes and perhaps some vascular compromise, this patient is relatively young and his surgery lasted less than 2 hours. He probably was in the supine position, which provides greatest safety. Long surgical procedures (more than 2 hours), obesity or extreme thinness, vascular impairment from diabetes, peripheral vascular disease, or movement-limiting problems like arthritis or artificial joints are most associated with damage to body tissue. (Cole DJ, Schlunt M: *Adult perioperative*

anesthesia: the requisites in anesthesiology, St. Louis, 2004, Mosby; Drain C, editor: *Perianesthesia nursing: a critical care approach,* ed 4, Philadelphia, 2003, Saunders; Rothrock J, editor: *Alexander's care of the patient in surgery,* ed 12, St. Louis, 2003, Mosby.)

8.11. Correct Answer: **b**
Expect labile and exaggerated blood pressures after surgical manipulation of the carotid artery. Baroreceptors in a diseased carotid artery grew accustomed to adjusting blood pressure through a veil of plaque. Manipulation or removal of this plaque that coats the carotid artery's intima exposes pressure-sensitive baroreceptors to unfiltered pressure. Baroreceptors are primary feedback mechanisms that sense and alter blood pressure and blood flow. Theoretically true pressures can be temporarily "misinterpreted" and the neurologic responses exaggerated. Functional damage to the vagus nerve would be seen as difficulty swallowing, hoarseness, speech problems, or loss of gag reflex. The goal of blood pressure regulation after carotid endarterectomy is a systolic blood pressure between 120 and 170 mmHg. Common sites of third spacing include the pleural cavity, peritoneal cavity, and pericardial sac. (Black J, Hokanson Hawks J: *Medical-surgical nursing: clinical management for positive outcomes,* ed 7, Philadelphia, 2005, Saunders; Macari-Hinson M, Moore C, Morley M: Carotid artery stenting: new hope for blocked vessels, *Nurs Manage* Spring[suppl]:14, 16, 18, 2006; Morton PG et al: *Critical care nursing: a holistic approach,* ed 8, Philadelphia, 2005, Lippincott Williams & Wilkins; Palmieri R: Cerebral artery stenosis paves the way for a stroke, *Nursing* 36[6]:36-41, 2006; Woods A:

Loosening the grip of hypertension, *Nursing* 34[12]:36-43, 2004.)

8.12. Correct Answer: **d**

The trigeminal nerve (cranial nerve V) moves the jaw and provides sensation to the face, scalp, cornea, and interior nose and mouth. After resection of a cerebellar tumor or acoustic neuroma, one postoperative assessment is determining proper motor function of jaw muscles. The motor function of the trigeminal nerve is monitored by the masseter and other chewing muscles. An abnormality is recognized if the patient is unable to clench teeth on one side of the face. (ASPAN: *Redi-Ref*, Cherry Hill, NJ, 2004, ASPAN; Assessing the cranial nerves, *Nursing* 36[11]:47-49, 2006; Quinn D, Schick L, editors: *ASPAN's perianesthesia nursing core curriculum: preoperative, Phase I and Phase II PACU nursing*, Philadelphia, 2004, Saunders; Jarvis C: *Physical examination and health assessment*, ed 4, Philadelphia, 2004, Saunders.)

8.13. Correct Answer: **c**

Malignant hyperthermia (MH) appears more commonly in the 1- to 30-year age-group, in all racial groups. Infants are seldom affected; boys and girls are equally susceptible until puberty, and then men seem affected twice as often as adult women. MH rarely occurs in patients older than 50 years. Preexisting muscular diseases, history of anesthetic complications, intraoperative death of a relative, or unexplained perioperative fever are "red flags" that alert health care providers to an MH-susceptible patient. (Atlee JL: *Complications in anesthesia*, ed 2, Philadelphia, 2007, Saunders; Quinn D, Schick L, editors: *ASPAN's perianesthesia nursing core curriculum: preoperative, Phase I and Phase II PACU*

nursing, Philadelphia, 2004, Saunders; Malignant Hyperthermia Association of the United States (MHAUS). Website: www.mhaus.org/index.cfm/fuseaction/Content.Display/PagePK/Home.cfm. Accessed June 5, 2007; Roizen M, Fleisher L: *Essence of anesthesia practice*, ed 2, Philadelphia, 2002, Saunders.)

8.14. Correct Answer: **b**

Prior to *any* medication for his restlessness, this patient must be assessed for contributing reasons. Hypoxia and pain are suspect causes and must be addressed before administering a sedative. Midazolam is a highly potent benzodiazepine that quickly causes respiratory depression and hemodynamic alterations. A 3-mg IV dose is too large and must be questioned. Elderly, frail, debilitated patients, children, or patients who have received narcotics receive one-half to two-thirds dose reductions. The nurse slowly titrates incremental 0.5- to 1-mg midazolam doses to clinical effect. (Burden N et al: *Ambulatory surgical nursing*, ed 2, Philadelphia, 2000, Saunders; Kost M: *Moderate sedation/analgesia: core competencies for practice*, ed 2, Philadelphia, 2004, Saunders; Odom-Forren J, Watson DS: *Practical guide to moderate sedation/analgesia*, ed 2, St. Louis, 2005, Mosby; Quinn D, Schick L, editors: *ASPAN's perianesthesia nursing core curriculum: preoperative, Phase I and Phase II PACU nursing*, Philadelphia, 2004, Saunders.)

8.15. Correct Answer: **a**

Hypotension is estimated to occur in about one third of patients receiving spinal anesthesia. The hypotension results from a sympathetic block that decreases venous return to the heart and decreases cardiac output and/or decreases systemic vascular resistance. The local anesthetic medication acts on spinal nerves to prevent vasoconstriction below the level of injection. The size of the vascular compartment expands for the duration of the block's effect, particularly above the T10 dermatome. Filling this compartment with additional IV fluid minimizes or prevents significant hypotension. PDPH is from a persistent leak of spinal fluid through the dural puncture site. The defining feature is a severe, pounding headache that worsens as the head is elevated. Euphoria is usually from the medications including narcotics given to the patient during the procedure. Diaphoresis is centrally controlled by the sympathetic nervous system and is primarily a thermoregulatory mechanism. Respiratory stimulation will blow off carbon dioxide, making the patient more alkalotic. A patient with alkalosis can hypoventilate to stimulate the medullary chemoreceptors and offset decreased alveolar ventilation. Vasoconstrictor usage with spinal anesthetics prolongs the duration of the anesthetic. With spinal anesthesia, there is a tendency for bradycardia from a high sympathetic blockade of the cardioaccelerator fibers slowing the heart rate secondary to a drop in venous return. (Rathmell JP, Neal JM, Viscomi CM: *Regional anesthesia: the requisites in anesthesiology*, St. Louis, 2004, Mosby; Robertson KM et al: *Anesthesiology board review*, ed 2, New York, 2006, McGraw-Hill; Stoelting RK, Miller RD: *Basics of anesthesia*, ed 5, London, 2007, Churchill Livingstone.)

8.16. Correct Answer: **c**
Gentamycin (and other "mycin" antibiotics) affect the neuromuscular junction. These medications can increase muscle weakness by reversing the cholinergic effects of the anticholinesterase (pyridostigmine) used to treat the patient's myasthenia gravis. Neostigmine is sometimes used during acute illness to manage myasthenia symptoms. Narcotics and sedatives may have exaggerated effects, so doses should be reduced. Myasthenia gravis gradually destroys acetylcholine receptors. Corticosteroids and short-acting anticholinesterase compounds are the two pharmacologic interventions used with patients diagnosed with myasthenia gravis. Corticosteroids may temporarily worsen manifestations; however, this is followed by gradual improvement in muscle strength. Ketorolac is not contraindicated for pain in patients with myasthenia gravis. (Atlee JL: *Complications in anesthesia*, ed 2, Philadelphia, 2007, Saunders; Black J, Hokanson Hawks J: *Medical-surgical nursing: clinical management for positive outcomes*, ed 7, Philadelphia, 2005, Saunders; Burden N et al: *Ambulatory surgical nursing*, ed 2, Philadelphia, 2000, Saunders; Karlet MC: *Nurse anesthesia secrets*, St. Louis, 2005, Mosby.)

8.17. Correct Answer: **d**
Inadequate amounts of anticholinesterase medication in the system produce myasthenic crisis. Symptoms include progressive respiratory failure, ptosis, diplopia, increased secretions, and hypertension. Absence of nausea, diarrhea, miosis, and bradycardia distinguish myasthenic crisis from its opposite, cholinergic crisis. In the PACU, a myasthenia gravis patient could develop increasing muscle weakness when anticholinesterases are withheld or as an effect of neuromuscular blocking medications. Both produce anticholinesterase deficiency. (Atlee JL: *Complications in*

anesthesia, ed 2, Philadelphia, 2007, Saunders; Burden N et al: *Ambulatory surgical nursing*, ed 2, Philadelphia, 2000, Saunders; Cole DJ, Schlunt M: *Adult perioperative anesthesia: the requisites in anesthesiology*, St. Louis, 2004, Mosby; Drain C, editor: *Perianesthesia nursing: a critical care approach*, ed 4, Philadelphia, 2003, Saunders; Roizen M, Fleisher L: *Essence of anesthesia practice*, ed 2, Philadelphia, 2002, Saunders.)

8.18. Correct Answer: **b**
Hypertension, edema, distended neck veins, or increased central venous pressure and a heart gallop indicated by an S3 sound suggest fluid volume excess. Temporarily, the patient's intravascular space increased because of moderate blood loss and vasodilation from spinal anesthetic. The space was filled intraoperatively with blood, colloid, and crystalloid. As the spinal effect recedes and capacity of arterioles to vasoconstrict returns postoperatively, this increased total body volume circulates through a smaller space and overloads the cardiovascular system. Usual blood loss replacement is mL per mL loss when replaced with blood and 3 mL per mL loss when replaced with crystalloids. (Drain C, editor: *Perianesthesia nursing: a critical care approach*, ed 4, Philadelphia, 2003, Saunders; Quinn D, Schick L, editors: *ASPAN's perianesthesia nursing core curriculum: preoperative, Phase I and Phase II PACU nursing*, Philadelphia, 2004, Saunders.)

8.19. Correct Answer: **a**
Hypotension, tachycardia, nausea, substernal chest pain, or flank pain occurs early during a transfusion as the patient's antibodies destroy incompatible red blood cells in the transfused blood. Fever and chills

develop later, along with hemoglobinuria, which leads to oliguria. An acute hemolytic reaction is caused by ABO-type incompatibility between the blood donor's red blood cell antigens and the recipient's antibodies. Blood-fluid incompatibility or sepsis from blood contamination also causes hemolysis. ABO incompatibility produces severe symptoms of hypotension with tachycardia, renal failure, and disseminated intravascular coagulation (DIC). (Springhouse: *Critical care nursing made incredibly easy!*, Philadelphia, 2004, Lippincott Williams & Wilkins; Drain C, editor: *Perianesthesia nursing: a critical care approach*, ed 4, Philadelphia, 2003, Saunders; Quinn D, Schick L, editors: *ASPAN's perianesthesia nursing core curriculum: preoperative, Phase I and Phase II PACU nursing*, Philadelphia, 2004, Saunders.)

8.20. Correct Answer: **d**
A postoperative spinal surgery patient must avoid twisting and malalignment. The technique of "log rolling" ensures spinal alignment, decreases spinal muscle spasms, and limits twisting of the back while repositioning. (Drain C, editor: *Perianesthesia nursing: a critical care approach*, ed 4, Philadelphia, 2003, Saunders; Quinn D, Schick L, editors: *ASPAN's perianesthesia nursing core curriculum: preoperative, Phase I and Phase II PACU nursing*, Philadelphia, 2004, Saunders.)

8.21. Correct Answer: **a**
Blood is highly irritating to neural tissue and produces severe pain. Hematoma formation in the spine compresses nerves and augments neurologic deficits, decreasing sensation and increasing motor weakness below the hematoma. The combination of severe incisional

pain and decreased motor and sensory function suggests a hematoma. Though most primary spinal tumors are benign, resecting an intramedullary tumor (one that develops within the spinal cord) is technically difficult and can damage nerve structures. A dural tear occurs when a fracture of the cranial base results in leakage of CSF. Spinal muscle spasms are associated with traumatic complete transverse spinal cord lesions and range in intensity from mild muscular twitching to vigorous mass reflexogenic states. The spasms are involuntary and do not mean voluntary movement is returning. Nerve entrapment is injury or inflammation of single nerves caused by pressure from surrounding tissues. (Black J, Hokanson Hawks J: *Medical-surgical nursing: clinical management for positive outcomes*, ed 7, Philadelphia, 2005, Saunders; Drain C, editor: *Perianesthesia nursing: a critical care approach*, ed 4, Philadelphia, 2003, Saunders; Hickey JV: *The clinical practice of neurological and neurosurgical nursing*, ed 5, Philadelphia, 2003, Lippincott Williams & Wilkins; Moore KL, Dalley AF: *Clinically oriented anatomy*, ed 5, Philadelphia, 2006, Lippincott Williams & Wilkins.)

8.22. Correct Answer: **c**
Bupivacaine and tetracaine are long-acting local anesthetics, with bupivacaine producing slightly more intense sensory anesthesia and tetracaine having a more pronounced motor block. Chemical structure, dose, and lipid solubility alter duration. Injected volume and concentration of the anesthetic solution determine the dose. Tetracaine with epinephrine has the longest duration of action of the available spinal anesthetic agents. Procaine 10% is a low-potency, short-acting medication with less than 60 minutes' effect. A lidocaine 5% solution has a moderate duration of action, approximately 60 minutes. Diluting a local anesthetic medication in dextrose increases its density relative to cerebrospinal fluid (CSF); adding dextrose helps extend the drug's spread across dermatomes but does not alter the block's duration. Adding a narcotic provides postoperative analgesia but does not lengthen motor and sensory block. (Drain C, editor: *Perianesthesia nursing: a critical care approach*, ed 4, Philadelphia, 2003, Saunders; Quinn D, Schick L, editors: *ASPAN's perianesthesia nursing core curriculum: preoperative, Phase I and Phase II PACU nursing*, Philadelphia, 2004, Saunders; Rathmell JP, Neal JM, Viscomi CM: *Regional anesthesia: the requisites in anesthesiology*, St. Louis, 2004, Mosby; Stoelting RK, Miller RD: *Basics of anesthesia*, ed 5, London, 2007, Churchill Livingstone.)

8.23. Correct Answer: **a**
Epinephrine or phenylephrine added to a local anesthetic solution prolongs the duration of effect. Anesthesia could continue up to 50% to 60% longer. Vasoconstriction and delayed elimination of medication mean neural tissue has contact with the local anesthetic medication for a longer time, extending the effect of the block. This prolonged effect increases the potential for hypotension, particularly in the setting of hypovolemia. The local anesthetic medication acts on spinal nerves to prevent vasoconstriction below the level of injection. The size of the vascular compartment expands for the duration of the block's effect, particularly above the T10 dermatome. Filling this compartment

with additional IV fluid minimizes or prevents significant hypotension. The effect of the spinal with epinephrine prolongs the block and the potential for hypotension. (Quinn D, Schick L, editors: *ASPAN's perianesthesia nursing core curriculum: preoperative, Phase I and Phase II PACU nursing*, Philadelphia, 2004, Saunders; Rathmell JP, Neal JM, Viscomi CM: *Regional anesthesia: the requisites in anesthesiology*, St. Louis, 2004, Mosby; Stoelting RK, Miller RD: *Basics of anesthesia*, ed 5, London, 2007, Churchill Livingstone.)

8.24. Correct Answer: **d**
Distribution of anesthetic block (spread) is influenced by the patient's position and the density (weight or baricity) of the solution. *Gravity* greatly affects movement of local anesthetic in spinal fluid. A patient who remains in a sitting position for 5 to 10 minutes after the administration of medication has a more localized block than the patient who is immediately placed in a supine position so the medication can spread to affect several dermatomes. Anesthetic *density* is influenced by the diluting solution. Hyperbaric solutions diluted in dextrose extend the block; isobaric solutions in saline affect only a small area. Baricity is an important consideration because it predicts the direction that local anesthetic solution will move after injection into the CSF. The anesthesiologist seeks to control both the direction and extent of local anesthetic movement in the subarachnoid space and resultant distribution of anesthesia. Spinal anesthesia is not ordinarily performed above the L2-L3 interspace because the caudal limitations in most adults lies between the L1 and L2 vertebrae. In approximately

2% of adults, the spinal cord extends to the third lumbar vertebrae. The incidence of post–dural puncture headaches (PDPHs) varies directly with the size of the needle. PDPHs are more likely to occur in younger patients. Adding a vasoconstrictor is probably unrelated to the height of the anesthetic block. (Drain C, editor: *Perianesthesia nursing: a critical care approach*, ed 4, Philadelphia, 2003, Saunders; Robertson KM et al: *Anesthesiology board review*, ed 2, New York, 2006, McGraw-Hill; Quinn D, Schick L, editors: *ASPAN's perianesthesia nursing core curriculum: preoperative, Phase I and Phase II PACU nursing*, Philadelphia, 2004, Saunders; Stoelting RK, Miller RD: *Basics of anesthesia*, ed 5, London, 2007, Churchill Livingstone.)

8.25. Correct Answer: **b**
Hypotension is a likely consequence of spinal blockade because of the anesthetic's vasodilating effects and paralysis of neurovascular response. Vasodilation increases the vascular space; circulating blood volume is suddenly insufficient in this enlarged compartment. Blocked peripheral blood vessels cannot constrict in response to decreased blood pressure. Thus increasing fluid volume, ensuring tissue oxygenation, and maintaining cerebral blood flow with a head-low position are appropriate. (Drain C, editor: *Perianesthesia nursing: a critical care approach*, ed 4, Philadelphia, 2003, Saunders; Quinn D, Schick L, editors: *ASPAN's perianesthesia nursing core curriculum: preoperative, Phase I and Phase II PACU nursing*, Philadelphia, 2004, Saunders; Rathmell JP, Neal JM, Viscomi CM: *Regional anesthesia: the requisites in anesthesiology*, St. Louis, 2004, Mosby; Stoelting RK,

Miller RD: *Basics of anesthesia*, ed 5, London, 2007, Churchill Livingstone.)

8.26. Correct Answer: **b**
A patient who can lift a knee from the bed surface has regained motor function to approximately the L2 or L3 dermatome. Ability to plantar flex toes indicates the block has receded to the S1 to S2 dermatomes. Risk of hypotension is high when blockade is at the T5 dermatome and significantly decreases with block resolution to the level of the umbilicus (T10). (Drain C, editor: *Perianesthesia nursing: a critical care approach*, ed 4, Philadelphia, 2003, Saunders; Quinn D, Schick L, editors: *ASPAN's perianesthesia nursing core curriculum: preoperative, Phase I and Phase II PACU nursing*, Philadelphia, 2004, Saunders; Rathmell JP, Neal JM, Viscomi CM: *Regional anesthesia: the requisites in anesthesiology*, St. Louis, 2004, Mosby; Stoelting RK, Miller RD: *Basics of anesthesia*, ed 5, London, 2007, Churchill Livingstone.)

8.27. Correct Answer: **c**
As spinal anesthetic blockade resolves, motor function generally returns before either sensory function or sympathetic tone. Usually neurologic function returns in the reverse order from blockade. Evidence of sympathetic blockade can continue after both motor and sensory functions return. Sympathetic block causes vasodilation; symptoms are related to hypotension and the relative fluid volume deficit vasodilation creates. The nurse tests the patient's sensory block by assessing the patient's perception of cold, pinprick, or touch. (Drain C, editor: *Perianesthesia nursing: a critical care approach*, ed 4, Philadelphia, 2003, Saunders;

Quinn D, Schick L, editors: *ASPAN's perianesthesia nursing core curriculum: preoperative, Phase I and Phase II PACU nursing*, Philadelphia, 2004, Saunders; Stoelting RK, Miller RD: *Basics of anesthesia*, ed 5, London, 2007, Churchill Livingstone.)

8.28. Correct Answer: **a**
Level of consciousness is the single most important indicator of neurologic function and is the first change the patient presents with altered cerebral tissue perfusion. Consciousness is a dynamic state that is subject to change and can occur rapidly or slowly. Utilization of the Glasgow Coma Scale (GCS) measures the level of consciousness and severity of injury through pupillary changes, verbal responsiveness, and motor response. (Black J, Hokanson Hawks J: *Medical-surgical nursing: clinical management for positive outcomes*, ed 7, Philadelphia, 2005, Saunders; Hickey JV: *The clinical practice of neurological and neurosurgical nursing*, ed 5, Philadelphia, 2003, Lippincott Williams & Wilkins.)

8.29. Correct Answer: **b**
Sudden and intense headache, neck pain or stiffness, and nausea with vomiting are classic indicators of subarachnoid bleeding. Seizures, visual impairment, confusion, disorientation, or complete loss of consciousness may coincide. This patient has a high risk for a subarachnoid hemorrhage; his already leaking aneurysm can spontaneously rupture at any time, filling the subarachnoid space with blood. The brain loses its autoregulatory ability and cerebral perfusion pressure plummets as intracranial pressure rapidly increases. Hemorrhage may spread through subarachnoid fluid and compress intracranial structures, producing other

neurologic deficits. Other danger signs that may indicate an enlarging aneurysm include unilateral enlarged pupil, slowed pulse rate, hypoventilation, and increased blood pressure. (Abram SE: *Pain medicine: the requisites in anesthesiology*, St. Louis, 2006, Mosby; Springhouse: *Critical care nursing made incredibly easy!* Philadelphia, 2004, Lippincott Williams & Wilkins; Henry MH, Thompson JN: *Clinical surgery*, ed 2, Philadelphia, 2005, Saunders; Papadakos PJ: *Critical care: the requisites in anesthesiology*, St. Louis, 2005, Mosby.)

8.30. Correct Answer: **b**
Place the patch on a flat area of the upper torso after a *water* wash and *clipping* body hair. Heat and skin nicks increase absorption of any transdermal drug. Do not scrub or shave hair. Patients often need premedication with IV medication before the fentanyl patch has effect; however, a 3-mL (150-mcg) single dose of IV fentanyl is excessive and likely will alter consciousness and breathing. (Skidmore-Roth L: *Mosby's 2006 nursing drug reference*, St. Louis, 2006, Mosby; St. Marie B, editor: *Core curriculum for pain management nursing*, Philadelphia, 2002, Saunders.)

8.31. Correct Answer: **c**
A drowsy patient who rouses to follow simple commands when stimulated is *lethargic*. An *awake* patient becomes fully oriented and appropriate when stimulated, whereas a *stuporous* patient is very difficult to rouse and only with strong stimuli. Descriptions of nursing observations are best to describe a patient's level of consciousness, because any distinctions among these states are subjective. (Lagerquist SL: *Davis's*

NCLEX-RN success with CD ROM, Philadelphia, 2001, FA Davis; Quinn D, Schick L, editors: *ASPAN's perianesthesia nursing core curriculum: preoperative, Phase I and Phase II PACU nursing*, Philadelphia, 2004, Saunders; Springhouse: *Pathophysiology: a 2-in-1 reference for nurses*, Philadelphia, 2004, Lippincott Williams & Wilkins.)

8.32. Correct Answer: **b**
Hypocapnia is desirable to help reduce cerebral blood flow and intracranial volume, thereby minimizing intracranial pressure fluctuations. The patient's postoperative drowsiness and suppressed level of consciousness can represent residual effects of anesthetic medications or physiologic imbalances like hypothermia, inadequate ventilation with hypoxemia and hypercarbia, or an acid-base, chemical (hypoglycemia), or electrolyte imbalance. In the immediate post-anesthesia period, these factors must be considered while evaluating the possibility of increased intracranial pressure related to neurologic damage. (Atlee JL: *Complications in anesthesia*, ed 2, Philadelphia, 2007, Saunders; Lagerquist SL: *Davis's NCLEX-RN success with CD ROM*, Philadelphia, 2001, FA Davis.)

8.33. Correct Answer: **a**
Reporting to the neurosurgeon the patient's decrease in sensorium from lethargic to stuporous is appropriate—and essential. Even a subtle alteration in level of consciousness, the "most sensitive indicator of neurologic function," is one early clue of intracranial changes. Neurologic changes occur quickly, within 15 minutes. Signs indicating intracranial pressure increases progress in a rostral (top/front end) to caudal (down/lower part) direction within

the brain or from cerebrum to brainstem. Therefore brainstem signs like respiratory and pupillary changes suggest that either early changes were undetected or intracranial hypertension occurred quickly. Respiratory depression, perhaps from re-narcotization, is another possible reason for the patient's lethargy, though the suggested naloxone dose (0.8 mg) is excessive. Naloxone is more appropriately titrated in small increments to the patient's level of response to avoid treatment-related intracranial pressure increases. (Springhouse: *Critical care nursing made incredibly easy!*, Philadelphia, 2004, Lippincott Williams & Wilkins; Drain C, editor: *Perianesthesia nursing: a critical care approach*, ed 4, Philadelphia, 2003, Saunders; Quinn D, Schick L, editors: *ASPAN's perianesthesia nursing core curriculum: preoperative, Phase I and Phase II PACU nursing*, Philadelphia, 2004, Saunders; Skidmore-Roth L: *Mosby's 2006 nursing drug reference*, St. Louis, 2006, Mosby; Springhouse: *Pathophysiology: a 2-in-1 reference for nurses*, Philadelphia, 2004, Lippincott Williams & Wilkins.)

8.34. Correct Answer: **d**
The patient has observable responses only to an unpleasant (noxious) stimulus. The Glasgow Coma Scale is a widely accepted and objective assessment tool used to document trends in several neurologic functions. Applying this scale, the patient's best eye-opening response occurs only to pain; his best verbal response is none; and his best motor response is left arm flexion. These responses are each assessed when the patient is considered maximally stimulated by voice, touch, or painful stimulus. Both left- and right-sided responses are

scored. (Atlee JL: *Complications in anesthesia*, ed 2, Philadelphia, 2007, Saunders; Lagerquist SL: *Davis's NCLEX-RN success with CD ROM*, Philadelphia, 2001, FA Davis; Drain C, editor: *Perianesthesia nursing: a critical care approach*, ed 4, Philadelphia, 2003, Saunders; Henry MH, Thompson JN: *Clinical surgery*, ed 2, Philadelphia, 2005, Saunders.)

8.35. Correct Answer: **b**
Pressure pain to the toe, fingernails, or knuckles is a legitimate assessment technique; strong pinches or tissue twisting, direct eyeball pressure, and breast or genital touch are not. A multi-institution study of motor responses to painful stimuli yielded the most consistent responses when pressure was applied to the nailbed. A painful, noxious stimulus may elicit a physical response or increase awareness of a patient with decreased level of consciousness. The patient's skin must be protected from bruises, abrasions, or breaks in integrity. Pressure may be applied to the area *above* the eye (supraorbital ridge). (Morton PG et al: *Critical care nursing: a holistic approach*, ed 8, Philadelphia, 2005, Lippincott Williams & Wilkins; Quinn D, Schick L, editors: *ASPAN's perianesthesia nursing core curriculum: preoperative, Phase I and Phase II PACU nursing*, Philadelphia, 2004, Saunders.)

8.36. Correct Answer: **c**
The patient's response to pain is *decortication*, indicating interrupted corticospinal pathways with a "functional disconnection" of inhibiting impulses. Decorticate posturing indicates that function has been cut off at a lower level. A lesion or pressure affects neurologic function at the level of the cerebrum or thalamus. Greater deterioration to the

midbrain or pons level produces decerebration with rigid extension of all extremities. Asynchronous reflex is when the response is not simultaneous with the activity. Withdrawal reaction occurs when the patient pulls away from the noxious stimulus rather than attempts to remove it. (Drain C, editor: *Perianesthesia nursing: a critical care approach*, ed 4, Philadelphia, 2003, Saunders; Hickey JV: *The clinical practice of neurological and neurosurgical nursing*, ed 5, Philadelphia, 2003, Lippincott Williams & Wilkins; Morton PG et al: *Critical care nursing: a holistic approach*, ed 8, Philadelphia, 2005, Lippincott Williams & Wilkins; Quinn D, Schick L, editors: *ASPAN's perianesthesia nursing core curriculum: preoperative, Phase I and Phase II PACU nursing*, Philadelphia, 2004, Saunders.)

8.37. Correct Answer: **a**
The patient's symptoms indicate a dire emergency to prevent herniation of brain tissue into linings of the cranial cavity. Herniation with brainstem compression is called *central herniation*. Compensatory adaptations that adjust CSF and blood flow (autoregulation) have been exhausted. The closed cranial cavity cannot expand to accommodate long-term increases in brain tissue, CSF volume, or blood flow. Compression of intracranial structures occurs instead—until the pressure exceeds cranial capacity and contents push through the most available, least resistant opening. Hydrocephalus indicates an imbalance between the production and absorption of the CSF. An obstruction of the normal CSF drainage pathways results in the CSF being shunted. (Atlee JL: *Complications in anesthesia*, ed 2, Philadelphia, 2007, Saunders; Hickey JV: *The clinical practice of neurological and neurosurgical nursing*, ed 5, Philadelphia, 2003, Lippincott Williams & Wilkins; Morton PG et al: *Critical care nursing: a holistic approach*, ed 8, Philadelphia, 2005, Lippincott Williams & Wilkins.)

8.38. Correct Answer: **c**
A lesion or increased pressure predominately in the *left* cerebral hemisphere will produce same-sided, or *ipsilateral*, changes in the *left* pupil. Right-sided cranial lesions likely affect the right pupil. Cranial nerve III nuclei responsible for controlling pupil size are located in the brainstem. By the time pupillary changes occur, pressure from herniating brain structures has already compressed cranial nerve III and prevented constriction, so pupils become unequal (anisocoria). When observed in the less-than-alert patient, particularly one with documented trauma or intracranial lesion, one dilated, or "blown," pupil is a true neurologic emergency. (Hickey JV: *The clinical practice of neurological and neurosurgical nursing*, ed 5, Philadelphia, 2003, Lippincott Williams & Wilkins.)

8.39. Correct Answer: **a**
Decreasing pCO_2 by manually hyperventilating the patient after reintubation reduces blood flow and may prevent further rises in intracranial pressure (ICP). Prolonged hyperventilation has been shown to worsen the outcome of patients with severe head injuries (pCO_2 of less than 25 mmHg). When hyperventilation is discontinued, ventilation rates should be returned to normal gradually to avoid the rebound effect of vasodilation. Immediate CT scanning may pinpoint intracranial bleeding for a likely surgical re-exploration. Subdural veins bleed

quickly and cause acute hematoma, compression of intracranial contents, and potential for rapid herniation. Meanwhile, mannitol may temporarily decrease ICP. Suctioning, stir-up activities, and positions that increase cerebral blood flow (flat) or flex the neck further stress labile patients who have limited intracranial adaptive reserves. (Faust RJ, editor: *Anesthesiology review*, ed 3, London, 2002, Churchill Livingstone; Miller RD et al, editors: *Anesthesia* (2-vol set with CD-ROM for Windows & Macintosh), ed 5, London, 2000, Churchill Livingstone; Morton PG et al: *Critical care nursing: a holistic approach*, ed 8, Philadelphia, 2005, Lippincott Williams & Wilkins.)

8.40. Correct Answer: **b**
Dexamethasone (Decadron) may decrease edema in cerebral tissues, thereby reducing the intracranial volume. Tissue edema occurs with surgical manipulation. The adaptive capacity that compensates for shifting blood flow, cerebrospinal fluid volume, and brain tissue mass may improve. This medication is a synthetic adrenocorticoid with intense antiinflammatory activity and a long duration of effect. Decadron is not used for supporting physiologic responses or decreasing seizure threshold. (Donohoe Dennison D: *Pass CCRN*, ed 2, St. Louis, 2000, Mosby; Drain C, editor: *Perianesthesia nursing: a critical care approach*, ed 4, Philadelphia, 2003, Saunders.)

SET 2

ANSWER KEY

8.41.	b		**8.57.**	c
8.42.	c		**8.58.**	d
8.43.	b		**8.59.**	b
8.44.	a		**8.60.**	d
8.45.	a		**8.61.**	d
8.46.	d		**8.62.**	c
8.47.	b		**8.63.**	a
8.48.	b		**8.64.**	b
8.49.	d		**8.65.**	d
8.50.	c		**8.66.**	a
8.51.	d		**8.67.**	b
8.52.	a		**8.68.**	a
8.53.	c		**8.69.**	a
8.54.	d		**8.70.**	c
8.55.	c		**8.71.**	c
8.56.	a		**8.72.**	b

SET 2

RATIONALES AND REFERENCES

8.41. Correct Answer: **b**
Respiratory depression often follows pain relief with fentanyl. Kappa receptor stimulation produces constricted, pinpoint-size pupils. Fentanyl is a highly potent opioid agonist with mu receptor effects that are similar to morphine. It is approximately 80 to 125 times as potent as morphine, acts quickly (within 5 to 6 minutes), and provides analgesia of moderate duration. This short duration of action reflects its rapid redistribution to inactive tissues, such as fat and skeletal muscles, with a decrease in plasma concentration of the drug. Patients who receive high doses of fentanyl may develop a "delayed-onset respiratory depression," which may occur about 45 minutes after administration of the drug when the drug is recycled from the inactive tissues into the plasma. (Drain C, editor: *Perianesthesia nursing: a critical care approach*, ed 4, Philadelphia, 2003, Saunders; Stoelting RK, Miller RD: *Basics of anesthesia*, ed 5, London, 2007, Churchill Livingstone.)

8.42. Correct Answer: **c**
This patient needs adequate arm support so that his fingers are elevated above his heart level to promote venous return. Ideally this position also promotes comfort. After replantation of an amputated body part, medical and nursing goals focus on promoting circulation and decreasing any factors that may cause vasoconstriction. Frequent neurovascular assessment is critical to quickly detect any circulatory compromise. The surgeon may request temperature monitoring or pulse detection to monitor blood flow. Warmth and adequate hydration promote blood flow. Analgesics promote comfort and interrupt the physiologic stress response that also produces peripheral vasoconstriction. (Quinn D, Schick L, editors: *ASPAN's perianesthesia nursing core curriculum: preoperative, Phase I and Phase II PACU nursing*, Philadelphia, 2004, Saunders; Oman KS, Koziol-McLain J: *Emergency nursing secrets*, ed 2, St. Louis, 2007, Mosby.)

8.43. Correct Answer: **b**
The reticular activating system (RAS) originates at the midbrain in an organized group of functional neurons, the reticular formation. Axons extend upward through to the thalamus and cortex to bring cerebral awareness of sensory and chemical input from environmental stimuli to conscious attention. The RAS is sensitive to depression by medication, hypoxia- or hypoglycemia-induced metabolic alterations, and even small changes in brainstem pressure. The RAS helps maintain consciousness and is active during awakening from sleep. The limbic-pyramidal system provides a neural substrate for emotions. This is the area where the neural pathways provide a connection between higher brain functioning and endocrine or autonomic activities. The corpus callosum connects the two cerebral hemispheres and is essential in the coordination of activities between the hemispheres. The thalamus functions as a sensory and motor relay center. (Black J, Hokanson Hawks J: *Medical-surgical nursing: clinical management for positive outcomes*, ed 7, Philadelphia, 2005, Saunders; McCance KL,

Huether SE: *Pathophysiology: the biologic basis for disease in adults and children*, ed 4, St. Louis, 2002, Mosby; Tortora GJ, Derrickson BH: *Principles of anatomy and physiology*, ed 11, Hoboken, NJ, 2006, John Wiley & Sons.)

8.44. Correct Answer: **a**
The corpus callosum connects the two cerebral hemispheres and is essential in the coordination of activities between hemispheres. The longitudinal fissure separates cortical hemispheres, the lateral ventricle gyri are the winding convolutions in the cavity in the cerebral hemisphere that communicates with the third ventricle through the interventricular foramen, and the central sulcus is the fissure separating the parietal and frontal lobes. Gyri are folds; sulci are grooves, and fissures are clefts within the cerebral cortex of the brain. (Drain C, editor: *Perianesthesia nursing: a critical care approach*, ed 4, Philadelphia, 2003, Saunders; Black J, Hokanson Hawks J: *Medical-surgical nursing: clinical management for positive outcomes*, ed 7, Philadelphia, 2005, Saunders; Moore KL, Dalley AF: *Clinically oriented anatomy*, ed 5, Philadelphia, 2006, Lippincott Williams & Wilkins; *Mosby's medical, nursing, & allied health dictionary*, ed 6, St. Louis, 2002, Mosby.)

8.45. Correct Answer: **a**
Hypoglycemia, a measured glucose of less than 50 mg/dL, can cause irreversible damage to the nervous system. Preoperative fasting, symptom-masking sedative and anesthetic medications, excessive insulin doses, and renal failure (a likelihood for the insulin-dependent patient who is older than 30 years) can mask recognition and prevent treatment of low glucose levels. An infection after multiple glucose

samplings is unlikely to happen immediately after surgery. Rapid infusion of blood products decreases ionized calcium caused by binding with the citrate; therefore hypocalcemia occurs. Antibiotic therapy is usually started preoperatively on patients having hip arthroplasty so altered intestinal flora should not impact the patient immediately postoperatively. (Miller RD et al, editors: *Anesthesia* (2-vol set with CD-ROM for Windows & Macintosh), ed 5, London, 2000, Churchill Livingstone; Papadakos PJ: *Critical care: the requisites in anesthesiology*, St. Louis, 2005, Mosby.)

8.46. Correct Answer: **d**
Mannitol is an osmotic diuretic that increases the serum osmolarity. Solute or particle concentration is then greater in circulating blood than in tissue, creating a pressure disparity. Mannitol is a "staple" medication in neurosurgery; the osmotic pressure gradient pulls water from intracellular (brain) tissue into the vascular compartment for excretion through the kidneys. Reducing cerebral edema decreases intracranial pressure. (Drain C, editor: *Perianesthesia nursing: a critical care approach*, ed 4, Philadelphia, 2003, Saunders; Skidmore-Roth L: *Mosby's 2006 nursing drug reference*, St. Louis, 2006, Mosby.)

8.47. Correct Answer: **b**
A single dose of epidural morphine (Duramorph) can depress respirations early, within the first hour or two after injection, and again several hours later. The patient's greatest hypoventilation risk continues for another 8 to 12 hours (up to 16 hours after injection). Morphine spreads slowly and gradually up (cephalad) through the cerebrospinal fluid, eventually

reaching the brain's respiratory centers. This migration is termed *rostral spread*. Protocols for post-epidural monitoring often recommend close consciousness and respiratory observation for up to 24 hours. Fentanyl is sometimes used as an epidural analgesic because its clearance from the body is more rapid, with less opportunity for spread through CSF to alter ventilation. Side effects of epidural opioids are respiratory depression, nausea and vomiting, urinary retention, and pruritus. Naloxone carefully titrated may suppress the side effects while leaving the analgesic effect intact. (Abram SE: *Pain medicine: the requisites in anesthesiology*, St. Louis, 2006, Mosby; Rathmell JP, Neal JM, Viscomi CM: *Regional anesthesia: the requisites in anesthesiology*, St. Louis, 2004, Mosby; Stoelting RK, Miller RD: *Basics of anesthesia*, ed 5, London, 2007, Churchill Livingstone.)

8.48. Correct Answer: **b**
During seizures, the clonic phase follows the tonic phase during which time the patient loses consciousness, has apnea, cries out, and develops generalized stiffness. During the clonic phase of a seizure, the patient will have jerking of the limbs and salivary frothing. Initially there is rhythmic, jerky contraction and relaxation of all body muscles, particularly those of the extremities. Patients are usually incontinent and may bite their lip, tongue, and inside of their mouth. (Black J, Hokanson Hawks J: *Medical-surgical nursing: clinical management for positive outcomes*, ed 7, Philadelphia, 2005, Saunders; Swearingen PL: *Manual of medical-surgical nursing care: nursing interventions and collaborative management*, ed 5, St. Louis, 2003, Mosby.)

8.49. Correct Answer: **d**
Observing a single, dilated pupil in this young patient likely reflects brain edema or rebleeding at the surgical site that displaces brain tissue. First, though, the nurse should distinguish new anisocoria (unequal pupils) from a pupil that is dilated from a congenital condition, from medications, or from prior eye surgery. The perianesthesia nurse needs to document pupil status, prior eye surgery, and use of mydriatic (dilating) ocular medications preoperatively to provide an important postoperative reference. Uncal displacement, the movement of part of the cerebrum's temporal lobe through the tentorium, is the most common herniation syndrome. Brain compression has occurred, and contents press on nuclei of cranial nerve III in the brainstem. Meningeal irritation signs include generalized throbbing headache and photophobia that become very severe, nuchal rigidity, Kernig sign, and Brudzinski sign. (Black J, Hokanson Hawks J: *Medical-surgical nursing: clinical management for positive outcomes*, ed 7, Philadelphia, 2005, Saunders; McCance KL, Huether SE: *Pathophysiology: the biologic basis for disease in adults and children*, ed 4, St. Louis, 2002, Mosby; Quinn D, Schick L, editors: *ASPAN's perianesthesia nursing core curriculum: preoperative, Phase I and Phase II PACU nursing*, Philadelphia, 2004, Saunders.)

8.50. Correct Answer: **c**
The procedure was probably performed while the patient was in the prone position. Specific attention ensures that bony prominences were adequately padded and body weight did not unduly compress soft tissues. Eye abrasions, especially during turning, and inadvertent ear bending can cause damage. Body weight might rest

against the rib cage and iliac crests, causing skin redness or open breaks in skin integrity during the hours of surgery. The nurse should document and report apparent injury and improvement in skin condition during the PACU stay. A sciatic nerve stretch test is done by raising the patient's leg until pain is elicited. The leg is then lowered to a comfortable level where the examiner dorsiflexes the foot to stretch the sciatic nerve. If pain occurs with dorsiflexion, the test is positive for sciatic nerve involvement. Sciatica is usually associated with intervertebral disk herniation and hyperflexion of the hip during surgery. (Morton PG et al: *Critical care nursing: a holistic approach*, ed 8, Philadelphia, 2005, Lippincott Williams & Wilkins; Rothrock J, editor: *Alexander's care of the patient in surgery*, ed 12, St. Louis, 2003, Mosby; Stoelting RK, Miller RD: *Basics of anesthesia*, ed 5, London, 2007, Churchill Livingstone; Swearingen PL: *Manual of medical-surgical nursing care: nursing interventions and collaborative management*, ed 5, St. Louis, 2003, Mosby.)

8.51.   Correct Answer: **d**
Supplemental doses of IV narcotics provide analgesia until concentrations of epidurally infused narcotics reach therapeutic levels. In this situation, small (2-3 mg) doses of IV morphine sulfate provide pain relief within 7 minutes while the pharmacy and nursing staff promptly ready the fentanyl solution and epidural infusion pump. As a single postoperative dose in the PACU, intravenous fentanyl 150 mcg and intramuscular morphine sulfate 15 mg is excessive. (St. Marie B, editor: *Core curriculum for pain management nursing*, Philadelphia, 2002, Saunders; Stoelting RK, Miller RD: *Basics of*

anesthesia, ed 5, London, 2007, Churchill Livingstone.)

8.52.   Correct Answer: **a**
Before any infusion is initiated, the epidural catheter *must* be gently aspirated to determine catheter contents; the PACU nurse must also document that catheter tubing is securely taped. Aspirating bloody fluid may reflect entry into the dura during spinal surgery or may signal catheter migration into an epidural blood vessel; a bolus of fentanyl could be inadvertently injected into the circulation. Easy aspiration of clear fluid may indicate catheter movement across the dura into the subarachnoid space to obtain cerebrospinal fluid. When sanctioned by state law, facility policy, and unit protocols, the nurse's responsibility includes pain and epidural catheter management. Whenever catheter movement is suspected or unexpected fluid is aspirated, the anesthesia provider must be informed and the infusion deferred. (ASPAN: *2006-2008 Standards of perianesthesia nursing practice*, Cherry Hill, NJ, 2006, ASPAN; Stoelting RK, Miller RD: *Basics of anesthesia*, ed 5, London, 2007, Churchill Livingstone.)

8.53.   Correct Answer: **c**
A purely *narcotic* epidural solution that contains no local anesthetic seldom causes profound hypotension. Narcotics do not directly block sympathetic fibers that control vascular constriction and dilation. Over time, a moderate blood pressure decrease may reflect increased comfort. Potential for respiratory depression must be a primary concern during continuous narcotic infusion as fentanyl circulates and affects the brain's respiratory center. Nausea, itching, and urinary retention are also common. The patient should be

able to move her legs; sensory or motor loss is unlikely with a purely narcotic infusion. (Drain C, editor: *Perianesthesia nursing: a critical care approach*, ed 4, Philadelphia, 2003, Saunders; Stoelting RK, Miller RD: *Basics of anesthesia*, ed 5, London, 2007, Churchill Livingstone.)

8.54. Correct Answer: **d**
Transfer from the PACU should be delayed pending further nursing observation and notification and evaluation by the physician. These symptoms are new and raise concern and do not relate to her surgical procedure. Severe pain unrelated to the surgical site or incision is significant and requires further investigation. Backache and neurologic changes may result from epidural hematoma, whereas thrombosis in an abdominal artery can produce weakness and buttock or leg pain. Answers **a, b**, and **c** are inappropriate because the *changes in the patient's condition are not related to her surgical procedure but to the epidural catheter in place*. The patient's neurologic assessment has deteriorated from when she arrived in the PACU. Repositioning the leg and increasing the epidural infusion will increase the patient's discomfort and add to the complication of increased bleeding in the epidural space. (Atlee JL: *Complications in anesthesia*, ed 2, Philadelphia, 2007, Saunders; Rathmell JP, Neal JM, Viscomi CM: *Regional anesthesia: the requisites in anesthesiology*, St. Louis, 2004, Mosby.)

8.55. Correct Answer: **c**
In this young and healthy patient, prolonged muscle relaxation probably results from atypical pseudocholinesterase, a genetically determined inability to metabolize succinylcholine.

Pseudocholinesterase may be deficient in either amount or effectiveness. The patient remains weak, and vigilant nursing observation and possibly respiratory support will be necessary until succinylcholine's effects naturally dissipate. Pseudocholinesterase deficiency can also be acquired. Normally the enzyme *pseudocholinesterase* rapidly destroys succinylcholine, the depolarizing muscle relaxant, in the plasma. (Burden N et al: *Ambulatory surgical nursing*, ed 2, Philadelphia, 2000, Saunders; Drain C, editor: *Perianesthesia nursing: a critical care approach*, ed 4, Philadelphia, 2003, Saunders; Stoelting RK, Miller RD: *Basics of anesthesia*, ed 5, London, 2007, Churchill Livingstone.)

8.56. Correct Answer: **a**
The device is too tight and the pressure is compressing the nerves and causing damage. Because of its softness, the A-frame itself would not cause pressure that leads to decreased circulation. Postoperative pain can cause the patient to not want to move but will not cause the patient to experience weakness. Pain control will alleviate the patient's desire to not move. Nerve damage is very rare, but the symptoms would generally be seen on admission, not 30 minutes after admission. (Litwack K, editor: *Core curriculum for perianesthesia nursing practice*, ed 4, Philadelphia, 1999, Saunders.)

8.57. Correct Answer: **c**
Rapid development of the patient's symptoms strongly suggests local anesthetic toxicity, which quickly penetrates the blood-brain barrier to produce dizziness, tingling, and tinnitus. Toxic effects may soon result in muscle twitching, tremors, and generalized seizure. Depending upon the amount of circulating local

anesthetic, vasodilation, hypotension, and delayed intracardiac conduction could also occur with toxicity; providing adrenergic antagonism with labetalol is probably unnecessary. Significance of the patient's symptoms is determined by the dose of local anesthetic absorbed. Oxygen, close nursing observation, and physician notification are primary first interventions. The toxicity occurs when a local anesthetic rapidly enters the circulation, either by rapid or unanticipated injection. (Burden N et al: *Ambulatory surgical nursing*, ed 2, Philadelphia, 2000, Saunders; Stoelting RK, Miller RD: *Basics of anesthesia*, ed 5, London, 2007, Churchill Livingstone.)

8.58. Correct Answer: **d**
Adequate capillary refill (within 3 seconds) and skin color indicate the circulatory status in the patient's casted extremity. Train-of-four (TOF) is used to monitor appropriate muscle relaxation after the use of muscle relaxants. After 6 hours, the patient's brachial plexus block has probably resolved; return of motor and sensory function is not usually a discharge requirement after a regional block. She must know how to protect her arm until these functions do return. Her discharge instructions will include use of her analgesic prescription and how to regularly assess her hand circulation. (Drain C, editor: *Perianesthesia nursing: a critical care approach*, ed 4, Philadelphia, 2003, Saunders; Papadakos PJ: *Critical care: the requisites in anesthesiology*, St. Louis, 2005, Mosby; Quinn D, Schick L, editors: *ASPAN's perianesthesia nursing core curriculum: preoperative, Phase I and Phase II PACU nursing*, Philadelphia, 2004, Saunders.)

8.59. Correct Answer: **b**
The patient's plaster cast will not dry for up to 24 hours and so is at risk for damage and deformity from dents, pressure, and hard surfaces. A deformed cast can increase pressure against her arm, compressing blood flow and impairing nerve and muscle function. Ice may help reduce pain and arm edema. To prevent skin breaks and possible infection, nothing should be inserted between the cast and her skin even though her skin may itch. (Black J, Hokanson Hawks J: *Medical-surgical nursing: clinical management for positive outcomes*, ed 7, Philadelphia, 2005, Saunders; Quinn D, Schick L, editors: *ASPAN's perianesthesia nursing core curriculum: preoperative, Phase I and Phase II PACU nursing*, Philadelphia, 2004, Saunders.)

8.60. Correct Answer: **d**
The patient's cast may still feel warm as it dries although the normal initial "burning" sensation probably has abated; the exterior surface may now feel cool. She should report fever, unrelenting pain, and cast odor to her surgeon as indicators of possible infection or compartment syndrome. The purplish hand color may be bruising but could also indicate venous congestion and impaired circulation from a cast that is too tight. Always compare the right and left fingers, hands, and arms for similarity in color, degree of swelling, temperature, pulses (if discernible), sensation, and capillary refill. (Black J, Hokanson Hawks J: *Medical-surgical nursing: clinical management for positive outcomes*, ed 7, Philadelphia, 2005, Saunders; Quinn D, Schick L, editors: *ASPAN's perianesthesia nursing core curriculum: preoperative, Phase I and Phase II PACU nursing*, Philadelphia, 2004, Saunders.)

8.61. Correct Answer: **d**
The primary purpose of the occipital lobes is to receive and understand visual images. The occipital lobe is located in the cortex of the brain, which also consists of the frontal, parietal and temporal lobes. The purpose of the frontal lobe is reasoning, emotions, and problem-solving. The purpose of the parietal lobe is movement, orientation, and perception. The purpose of the temporal lobe includes auditory, memory and speech. (Black J, Hokanson Hawks J: *Medical-surgical nursing: clinical management for positive outcomes*, ed 7, Philadelphia, 2005, Saunders; Springhouse: *Critical care nursing made incredibly easy!*, Philadelphia, 2004, Lippincott Williams & Wilkins; Morton PG et al: *Critical care nursing: a holistic approach*, ed 8, Philadelphia, 2005, Lippincott Williams & Wilkins; Quinn D, Schick L, editors: *ASPAN's perianesthesia nursing core curriculum: preoperative, Phase I and Phase II PACU nursing*, Philadelphia, 2004, Saunders.)

8.62. Correct Answer: **c**
Maintaining hip alignment is essential for the patient. After repair of a fracture to the femoral neck, adduction, hip flexion, and often positioning on the operative side are specifically avoided. She also still has spinal anesthetic effects and no motor control of her legs; the legs will naturally externally rotate and adduct. Limiting leg movement, securing an abduction pillow between her thighs, perhaps placing a trochanter roll next to the left thigh, and maintaining a flat position without hip flexion promote hip safety. Ice may reduce swelling and pain. Avoid placing pillows behind her knees that could impair circulation and compress nerves; observe for hip drainage that could seep from the dressing and pool beneath the patient. (Drain C, editor: *Perianesthesia nursing: a critical care approach*, ed 4, Philadelphia, 2003, Saunders; Quinn D, Schick L, editors: *ASPAN's perianesthesia nursing core curriculum: preoperative, Phase I and Phase II PACU nursing*, Philadelphia, 2004, Saunders.)

8.63. Correct Answer: **a**
The patient's ability to form the words to state her name indicates that she can speak. An intact left cortical hemisphere is essential to both spoken language and comprehension. The dominant frontal lobe area at the inferior portion of the third gyrus controls motor speech. Damage to this area renders the patient able to understand written and oral language but unable to produce words. Located within the temporal lobe area is the primary auditory reception area and Wernicke's area, which is associated with language comprehension. The parietal lobe is the primary center for sensation. The occipital lobe is the primary visual receptor center. Damage to any of these specific cortical areas produces a corresponding loss of function. (Springhouse: *Critical care nursing made incredibly easy!*, Philadelphia, 2004, Lippincott Williams & Wilkins; Morton PG et al: *Critical care nursing: a holistic approach*, ed 8, Philadelphia, 2005, Lippincott Williams & Wilkins; Quinn D, Schick L, editors: *ASPAN's perianesthesia nursing core curriculum: preoperative, Phase I and Phase II PACU nursing*, Philadelphia, 2004, Saunders.)

8.64. Correct Answer: **b**
A lesion at *Broca's area*, at the third convolution of the person's dominant frontal lobe (usually the left), impairs the ability to speak and

causes motor (expressive) aphasia. Producing words is difficult even though muscles controlling the mouth move adequately and ability to understand remains intact. Understanding spoken words, assuming auditory capability is intact, is governed by Wernicke's area. Damage here produces sensory aphasia. (Black J, Hokanson Hawks J: *Medical-surgical nursing: clinical management for positive outcomes*, ed 7, Philadelphia, 2005, Saunders; Morton PG et al: *Critical care nursing: a holistic approach*, ed 8, Philadelphia, 2005, Lippincott Williams & Wilkins; Quinn D, Schick L, editors: *ASPAN's perianesthesia nursing core curriculum: preoperative, Phase I and Phase II PACU nursing*, Philadelphia, 2004, Saunders.)

8.65. Correct Answer: **d**
Coordinated (conjugate) eye movements with no jerking (nystagmus) and with pupils that constrict briskly to light and simultaneously (consensually) and upper eyelid elevation indicate proper oculomotor function. Cranial nerves III (oculomotor), IV (trochlear), and VI (abducens) team to control optic function identified in the neurologic examination as the *PERRLA* (pupils equal, round, react to light and accommodation). Pupil size inequity, nonsymmetric pupillary response to light, or extraocular movements can indicate extreme pressure on brainstem structures (midbrain and pons) that contain the nuclei of these cranial nerves. In the postcraniotomy patient, such unilateral changes are critical events. (Black J, Hokanson Hawks J: *Medical-surgical nursing: clinical management for positive outcomes*, ed 7, Philadelphia, 2005, Saunders; Morton PG et al: *Critical care nursing: a holistic approach*, ed 8, Philadelphia, 2005, Lippincott

Williams & Wilkins; Quinn D, Schick L, editors: *ASPAN's perianesthesia nursing core curriculum: preoperative, Phase I and Phase II PACU nursing*, Philadelphia, 2004, Saunders.)

8.66. Correct Answer: **a**
Upper arm muscle strength and tone are assessed when both arms are extended with palms facing up. The patient's eyes are closed during assessment. Loss of strength causes a weak arm to rotate and begin to fall (termed *pronator drift*). Increasing intracranial pressure likely produces noticeable upper extremity weakness before the lower arm is affected. Therefore a traditional "squeeze my hand" command and "hyperextending one's hand and wrist" do not provide reliable information to detect small, early changes in the relationships among cerebral function and muscle control, strength, and tone that occur long before consciousness changes. Adducting one's shoulder is a function of cranial nerve XI (spinal accessory nerve), which penetrates and innervates the sternocleidomastoid and trapezius and not the upper arm. Even decerebrate patients can seem to squeeze a hand, though not to command. (Black J, Hokanson Hawks J: *Medical-surgical nursing: clinical management for positive outcomes*, ed 7, Philadelphia, 2005, Saunders; Moore KL, Dalley AF: *Clinically oriented anatomy*, ed 5, Philadelphia, 2006, Lippincott Williams & Wilkins; Morton PG et al: *Critical care nursing: a holistic approach*, ed 8, Philadelphia, 2005, Lippincott Williams & Wilkins; Quinn D, Schick L, editors: *ASPAN's perianesthesia nursing core curriculum: preoperative, Phase I and Phase II PACU nursing*, Philadelphia, 2004, Saunders.)

8.67. Correct Answer: **b**
Capillaries in the choroid plexus of the lateral and third ventricles produce 500 to 600 mL of CSF each day. Osmotic pressure and active transport systems contribute to production. Subarachnoid spaces contain most (about 100 mL) of the approximately 100 to 160 mL of CSF continuously circulating through the brain's ventricular system and subarachnoid space. (Black J, Hokanson Hawks J: *Medical-surgical nursing: clinical management for positive outcomes*, ed 7, Philadelphia, 2005, Saunders; Quinn D, Schick L, editors: *ASPAN's perianesthesia nursing core curriculum: preoperative, Phase I and Phase II PACU nursing*, Philadelphia, 2004, Saunders.)

8.68. Correct Answer: **a**
Systolic blood pressure increases, diastolic blood pressure decreases, and profound bradycardia develops as the brain's adaptive capacity succumbs to continuous increases in intracranial pressure. A patient presenting these three signs of Cushing's triad faces imminent death. Clinicians ***must act*** earlier to reverse more subtle signs of increasing intracranial pressure and potential herniation long before continued ischemia and medullary pressure produce this triad of signs and herald irreversible neurologic damage. (Black J, Hokanson Hawks J: *Medical-surgical nursing: clinical management for positive outcomes*, ed 7, Philadelphia, 2005, Saunders; Drain C, editor: *Perianesthesia nursing: a critical care approach*, ed 4, Philadelphia, 2003, Saunders; Morton PG et al: *Critical care nursing: a holistic approach*, ed 8, Philadelphia, 2005, Lippincott Williams & Wilkins; Quinn D, Schick L, editors: *ASPAN's perianesthesia nursing core curriculum:*

preoperative, Phase I and Phase II PACU nursing, Philadelphia, 2004, Saunders.)

8.69. Correct Answer: **a**
Most connections between the higher and lower brain structures (tracts) emerge from the medulla (brainstem) after the pyramids decussate, or cross, to the opposite side. Voluntary muscle activity is controlled by the pyramidal system, which arises in the frontal lobes and descends through the brainstem. The right lateral pyramidal tract, therefore, carries impulses to control left contralateral functions. (Drain C, editor: *Perianesthesia nursing: a critical care approach*, ed 4, Philadelphia, 2003, Saunders; Morton PG et al: *Critical care nursing: a holistic approach*, ed 8, Philadelphia, 2005, Lippincott Williams & Wilkins.)

8.70. Correct Answer: **c**
Hemoglobin is generally measured early in the postoperative period and regularly thereafter. Surgical intervention for scoliosis is associated with potential for major blood loss, and replacing lost blood cells may be necessary to ensure adequate tissue oxygenation. Patients with significant scoliosis may have altered lung capacity; deep breathing is essential to help maintain lung tissue expansion. To prevent instrument displacement, the patient should *not* use her arms to reposition herself or be lifted under her arms by others. Facial edema *is* likely from gravity-induced migration of fluid to lips, eyes, nose, and cheeks during several intraoperative hours in a prone position; these fluids gradually re-shift over days. Gastric distention and potential for ileus are best relieved by nasogastric tube, not position. (Black J, Hokanson Hawks J: *Medical-surgical nursing: clinical*

management for positive outcomes, ed 7, Philadelphia, 2005, Saunders; Quinn D, Schick L, editors: *ASPAN's perianesthesia nursing core curriculum: preoperative, Phase I and Phase II PACU nursing*, Philadelphia, 2004, Saunders.)

8.71. Correct Answer: **c**

"Salvage" of intraoperative blood loss, washing away many contaminants and then re-infusing, provides the patient with immediately available blood. Viability, function and numbers of platelets, and specific clotting factors remain near normal for up to 24 hours; these factors diminish as blood is banked and stored. Processing of shed blood washes away most but not all of the citrate that can alter function of coagulation factors. Blood must be reinfused within 6 hours through tubing with microaggregate filters. (Atlee JL: *Complications in anesthesia*, ed 2, Philadelphia, 2007, Saunders; Cole DJ, Schlunt M: *Adult perioperative anesthesia: the requisites in anesthesiology*, St. Louis, 2004, Mosby.)

8.72. Correct Answer: **b**

No medications, including patient-controlled analgesia (PCA) narcotics, should infuse with blood. Evidence of hemolysis (hematuria), transfusion reaction (fever, chills, nausea, flank pain, oliguria), particulate microembolism, and sepsis *can* occur with autotransfusion. Procedures for reinfusing processed, shed intraoperative blood resemble procedures for transfusion of banked blood: infuse within 4 hours, follow established facility protocols for tubing requirements and patient identification, and closely monitor temperature, vital signs, and the patient response. Cramping, tingling, or new cardiac dysrhythmias may indicate altered calcium balance or acidosis; increased wound drainage can indicate developing coagulopathy. (Springhouse: *IV Therapy Made Incredibly Easy!* Philadelphia, 1998, Lippincott Williams & Wilkins.)

SET 3

ANSWER KEY

8.73.	c		**8.87.**	a
8.74.	d		**8.88.**	c
8.75.	c		**8.89.**	d
8.76.	d		**8.90.**	a
8.77.	d		**8.91.**	b
8.78.	a		**8.92.**	b
8.79.	a		**8.93.**	c
8.80.	c		**8.94.**	d
8.81.	c		**8.95.**	a
8.82.	b		**8.96.**	c
8.83.	c		**8.97.**	d
8.84.	d		**8.98.**	c
8.85.	b		**8.99.**	d
8.86.	b			

SET 3

8.73. Correct Answer: **c**

This would not be an appropriate block for this type of surgery. Interscalene blocks do not totally numb the hand adequately to do surgery. To adequately perform surgery on the hand would require additional blocking of the ulnar nerve. The uses for the interscalene blocks are shoulder procedures and some arm/hand surgeries (if a tourniquet is to be used, must also block the intercostobrachial nerve). (Graber R: *Interscalene block.* Website: www.uhcanesthesia.com/ClinDiv/Anesthesiology/Regional-%20Anesthesia/ISB/view. Accessed May 2, 2007; Litwack K, editor: *Core curriculum for perianesthesia nursing practice,* ed 4, Philadelphia, 1999, Saunders; Perry AG, Potter PA: *Clinical nursing skills and techniques,* ed 6, St. Louis, 2006, Mosby.)

8.74. Correct Answer: **d**

Numbness right after the surgery is likely caused by the block. The status needs to be observed for length of numbness to assess for any complications. Complications can occur with interscalene blocks. Postoperative paresthesias or nerve deficit is one complication from an interscalene block. This is thought to be caused by nerve damage from needle placement and will generally resolve within 3 months. This complication could also be caused by trauma from the surgery or positioning. Toxic local anesthetic levels can occur either from direct injection of the local anesthetic into the vascular system, from slow absorption of the local anesthetic, or from poor technique. This complication can result in seizures and unconsciousness. Phrenic nerve palsy can also be a complication with this block since the phrenic nerve roots are anesthetized as they pass through the interscalene sheath. This complication, however, would manifest as the inability to take a deep breath, which develops as the block onsets. Nurses should be aware of this complication, particularly with patients with a preexisting condition of chronic obstructive pulmonary disease (COPD). Recurrent laryngeal nerve palsy presents as hoarseness and tends to occur mainly on the right side where the laryngeal nerve loops around the right subclavian artery. One other complication from interscalene blocks is Horner's syndrome, which is caused by secondary blockade of the sympathetic chain in the neck. Horner's syndrome manifests as myosis, ptosis, enophthalmos, unilateral flushing of the conjunctiva, and nasal congestion. Pneumothorax may also occur when a more supraclavicular approach is used. With this complication, dyspnea generally develops over time and if dyspnea develops immediately, then the nurse should question phrenic nerve palsy. Puncture of the subclavian artery can occur during a subclavian perivascular technique. A hematoma will form, but there is no neurologic sequela. (Graber R: *Interscalene block.* Website: www.uhcanesthesia.com/ClinDiv/Anesthesiology/Regional%20Anesthesia/ISB/view. Accessed May 2, 2007; Perry AG, Potter PA: *Clinical nursing skills and techniques,* ed 6, St. Louis, 2006, Mosby.)

8.75. Correct Answer: **c**

Nitroprusside can actually increase intracranial pressure (ICP) even when the effect on blood pressure is small. Normal ICP is 0 to 15 mmHg. To maintain ICP within normal parameters, attention to specific details of patient management is necessary. Hyperventilation maintains pCO_2 in the hypocapnic range of 30 to 35 mmHg; a head-elevated position of 15 to 30 degrees with *no* knee flexion and straightly aligned neck encourages venous drainage from the head; a 20% mannitol solution initiated within the first hour effectively decreases ICP by 15 to 20 mmHg. (Black J, Hokanson Hawks J: *Medical-surgical nursing: clinical management for positive outcomes*, ed 7, Philadelphia, 2005, Saunders; Morton PG et al: *Critical care nursing: a holistic approach*, ed 8, Philadelphia, 2005, Lippincott Williams & Wilkins.)

8.76.   Correct Answer: **d**
Three waveforms—*A, B*, and *C*—are used to monitor intracranial pressure. *A* waves are an ominous sign of intracranial decompensation and poor compliance. *B* waves correlate with changes in respiration, and *C* waves correlate with changes in arterial pressure. Plateau waves, or *A* waves, indicate a trend toward above-normal intracranial pressure (ICP) and correlate with cerebral ischemia. Patient management includes interventions to reduce pressure. Patients with invasive ICP catheters or bolts have significantly increased risk of infection; use of steroids suppresses immunity and further increases infection potential. Aseptic technique and reporting any drainage are essential. *Never* "flush" the monitoring system! Though nursing actions certainly are planned according to changes and trends in intracranial pressure, calculating intracranial compliance is the physician's responsibility. (Black J, Hokanson

Hawks J: *Medical-surgical nursing: clinical management for positive outcomes*, ed 7, Philadelphia, 2005, Saunders; Springhouse: *Critical care nursing made incredibly easy!* Philadelphia, 2004, Lippincott Williams & Wilkins; Morton PG et al: *Critical care nursing: a holistic approach*, ed 8, Philadelphia, 2005, Lippincott Williams & Wilkins.)

8.77.   Correct Answer: **d**
The Monro-Kellie hypothesis reflects the principles of intracranial volume. This volume is a dynamic relationship equal to the volume of the brain plus volume of cerebral blood plus cerebrospinal fluid volume. Altering any one of these factors affects the others. Usually, when brain volume increases, autoregulatory processes decrease cerebral blood flow to maintain a constant intracranial volume. Volume translates to pressure. As autoregulatory mechanisms fail, the volume of intracranial contents increases; because the skull cannot expand to accommodate the increased volume, pressure increases. (Black J, Hokanson Hawks J: *Medical-surgical nursing: clinical management for positive outcomes*, ed 7, Philadelphia, 2005, Saunders; Morton PG et al: *Critical care nursing: a holistic approach*, ed 8, Philadelphia, 2005, Lippincott Williams & Wilkins; Quinn D, Schick L, editors: *ASPAN's perianesthesia nursing core curriculum: preoperative, Phase I and Phase II PACU nursing*, Philadelphia, 2004, Saunders.)

8.78.   Correct Answer: **a**
A cerebral perfusion pressure (CPP) of only 43 mmHg in a non-anesthetized patient indicates inadequate blood flow and ischemia. To adequately perfuse the brain, CPP must be at least 60 mmHg; normal CPP is 70 to 100 mmHg. CPP is the

calculated difference between mean arterial pressure (MAP)—blood entering the brain—and intracranial pressure (ICP)—resistance to this flow. Therefore CPP = MAP − ICP. (Black J, Hokanson Hawks J: *Medical-surgical nursing: clinical management for positive outcomes*, ed 7, Philadelphia, 2005, Saunders; Drain C, editor: *Perianesthesia nursing: a critical care approach*, ed 4, Philadelphia, 2003, Saunders; Morton PG et al: *Critical care nursing: a holistic approach*, ed 8, Philadelphia, 2005, Lippincott Williams & Wilkins; Quinn D, Schick L, editors: *ASPAN's perianesthesia nursing core curriculum: preoperative, Phase I and Phase II PACU nursing*, Philadelphia, 2004, Saunders; Stoelting RK, Miller RD: *Basics of anesthesia*, ed 5, London, 2007, Churchill Livingstone.)

8.79. Correct Answer: **a**
The vascularity of meningiomas makes bleeding a high-potential intraoperative complication; blood is usually crossmatched for possible use. Meningiomas are typically slow-growing, usually benign, and often vascular tumors and represent up to 20% of all intracranial tumors. Incidence is age-related and highest among adult men. Location in the brain determines symptoms. As the tumor size increases, surrounding brain structures are *compressed* rather than invaded. Though well-encapsulated, size and tumor location complicate resection. (Black J, Hokanson Hawks J: *Medical-surgical nursing: clinical management for positive outcomes*, ed 7, Philadelphia, 2005, Saunders; Morton PG et al: *Critical care nursing: a holistic approach*, ed 8, Philadelphia, 2005, Lippincott Williams & Wilkins.)

8.80. Correct Answer: **c**
CSF contains glucose. Yellowish drainage from the surgical site, ear, eye, or nose could be CSF, indicating dural tear. Potential for infection rises. Do not suction drainage! Do not "pack" dressings into any site when CSF leak is suspected! Confirm glucose presence, and report to the physician. (Black J, Hokanson Hawks J: *Medical-surgical nursing: clinical management for positive outcomes*, ed 7, Philadelphia, 2005, Saunders; Quinn D, Schick L, editors: *ASPAN's perianesthesia nursing core curriculum: preoperative, Phase I and Phase II PACU nursing*, Philadelphia, 2004, Saunders; Swearingen PL: *Manual of medical-surgical nursing care: nursing interventions and collaborative management*, ed 5, St. Louis, 2003, Mosby.)

8.81. Correct Answer: **c**
Difficulty in maintaining airway patency or the presence of an abnormal breathing pattern heralds a complication requiring that the PACU nurse notify the surgeon, particularly after an infratentorial approach. Edema or postoperative bleeding in the posterior fossa, the area below the tentorium, compresses brainstem structures. Altered respiratory status, cardiovascular stability, and function of cranial nerves with nuclei in the medulla result. The cerebellum, located in the infratentorium, coordinates, not initiates, movement; fine motor incoordination more likely indicates postoperative cerebellar dysfunction than does paralysis. Receptive aphasia, a sign of temporal lobe involvement, is when language is not understood. Serosanguineous nasal drainage (rhinorrhea) occurs when CSF drainage occurs because of a fracture in the anterior fossa with "raccoon eyes" being a late sign of this type of fracture. (Black J, Hokanson Hawks

280

J: *Medical-surgical nursing: clinical management for positive outcomes*, ed 7, Philadelphia, 2005, Saunders; Hickey JV: *The clinical practice of neurological and neurosurgical nursing*, ed 5, Philadelphia, 2003, Lippincott Williams & Wilkins; Morton PG et al: *Critical care nursing: a holistic approach*, ed 8, Philadelphia, 2005, Lippincott Williams & Wilkins.)

8.82. Correct Answer: **b**
Interventions that move the patient's body as a unit (without bends or twists) minimize neck flexion, extension, or malalignment. "Log-roll" turns avoid brainstem pressure or circulatory impairment that potentially compromises respiratory function by reducing stasis of fluids in the lungs. Coughing and suction are avoided when possible. Suctioning should be approached thoughtfully to avoid hypoxemia as well as increased intrathoracic pressure. By limiting the duration of suctioning to no more than 10 seconds at a time, one avoids stimulating the cough reflex and decreases the incidence of increased intrathoracic and intracranial pressure. PEEP increases intrathoracic pressure, reduces venous return, and therefore increases intracranial pressure. By achieving a functional Phase II block the result is the patient being ventilated until the return of the normal neuromuscular transmission. (Drain C, editor: *Perianesthesia nursing: a critical care approach*, ed 4, Philadelphia, 2003, Saunders; Morton PG et al: *Critical care nursing: a holistic approach*, ed 8, Philadelphia, 2005, Lippincott Williams & Wilkins; Quinn D, Schick L, editors: *ASPAN's perianesthesia nursing core curriculum: preoperative, Phase I and Phase II PACU nursing*, Philadelphia, 2004, Saunders.)

8.83. Correct Answer: **c**
Supratentorial is the area above the tentorium that includes the cerebrum. The supratentorial approach is used for frontal, temporal, parietal, and occipital lesions. Right-sided deficits below the brainstem must raise nursing concern for this patient's neurologic health. For this patient, dilation of the right pupil probably has less ominous significance than motor dysfunction on the left side. Corticospinal tracts connecting this patient's left cerebral cortex with spinal cord cells in the anterior horn decussate, or cross, to control function on his right side. Control of pupillary constriction occurs at the midbrain, above the area where pyramidal tracts cross. (Hickey JV: *The clinical practice of neurological and neurosurgical nursing*, ed 5, Philadelphia, 2003, Lippincott Williams & Wilkins; Morton PG et al: *Critical care nursing: a holistic approach*, ed 8, Philadelphia, 2005, Lippincott Williams & Wilkins.)

8.84. Correct Answer: **d**
For each patient, the physician determines the rate and volume of cerebrospinal fluid to be removed through the ventriculostomy. A ventriculostomy system is inserted to manage hydrocephalus (impaired cerebrospinal fluid circulation) that significantly dilates cerebral ventricles and increases intracranial pressure. Infection from this invasive system and ventricular collapse from excessive drainage are the greatest associated risks. The system must remain sterile, is generally "leveled" with the zero-point near the patient's ear (approximately the foramen of Monro), and often is positioned by the neurosurgeon. Negative pressure is *never* applied to the system. (Springhouse: *Critical care nursing made incredibly easy!* Philadelphia,

2004, Lippincott Williams & Wilkins; McCance KL, Huether SE: *Pathophysiology: the biologic basis for disease in adults and children*, ed 4, St. Louis, 2002, Mosby; Morton PG et al: *Critical care nursing: a holistic approach*, ed 8, Philadelphia, 2005, Lippincott Williams & Wilkins.)

8.85. Correct Answer: **b**
This patient easily moves her right leg and can raise her knee, indicating the strength to overcome gravity. She cannot, however, maintain her own muscle strength against resistance applied by the nurse-examiner. Physician expectations are important to determine. The patient's weakness may be similar to her preoperative weakness and of little current concern. Inform the surgeon of new or increasing weakness. Strength of the patient's arms and left leg muscles is normal. Observations of muscle activity are often rated on a scale (typically with grades 0 to 5) to objectively communicate muscle strength. Whether a rating scale is used or not, extremity muscle strength must be frequently documented—as clinically indicated in the PACU or as physician-ordered. (Hickey JV: *The clinical practice of neurological and neurosurgical nursing*, ed 5, Philadelphia, 2003, Lippincott Williams & Wilkins; McCance KL, Huether SE: *Pathophysiology: the biologic basis for disease in adults and children*, ed 4, St. Louis, 2002, Mosby; Morton PG et al: *Critical care nursing: a holistic approach*, ed 8, Philadelphia, 2005, Lippincott Williams & Wilkins.)

8.86. Correct Answer: **b**
To decrease edema after spinal trauma, "megadoses" of steroids have improved neurologic function. Though some consider this a controversial practice, some practitioners rapidly infuse methylprednisolone 30 mg/kg, followed by a smaller dose each hour for 23 hours. When initiated promptly after injury (surgical trauma with decreased neurologic function, in her situation), motor and sensory function have significantly improved for some patients. (Donohoe Dennison D: *Pass CCRN*, ed 2, St. Louis, 2000, Mosby; Hickey JV: *The clinical practice of neurological and neurosurgical nursing*, ed 5, Philadelphia, 2003, Lippincott Williams & Wilkins; Morton PG et al: *Critical care nursing: a holistic approach*, ed 8, Philadelphia, 2005, Lippincott Williams & Wilkins.)

8.87. Correct Answer: **a**
Symptoms of gastrointestinal irritability (nausea, vomiting, peptic ulcers) are likely consequences of steroid administration. Often, concurrent doses of medications to reduce gastric acidity are also provided. When caring for the patient, the PACU nurse must be mindful of her increasing infection risk because of the acute antiinflammatory influence of high-dose steroids. Eventually, a schedule of tapered steroid dose reduction will be needed to prevent adrenal crisis associated with abrupt withdrawal. (Donohoe Dennison D: *Pass CCRN*, ed 2, St. Louis, 2000, Mosby; Hickey JV: *The clinical practice of neurological and neurosurgical nursing*, ed 5, Philadelphia, 2003, Lippincott Williams & Wilkins.)

8.88. Correct Answer: **c**
Recurrent respiratory depression and re-sedation are likely; the effects of sufentanil likely will "outlive" any reversal provided by naloxone. Sufentanil (Sufenta) is often delivered by continuous

infusion, particularly for long surgical procedures. Sufenta is similar to fentanyl in action but 5 to 10 times more potent. Depression of ventilation and bradycardia may be more profound with sufentanil than with fentanyl. Inhaled anesthetics and sedatives further potentiate the effects. Relaxation of muscles is usually from the muscle relaxants used during the procedure and not from the Sufenta. Like fentanyl, patients receiving sufentanil may develop some chest wall rigidity. Usage of large doses may produce skeletal muscle rigidity that makes ventilation of the lungs difficult, resulting in more respiratory depression. (Drain C, editor: *Perianesthesia nursing: a critical care approach*, ed 4, Philadelphia, 2003, Saunders; Stoelting RK, Miller RD: *Basics of anesthesia*, ed 5, London, 2007, Churchill Livingstone.)

8.89. Correct Answer: **d**
Nystagmus is involuntary, disconjugate, jerking or oscillating movement of the eyes and an abnormal ocular response. The eyes of a normally alert person do not show involuntary movements. (Agnes M, editor: *Webster's New World College Dictionary*, ed 4, Hoboken, 2004, John Wiley & Sons; Black J, Hokanson Hawks J: *Medical-surgical nursing: clinical management for positive outcomes*, ed 7, Philadelphia, 2005, Saunders; Hickey JV: *The clinical practice of neurological and neurosurgical nursing*, ed 5, Philadelphia, 2003, Lippincott Williams & Wilkins.)

8.90. Correct Answer: **a**
The patient has normal reflex responses. Assessment of reflexes compares left and right responses for symmetry and reaction strength. Deep tendon (or muscle stretch) reflexes are commonly graded on a

0-to-4 scale; "2" is the normal response, "0" indicates no response to a reflex hammer tap. Brisk, hyperactive reflexes suggest disease or chemical imbalance and are scored as "4." Presence of a downward toe sign to plantar stroking (Babinski sign) is not numerically graded and always indicates positive results—and pathology. 0 = Absent; 1 = Diminished; 2 = Normal; 3 = Brisker than normal; 4 = Hyperactive (clonus). Superficial reflex grades: 0 = Absent; ± = Equivocal or barely present; + = Normally active. (Black J, Hokanson Hawks J: *Medical-surgical nursing: clinical management for positive outcomes*, ed 7, Philadelphia, 2005, Saunders; Springhouse: *Critical care nursing made incredibly easy!* Philadelphia, 2004, Lippincott Williams & Wilkins; Quinn D, Schick L, editors: *ASPAN's perianesthesia nursing core curriculum: preoperative, Phase I and Phase II PACU nursing*, Philadelphia, 2004, Saunders.)

8.91. Correct Answer: **b**
An autologous bone graft moves healthy bone pieces from one site in the patient's body to stabilize bone at another, usually for fusion of vertebrae or after fractures. Often bone from the iliac crest is used; pain from the donor site may be intense and require ice and narcotic analgesia. The Luque rods are stainless steel rods with sublaminar wires that are used for posterior spinal fusions. Steroids are used to suppress the immune system and, if used, will be in low doses. (Rothrock J, editor: *Alexander's care of the patient in surgery*, ed 12, St. Louis, 2003, Mosby; Swearingen PL: *Manual of medical-surgical nursing care: nursing interventions and collaborative management*, ed 5, St. Louis, 2003, Mosby.)

8.92. Correct Answer: **b**
Blood may drain unnoticed beneath the patient's leg; the accumulated drainage can be a significant volume. In addition, drainage collected in the wound drain can easily be more than 100 mL, particularly if a tourniquet was applied to the leg intraoperatively. The patient has increased potential for venous thrombosis; leg movement is encouraged. In addition, range-of-motion activities increase circulation while promoting joint mobility. Pillow pressure behind the knee (popliteal area) is avoided; a pillow inhibits knee movement and compromises limb circulation. (Quinn D, Schick L, editors: *ASPAN's perianesthesia nursing core curriculum: preoperative, Phase I and Phase II PACU nursing*, Philadelphia, 2004, Saunders; Swearingen PL: *Manual of medical-surgical nursing care: nursing interventions and collaborative management*, ed 5, St. Louis, 2003, Mosby.)

8.93. Correct Answer: **c**
Alternating compression and decompression pressures and soft, loose leg wraps of the 65-year-old man's sequential compression devices are least likely to restrict circulation. Patients with soft tissue or crush injuries, bleeding with hematoma into the skin, casted fractures, and prolonged compression by casts, weight, or pressure have high risk for compartment syndrome. When in lithotomy position for 3 hours, circulation in the anesthetized woman's posterior lower legs can be restricted; she is unable to feel the pain and alter her position to relieve pressure. Compartment syndrome occurs when extremity circulation and nerve function are compromised by greatly elevated pressures within the extremity. Greatest risk is within 6 hours after the precipitating event. (Atlee JL:

Complications in anesthesia, ed 2, Philadelphia, 2007, Saunders; McCance KL, Huether SE: *Pathophysiology: the biologic basis for disease in adults and children*, ed 4, St. Louis, 2002, Mosby; Quinn D, Schick L, editors: *ASPAN's perianesthesia nursing core curriculum: preoperative, Phase I and Phase II PACU nursing*, Philadelphia, 2004, Saunders; Swearingen PL: *Manual of medical-surgical nursing care: nursing interventions and collaborative management*, ed 5, St. Louis, 2003, Mosby.)

8.94. Correct Answer: **d**
Pain, paresthesia, pallor, paralysis, and decreased pulse ("the five Ps") are the hallmark signs of compartment syndrome. Circulatory impairment and nerve compression in an increasingly tight, high-pressure extremity segment (compartment) produces these symptoms. Burning indicates sensory damage (paresthesia); decreasing motor strength and decreasing pulse quality are relatively early signs of increasing compartment pressure. Pulse absence and true cyanosis (not pallor) develop much later, after significant tissue damage has occurred. (Atlee JL: *Complications in anesthesia*, ed 2, Philadelphia, 2007, Saunders; Quinn D, Schick L, editors: *ASPAN's perianesthesia nursing core curriculum: preoperative, Phase I and Phase II PACU nursing*, Philadelphia, 2004, Saunders; Swearingen PL: *Manual of medical-surgical nursing care: nursing interventions and collaborative management*, ed 5, St. Louis, 2003, Mosby.)

8.95. Correct Answer: **a**
Immobilizing the extremity, bivalving the cast, and continuous monitoring of the extremity are all part of the care plan for the patient experiencing compartment

syndrome. Position changes are needed to prevent immobility complications. The affected extremity should be kept at heart level because elevation above the heart level decreases local arterial perfusion, further compromising blood flow. Avoid cold applications in compartment syndrome because they can lead to vasoconstriction, which can further compromise circulation. (Atlee JL: *Complications in anesthesia*, ed 2, Philadelphia, 2007, Saunders; Black J, Hokanson Hawks J: *Medical-surgical nursing: clinical management for positive outcomes*, ed 7, Philadelphia, 2005, Saunders; Harvey CV: Complications, *Orthop Nurs* 25[6]:410-414, 2006; Quinn D, Schick L, editors: *ASPAN's perianesthesia nursing core curriculum: preoperative, Phase I and Phase II PACU nursing*, Philadelphia, 2004, Saunders; Swearingen PL: *Manual of medical-surgical nursing care: nursing interventions and collaborative management*, ed 5, St. Louis, 2003, Mosby.)

8.96. Correct Answer: **c**
The respiratory function and patterns of respiration are important in detecting worsening neurologic injury and the need for respiratory support. The cerebellum synchronizes and coordinates the muscular efforts while the cerebrum has some control over the rate and rhythm of respiration. The brainstem includes the lower midbrain, the pons, and the medulla oblongata. The brainstem is responsible for central neurogenic hyperventilation, apneustic, and cluster breathing patterns. As the patterns go from Cheyne-Stokes to central neurogenic hyperventilation to apneustic to cluster to finally ataxic breathing, the more serious the problem is for the patient. The hypothalamus controls visceral, autonomic, endocrine, and emotional functions. (Hickey JV: *The clinical practice of neurological and neurosurgical nursing*, ed 5, Philadelphia, 2003, Lippincott Williams & Wilkins; Morton PG et al: *Critical care nursing: a holistic approach*, ed 8, Philadelphia, 2005, Lippincott Williams & Wilkins; Urden LD et al: *Priorities in critical care nursing*, ed 4, St. Louis, 2004, Mosby.)

8.97. Correct Answer: **d**
The Glasgow Coma Scale (GCS) reflects a numeric expression of cognition, behavior, and neurologic function. The total of the three scores measure the level of consciousness and severity of injury through eye opening, verbal responsiveness, and motor response. The scores can range from a score of 15 (normal) and the lowest score of 3 (most severe). A score of 8 or below is indicative of the patient being in a coma. (Black J, Hokanson Hawks J: *Medical-surgical nursing: clinical management for positive outcomes*, ed 7, Philadelphia, 2005, Saunders; Swearingen PL: *Manual of medical-surgical nursing care: nursing interventions and collaborative management*, ed 5, St. Louis, 2003, Mosby.)

8.98. Correct Answer: **c**
All the listed assessments are appropriate for this respiratory rate of 28, and tracheal retraction can indicate respiratory difficulties. These findings in conjunction with the patient history of asthma should trigger the PACU nurse to complete a thorough respiratory assessment. (Litwack K, editor: *Core curriculum for perianesthesia nursing practice*, ed 4, Philadelphia, 1999, Saunders.)

8.99. Correct Answer: **d**
Demerol depresses pain impulse transmission at the spinal cord level by interacting with opioid

receptors. Demerol breaks down into the metabolite of normeperidine. This can occur in patients who have liver and/or renal dysfunction. This can lead to confusion in the elderly population. Morphine depresses pain impulse transmission at the spinal cord level by interacting with opioid receptors. Morphine is not contraindicated in the elderly but should be used with caution because of the respiratory depression that can result from its use. Dilaudid inhibits ascending pain pathways in the CNS, increases pain threshold, and alters pain perception. No precautions or contraindications are listed for use in the geriatric patient. Toradol inhibits prostaglandin synthesis by decreasing an enzyme needed for biosynthesis; it has analgesic, antiinflammatory, and antipyretic effects. Use in the elderly is not contraindicated but should be used with caution because of the aging process. Toradol should not be given to anyone with a bleeding disorder or renal insufficiency because the kidneys excrete the drug. (Litwack K, editor: *Core curriculum for perianesthesia nursing practice*, ed 4, Philadelphia, 1999, Saunders; Skidmore-Roth L: *Mosby's 2006 nursing drug reference*, St. Louis, 2006, Mosby.)

Chapter 9

Intraabdominal and Retroperitoneal Observations

Scenarios and items in this section focus on the *renal, genitourinary, gynecologic, hepatic*, and *gastrointestinal* systems. Though specific functions of these systems vary, these concepts are considered together because:

- Anatomically, the primary organs for these systems are located within the abdomen or retroperitoneum

- Nursing assessments related to potential post-surgical complications are similar
- The nursing process focuses include detecting hidden bleeding; restoring thermal, fluid, and electrolyte balance; promoting oxygenation and pulmonary function; and ensuring integrity of surgical drains, stomas, and anastomoses

ESSENTIAL CORE CONCEPTS	AFFILIATED CORE CURRICULUM CHAPTERS
Nursing Process	**Chapter 2**
Assessment	
Planning and Intervention	
Evaluation	
Renal and Genitourinary Systems	**Chapters 19, 44**
Anatomy, Structure, and Function	
Adrenals and Lymphatics	
Nephron, Cortex, and Medulla	
Sex-Related Variations	
Ureters, Bladder, Urethra, and Sphincters	
Physiologic Concerns	
Hormonal	
Prostaglandins and Erythropoietin	
Renin-Angiotensin	
Vitamin D	
Metabolic	
Fluid and Chemical Aldosterone and ADH	
Filtration and Clearance	
Pathology	
Acute Tubular Necrosis	
Acute vs. Chronic Renal Failure: Cause and Effect	

    Azotemia and Oliguria
    Blood Flow, Pressure, and Ischemia
    End-Stage Renal Disease (ESRD)
    Prerenal-Intrarenal-Postrenal Alterations
    Stones, Toxicity, Trauma, and Chemical
      Changes

Perianesthesia Priorities
    Hemorrhage, Fluid Shifts, Chemical
      Changes
    Stomas, Stents, and Catheters
    Strain (Urine), Drain (Wound), and Pain

Surgical Interventions
    Lasers, Shocks, and Scopes
    Position-Related Outcomes
    Resections, Suspensions, and Organ
      Removal

Gastrointestinal and Hepatic Systems   Chapters 19, 42, 55

Anatomy, Structure, and Organ
  Function
    Esophagus, Stomach, Intestine, and Colon
    Gallbladder, Liver, Pancreas, and Spleen
    Pathology
    Polyps, Tumors, and Stones
    Strictures, Obstructions, Trauma, and
      Adhesions
    Ulcers, Infarcts, and -itis's

Physiologic Balance
    Nutrition, Fluid, and Electrolytes
    Temperature, Hemostasis, and Sepsis

Perianesthesia Priorities
    Drains, Tubes, and Stomas
    Hydration, Clots, and Electrolytes
    Lungs, Circulation, and Distention
    Position, Pain, and Thrombus

Surgical Interventions
    Anastomoses and Pouches
    Biopsies, Scopes, and Scans
    -ectomy's, Bypasses, -plasty's and -otomy's
    Position-Related Outcomes

Gynecologic System   Chapter 45

Anatomy, Structure, and Organ
  Function
Pathologic Conditions
    -cele's, Hormones, Tumors, and Infections
    Ectopic Pregnancies and Abortions

Perianesthesia Priorities
    Catheters, Drains, and Tubes
    Embolus, Electrolytes, and Hydration
    Sepsis, Position, and Hemostasis
Surgical Interventions
    Aspirations, Dilations, and Ligations
    Hysterectomy, Oophorectomy, and
      Salpingectomy
    Lasers, -scope's, and Suspensions
    Position-Related Outcomes

Set 1

9.1. Oliguria refers to:
a. retention of nitrogenous waste products.
b. less than 400 mL daily urine production.
c. unrecognized obstruction of urinary catheter.
d. a syndrome of uremia, alkalosis, and absent urine.

NOTE: Consider the scenario and items 9.2-9.5 together.

After abdominoperineal resection, a male patient arrives in the PACU in supine, head-flat position. He is drowsily responsive, moans, and indicates abdominal cramping and nausea. The intermittent pneumatic compression leg wraps are functioning, and the nasogastric tube drains scant amounts of dark red fluid. One abdominal wound drain is in compressed position, and a perineal sump drain is attached to low suction.

9.2. The patient's *most* immediate postoperative risk is the potential for:
a. deep vein thrombosis.
b. dumping syndrome.
c. inhalation of aspirated particles.
d. malnutrition from impaired absorption syndrome.

9.3. During assessment of the patient's surgical condition, the PACU nurse is *most* concerned to observe:
a. 75 mL serosanguineous perineal drainage in 1 hour.
b. absent bowel sounds and a soft abdomen.
c. 45 mL tan nasogastric fluid and potassium = 4.7 mEq/L.
d. clear yellow urine and a light gray stoma.

NOTE: The scenario continues.

The patient received an inhalation anesthetic with intravenous (IV) opioid. The anesthesiologist placed an epidural catheter for postoperative pain management but did not inject any medication. The PACU nurse observes that the patient is "splinting" his respirations and chooses to begin the infusion promptly. The protocol for epidural bupivacaine and hydromorphone includes a bolus dose and parameters for titration.

9.4. Before initiating the epidural infusion, the nurse ensures that the anesthesiologist administers the test dose and that:
a. the patient rates his pain as "higher than 7" on the pain scale of 0 to 10.
b. an opioid agonist/antagonist is immediately available.
c. the IV catheter is patent and the site is without erythema.
d. the patient moves his feet, indicating the catheter rests in the intrathecal space.

9.5. After 1 hour of epidural medication, the patient rates his pain at a "7" on the 0-to-10 pain scale. With support of hospital protocols and physician collaboration, the PACU nurse should:
a. administer hydromorphone 2 mg intramuscularly while awaiting effect of epidural medication.
b. re-inject the epidural catheter with a small supplemental bolus.
c. double the infusion's opioid concentration and then expand dosing parameters.
d. reposition the catheter and then adjust the infusion rate.

9.6. After open cholecystectomy, a patient remains in the PACU for 4 hours because of an unanticipated high census on the nursing unit. During this period, the PACU nurse measures T-tube drainage

of 60 mL each hour. Dressings are dry, and the abdomen is soft and round with moderate incisional tenderness. The PACU nurse intervenes by:
a. documenting this normal hourly drainage volume.
b. stripping the tubing for patency.
c. informing the surgeon of the abdominal status.
d. attaching the T-tube to suction.

NOTE: Consider items 9.7-9.9 together.

9.7. After pancreaticoduodenectomy, a patient will *most likely* require regular:
a. serum glucose assessment.
b. glucocorticoid doses.
c. potassium supplementation.
d. platelet infusions.

9.8. With regard to this patient's gastrointestinal assessment, the *most* appropriate nursing plan of care includes:
a. irrigating the nasogastric tube with 30 mL normal saline each hour.
b. asking the surgeon to identify tube locations and expected drainage.
c. quickly reinserting the nasogastric tube removed by the agitated patient.
d. anticipating absent bowel sounds and a firm, tympanic abdomen.

9.9. This patient's surgery involves:
a. pancreatic reconstruction and removal of a liver lobe, duodenum, and gallbladder.
b. removing the spleen, biliary decompression with bile duct dilation, and creating an ileostomy.
c. cholecystectomy and diverting ascitic and pancreatic fluid into the superior vena cava.
d. resecting the pancreas, duodenum, lower stomach, and bile duct and constructing a gastrojejunostomy.

9.10. Decreased blood and renal perfusion pressures prompt:
a. renin release with renovascular constriction.
b. decreased urine excretion caused by ADH suppression.

c. aldosterone-induced sodium excretion.
d. renal vasodilation from angiotensin II effect.

NOTE: Consider the scenario and items 9.11-9.13 together.

A 55-year-old female patient has a long history of postoperative nausea and vomiting (PONV). The anesthetic plan during her vaginal hysterectomy includes preoperative placement of a scopolamine patch behind the left ear.

9.11. Scopolamine is classified as a/an:
a. class III antiemetic.
b. anticholinergic.
c. class II neuroleptic.
d. acetylcholinesterase.

9.12. The PACU nurse anticipates the scopolamine may affect the patient's PACU care by contributing to:
a. agitation and excitement.
b. malignant hyperthermia.
c. delayed awakening.
d. dizziness and excessive salivation.

9.13. Two hours postoperatively, the PACU nurse prepares the patient for transfer from PACU. With regard to the patient's surgical outcomes, the nurse is *most* concerned when nursing assessment reveals:
a. lumbar pain and occipital headache.
b. soft abdomen and menstrual-like cramps.
c. leg pain during foot dorsiflexion.
d. no sanguineous fluid in wound drain or on perineal pad.

9.14. Deficits related to intraoperative positioning are least affected by a patient's:
a. duration of surgery.
b. anesthetic technique.
c. geriatric age.
d. physical condition.

NOTE: Consider the scenario and items 9.15-9.17 together.

A 73-year-old woman arrives in the PACU after exploratory laparotomy and excision of a pelvic mass and lymph node dissection.

The patient is settled in PACU and is currently stable. Her health history includes rheumatoid arthritis and a recently resolved pneumonia. Medications include naproxen prn and prednisone 60 mg daily.

9.15. The PACU nurse scans the patient's record to determine the preoperative baseline oxygen saturation and verify the patient has:
a. no chemical addictions.
b. estrogen replacement therapy.
c. hydrocortisone coverage.
d. no risk factors for thromboembolism.

9.16. When aware of her surroundings, the patient is *best* positioned:
a. with her head elevated 30°.
b. however she wishes.
c. flat and on her left side.
d. in Fowler position with her feet elevated.

9.17. With regard to her chronic steroid use, the patient has increased postoperative risk for:
a. pulmonary edema.
b. wound infection.
c. diabetes insipidus.
d. fluid deficit.

9.18. When assessing the postoperative patient for acute renal failure (ARF), the perianesthesia nurse should be aware of potential nursing diagnoses such as Risk for Imbalanced Fluid Volume and:
a. realize that preoperative psychosocial assessment is not pertinent.
b. implement frequent fluid boluses.
c. reduced sensitivity to opioids.
d. review pertinent preoperative diagnostic data.

9.19. Intervention for oliguria from prerenal causes may include:
a. ureteral stent placement.
b. aminoglycoside antibiotics.
c. furosemide.
d. dopamine infusion at 3.5 mg/kg.

9.20. A patient is scheduled for a vasectomy, using a local anesthetic and moderate sedation with fentanyl and midazolam. A Phase I PACU nurse with extensive operating room experience monitors the patient's status during the procedure and has no other responsibilities. Cardiac and noninvasive blood pressure monitors and a pulse oximeter are attached to the patient. The surgeon arrives and demands the nurse remove the equipment because he believes such monitoring is unnecessary. The nurse's *most* effective response is to:
a. refuse to remain in the room during the procedure.
b. inform the surgeon of moderate sedation policy.
c. discontinue the monitors and auscultate respirations.
d. tactfully request the surgeon cancel the procedure.

9.21. 30 minutes after arriving in the PACU after a resection of 15 g of prostate tissue during a transurethral resection of the prostate (TURP) and placement of a suprapubic catheter, the patient experiences epigastric, suprapubic, and left shoulder pain and has a firm abdomen. Blood pressure is 94/50 and heart rate is 126 bpm. The patient is diaphoretic and nauseated. The nurse pages the physician and further assesses the patient for possible:
a. evolving myocardial infarction.
b. septic bacteremia.
c. perforated bladder.
d. bladder spasm with prostatic bleeding.

9.22. Patient education priorities after extracorporeal shock wave lithotripsy (ESWL) focus primarily on:
a. hematuria prevention.
b. forced hydration.
c. scheduled analgesia.
d. antibiotic effects.

NOTE: Consider the scenario and items 9.23-9.25 together.

After a 4-hour exploratory laparotomy, transverse colon and tumor resection, and creation of colostomy, a male patient has persistent hypotension in the PACU with blood pressure at 80/42. Cardiac rhythm is sinus with heart rate at 102 bpm. The patient has a preoperative history of seasonal allergy, migraine headaches, and osteoarthritis. No hemodynamic monitoring catheters were inserted. Urine volume remains 40 mL/hr, and 5% dextrose in 0.45% normal saline with 20 mEq of potassium chloride is infusing at 150 mL/hr. The patient's temperature is 37° C (98.6° F), and he is responsive to verbal stimuli, with moderate pain managed using morphine delivered with patient-controlled analgesia (PCA) technique. Hemoglobin is 12.5 g/dL, and potassium is 3.8 mEq/L.

9.23. The *most likely* potential explanation for the patient's hypotension is:
   a. extracellular fluid deficit from hypertonic intravenous infusions.
   b. perioperative myocardial infarction with shock.
   c. unrecognized preoperative gastrointestinal fluid loss.
   d. fluid relocation with altered capillary permeability.

9.24. Perianesthesia nursing and medical goals for the patient focus on:
   a. instituting renal replacement therapy.
   b. supporting cardiac output and renal perfusion.
   c. recirculating intraintestinal fluid.
   d. increasing osmotic pressure with whole blood.

NOTE: The scenario continues.

The patient ultimately receives 3000 mL of lactated Ringer's solution during a 3-hour stay in the PACU. When approved for discharge from Phase I PACU, the patient is alert, has moderate pain, has no audible rales, and denies dyspnea. Urine output remains 35 mL/hr; blood pressure is consistently 100/52, heart rate is 98 bpm with normal sinus rhythm, and oxygen saturation is 98%.

9.25. The PACU nurse communicates the patient's fluid status to the nurse on the surgical nursing unit and anticipates that:
   a. fluid reabsorption will occur when capillaries heal.
   b. spontaneous diuresis will begin within 6 hours.
   c. low-rate hypotonic fluids will prevent tissue edema.
   d. pain will increase cardiac tone and decrease afterload.

9.26. Renal failure from prerenal origins differs from acute tubular necrosis (ATN) by the amount of:
   a. urine production.
   b. concentrating ability.
   c. nephron damage.
   d. renin release.

Set 2

NOTE: Consider the scenario and items 9.27-9.28 together.

A female patient was scheduled for laparoscopy to evaluate recurrent abdominal pain. The surgeon anticipated a left salpingectomy and oophorectomy. The patient received succinylcholine for intubation, midazolam, and fentanyl. The surgeon's plan changed intraoperatively, and the patient's surgery ended quickly after lysis of adhesions and laser treatment of endometriosis. The patient arrives in the PACU apneic and not moving. Respiratory support is provided with a mechanical ventilator, a rash scatters across her chest and upper arm, and the patient shows no muscle response to nerve stimulator impulses.

9.27. The nurse considers the patient's response to intraoperative muscle relaxants and anticipates:
  a. a permanent paralysis from atypical response.
  b. any arm movements will precede intercostal action.
  c. abdominal muscle function will precede eye opening.
  d. brief sensory deficit from allergic reaction.

NOTE: The scenario continues.

Within 90 minutes, the patient is alert, demonstrates adequate muscle strength, and is extubated. By late afternoon, she is fully awake, sipping fluids, and slowly preparing for discharge home. The patient mentions pain when smiling, turning her head, and moving about.

9.28. This discomfort is probably related to:
  a. nerve compression during lithotomy position.
  b. intraabdominal tissue burn.
  c. muscle strain from postanesthetic vomiting.
  d. intraoperative muscle fasciculation.

9.29. A 38-year-old male patient is scheduled for a cystoscopy, ureteral stent placement, and extracorporeal shock wave lithotripsy (ESWL). The patient's preoperative history and physical assessment document allergies to fish, milk, and eggs and recent episodes of conjunctivitis, eye swelling, and itchy, red hands at work. The preanesthesia nurse consults the anesthesia provider to express her concern about this patient's increased risk to develop:
  a. bronchospasm during endotracheal intubation.
  b. anaphylaxis after propofol sedation.
  c. corneal abrasion from lateral position.
  d. upper quadrant pain with IV morphine sulfate.

9.30. The capacity of a normally functioning bladder is approximately:
  a. 250 mL of urine.
  b. 500 mL of urine.
  c. 1000 mL of urine.
  d. 1500 mL of urine.

NOTE: Consider the scenario and items 9.31-9.33 together.

After a motor vehicle accident, a comatose motorcyclist was admitted to the hospital with multiple injuries. Six hours later, a depressed skull fracture was surgically repaired. Now, 24 hours after injury, his abdomen has been explored, his spleen excised, and the patient had an open reduction and internal fixation of a left hip fracture.

9.31. During initial assessment, the PACU nurse would be *most* concerned about:
  a. platelets of $98,000/mm^3$.
  b. temperature of 39.8° C (103.6° F).
  c. urine output of 29 mL/hr.
  d. hemoglobin of 9.8 g/dL.

NOTE: The scenario continues.

During PACU admission procedures, this patient actively shivers, blood pressure is 100/50, and respiratory rate is 28 breaths/min. ECG indicates sinus tachycardia; shivering artifact makes initial SpO_2 measurement difficult.

9.32. The PACU nurse:
   a. automatically initiates analgesia protocol.
   b. applies active rewarming device.
   c. administers butorphanol to suppress shivering.
   d. documents skin warmth, dryness, and redness.

9.33. Classic indicators of early respiratory distress in an adult with septic shock are:
   a. hyperventilation with respiratory alkalosis and elevated lactate.
   b. hypoventilation with decreased pulse pressure and excess circulating corticosteroids.
   c. hyperventilation with peripheral cyanosis and acidosis.
   d. hypoventilation with elevated lactate and low serum glucose.

9.34. Risk of nephrotoxicity from aminoglycoside antibiotics may be reduced by providing concurrent:
   a. nonsteroidal antiinflammatory drugs (NSAIDs).
   b. adequate intravascular volume using isotonic crystalloid solutions.
   c. high-dose thiazide diuretics.
   d. potassium supplementation.

NOTE: Consider the scenario and items 9.35-9.36 together.

A healthy middle-aged woman had an uneventful abdominal hysterectomy that ended 2 hours ago; intraoperative blood loss was 100 mL. She is drowsy and states abdominal pain score is "6" (on a 0-to-10 numeric rating scale). Blood pressure is low-normal though generally only 10% less than her preoperative measures; in the PACU her blood pressure dipped to 88/48 twice. The patient's cardiac rhythm is sinus at a consistent rate of 128 bpm.

9.35. The PACU nurse's ongoing assessment of this patient considers this situation's *most likely* explanation is:
   a. fever-induced tachycardia related to hyperdynamic sepsis.
   b. neurogenic vasodilation related to untreated hypothermia.
   c. decreased venous return related to evolving silent myocardial infarction.
   d. reflex tachycardia related to intravascular volume deficit.

9.36. The *most* appropriate collaborative nurse-physician interventions for the patient's immediate care are:
   a. restrict fluids, and administer oxygen and phenylephrine 0.3 mg prn.
   b. rapid crystalloid infusion and measure hemoglobin.
   c. acetaminophen suppository and titrate esmolol infusion.
   d. active rewarming, labetalol 5 mg, and measure prothrombin time.

NOTE: Consider the scenario and items 9.37-9.42 together.

At 2 AM, an "on-call" PACU nurse is phoned to care for a 25-year-old female patient after an emergency laparoscopy and salpingectomy to remove an ectopic pregnancy.

9.37. According to ASPAN's *Standards of Perianesthesia Nursing Practice*, recommended postanesthesia care for the patient includes:
   a. observation in the ICU by a PACU nurse and an ICU nurse in the adjacent isolation room.
   b. care by a registered nurse and visitation in PACU by two family members.
   c. presence of two registered nurses in the PACU for duration of Phase I period.
   d. one registered nurse at the bedside and an anesthesiologist available by pager in the obstetric suite.

9.38. Before transfer to an inpatient hospital bed, the PACU nurse administers $Rh_o(D)$ immune globulin (Rho-GAM)

to the patient, who is Rh negative, to prevent:
a. hemolysis of maternal erythrocytes.
b. maternal Rh sensitivity and antibody formation.
c. antibody stimulation in a future Rh negative fetus.
d. maternal conversion to Rh positivity.

9.39. A preoperative intervention intended to reduce potential adverse outcomes related to the patient's position during laparoscopy would *most likely* include:
a. H_2 antagonists.
b. bladder distention.
c. antiembolic stockings.
d. beta blockers.

9.40. At 4:20 AM, 30 minutes after admission to the PACU, the nurse is *most* concerned when the patient's assessment reveals:
a. bradycardia and moderate vaginal bleeding.
b. severe right shoulder pain and nausea.
c. tachycardia and a flat, silent abdomen.
d. painful, firm abdomen and bloody bandages.

9.41. The PACU nurse discovers that the patient is unable to dorsiflex the great toe on her right foot. This deficit may indicate intraoperative:
a. sciatic nerve injury.
b. posterior tibial nerve compression.
c. femoral nerve pressure.
d. peroneal nerve dysfunction.

9.42. During laparoscopy, peripheral nerve injury is most often related to:
a. lithotomy position.
b. intramuscular injection.
c. retractor pressure.
d. prolonged hip extension.

NOTE: Consider items 9.43-9.45 together.

9.43. During a hemorrhoidectomy, sphincterotomy, and repair of a large rectal fistula, a male patient received cisatracurium. This medication is a:
a. short-acting, depolarizing muscle relaxant.

b. drug with the same onset time as succinylcholine.
c. depolarizing relaxant reversible with flumazenil.
d. nondepolarizing muscle relaxant of intermediate duration.

9.44. Potentiation of cisatracurium effects is *least* likely with:
a. postoperative neostigmine 2.5 mg.
b. isoflurane at 1.25 monitored anesthesia care to maintain anesthesia.
c. intraoperative gentamicin 80 mg.
d. concurrent administration of lidocaine 100 mg.

9.45. With regard to the patient's surgical procedure, the Phase I PACU nurse has the *most* concern when:
a. sanguineous drainage saturates dressings twice in 1 hour.
b. postoperative urination is difficult.
c. the patient reports significant perineal pressure and severe rectal pain.
d. no drainage and absent perineal sensation occur.

9.46. A female patient's Crohn's disease was surgically treated with a 4-hour total proctocolectomy and creation of a continent ileostomy. On the same day in the Phase I PACU, she mentions right heel pain and an aching back. At this time, the *most* appropriate nursing intervention is to:
a. request an anticoagulation protocol to monitor risk of deep vein thrombus.
b. reposition the patient's feet to limit contact with the stretcher.
c. further assess the patient for right leg compartment syndrome.
d. provide sedation and frequent analgesic so the patient will relax and doze.

9.47. A patient with a blood urea nitrogen (BUN) of 55 mg/dL and serum creatinine of 5.2 mg/dL is considered:
a. anuric.
b. cachectic.
c. oliguric.
d. azotemic.

SET 3

ITEMS 9.48–9.73

9.48. The patient's surgeon orders that the patient receive 1 g vancomycin before her low anterior resection. The preanesthesia nurse administers the vancomycin over at least 60 minutes to reduce the potential for:
a. postoperative ototoxicity.
b. bile duct spasm.
c. hypotensive response.
d. delayed muscle relaxant metabolism.

NOTE: Consider items 9.49-9.52 together.

9.49. A male patient's temperature is 34.9° C (94.8° F) when he is admitted to the PACU after general anesthesia for exploratory laparotomy and right colectomy. Physiologic consequences related to this temperature include:
a. rapid return to alertness and lower oxygen demand.
b. respiratory alkalosis with metabolic acidosis.
c. increased hepatic circulation and drug clearance.
d. peripheral vasoconstriction with dysrhythmia risk.

9.50. Initial nursing interventions to address the patient's hypothermia include all the following goals *except:*
a. reversing metabolic acidosis.
b. improving tissue perfusion.
c. preventing radiant heat loss.
d. suppressing muscle activity.

9.51. As the patient's core temperature approaches 35.5° C (95.9° F), he begins to shiver. Physiologic concerns during rewarming include:
a. fibrinogenesis and rewarming hypervolemia.
b. hypotension and carbon dioxide production.

c. bradycardia and preventing evaporative heat loss.
d. diuresis and metabolic alkalosis.

9.52. The PACU nurse visits the patient on his first postoperative day. To determine any adverse hypothermia-related outcomes, the nurse assesses the patient for:
a. epinephrine depletion.
b. overcompensated hypothermia.
c. generalized myalgia.
d. renewed paralysis.

9.53. The greatest priority in the Phase I PACU nurse's plan of care for the patient after a subtotal gastrectomy procedure is:
a. stimulating frequent deep breaths and position shifts.
b. monitoring reoccurrence of peritoneal ascites.
c. reporting 25 mL bright red nasogastric returns.
d. ensuring patency and traction on double-balloon gastric tube.

NOTE: Consider the scenario and items 9.54-9.56 together.

A 23-year-old man with a testicular mass is admitted to the PACU after a right orchiectomy. Blood pressure is 124/72, pulse is 62, respirations are 16, and pulse oximeter shows 98% SaO_2 on room air. The patient's inguinal incision is dry and intact. An ice pack has been applied. Pain is controlled with analgesics. The patient is quiet and appears distant.

9.54. When assessing this patient, the nurse considers that he is:
a. not outgoing and leaves him to his thoughts.
b. drowsy from anesthesia.

c. concerned about the pathology of his tumor and his altered body image.

d. experiencing emergence delirium.

NOTE: The scenario continues.

The perianesthesia nurse's plan of care for this patient includes pain management. The patient has been receiving fentanyl 25 mcg intravenously to keep his pain level below a "4" on a 1-to-10 numeric pain scale.

9.55. The perianesthesia nurse evaluates the patient's pain relief as well as assesses the patient for adverse effects, which include:

a. bradycardia.

b. tachypnea.

c. hypertension.

d. hypothermia.

9.56. While caring for this patient, the *greatest* potential infection risk to the PACU nurse is:

a. cytomegalovirus (CMV) from a vomitus spill onto a fresh skin abrasion.

b. hepatitis B virus (HBV) from spilled wound drainage onto the nurse's finger paper cut.

c. human immunodeficiency virus (HIV) from a mucus splash to upper lip during a cough.

d. hepatitis A virus (HAV) from a blood splash to the cornea during sampling for laboratory tests.

9.57. The nurse caring for the patient after a vaginal hysterectomy is most concerned when:

a. the patient mentions low back pain and tingling toes.

b. no tension is applied to the suprapubic catheter.

c. the patient reports abdominal pressure and cramping.

d. one perineal pad saturates with blood in an hour.

9.58. The obese patient is most likely to develop postoperative:

a. hyperventilation syndrome.

b. hypermetabolism of opioids.

c. hyperglycemia.

d. hypercarbia while asleep.

9.59. Upon arrival in PACU after a general anesthetic with sevoflurane and opioid analgesic, a middle-aged man repeatedly attempts to sit up, states he wants to get out of bed, removes his oxygen face tent, and picks at his abdominal dressing. The PACU nurse attempts to reassure and reorient this man and assesses him for the most likely causes of his restlessness, including hypoxia, pain, and:

a. recurrent angina.

b. halogenated-gas toxicity.

c. distended bladder.

d. renarcotization.

NOTE: Consider the scenario and items 9.60-9.62 together.

A 37-year-old male patient is undergoing evaluation for possible bariatric surgery. His body mass index (BMI) is 50. Surgical options include both restrictive and malabsorptive procedures. The patient typically enjoys sweets, milk shakes, and ice creams.

9.60. The patient may be recommended for a combination restrictive and malabsorptive-type procedure (e.g., Roux-en-Y gastric bypass operation) because:

a. a restrictive procedure (e.g., laparoscopic adjustable gastric banding) is more invasive with an increased risk of infection.

b. the patient may generate more acceptable weight loss because of his excessive weight and past eating habits.

c. eating sweets and drinking high-calorie liquids will be difficult after vertical banded gastroplasty.

d. the patient is at greater risk for developing obstructive sleep apnea postoperatively.

9.61. Preoperative education for the patient includes information about preparation and the surgical procedure. This education would also include postoperative instructions related to:

a. diet, lifestyle changes, and potential complications.

b. increasing dietary intake of high-calorie foods to provide energy while recovering.

c. decreasing activity to minimize risk of thrombophlebitis.

d. prolonged fasting and bowel rest to promote wound healing.

9.62. Postoperatively the patient will require continued monitoring of oxygen saturation and application of continuous positive airway pressure (CPAP) when he leaves the PACU. Oxygen saturation monitoring:

a. guides postoperative analgesic administration.

b. promotes ventilation.

c. measures oxygenation.

d. predicts adequate respiratory functioning.

9.63. Which of the following statements is *true* regarding the use of isoflurane as an inhalation agent?

a. Isoflurane has rare toxic effects.

b. Caution is advised in patients with known renal impairment.

c. Isoflurane may not be useful in patients with hepatic insufficiency.

d. Isoflurane is useful for mask inductions.

9.64. Oliguria from prerenal causes often improves after:

a. irrigation and traction to the urinary catheter.

b. 300 mL crystalloid bolus.

c. gentamicin 60 mg for a patient with myoglobinuria.

d. a flat and supine position.

9.65. The most sensitive indicator of renal function is serum:

a. urea nitrogen.

b. osmolality.

c. potassium.

d. creatinine.

NOTE: Consider the scenario and items 9.66-9.67 together.

A patient with acute renal failure (ARF) is admitted to the PACU for observation after a double-lumen subclavian catheter was surgically inserted for hemodialysis access. The patient received midazolam with intraoperative monitoring by the anesthesia provider.

9.66. This patient is *particularly* at risk to develop:

a. respiratory alkalosis.

b. intravascular sepsis.

c. nosocomial peritonitis.

d. serum potassium deficit.

9.67. The PACU nurse observes tall, peaked T waves on this patient's cardiac monitor. The QRS complex extended from 0.10 seconds to 0.14 seconds. The *most* likely source of this observation is:

a. ventricular hypertrophy.

b. hyperkalemia.

c. hypocalcemia.

d. myocardial ischemia.

NOTE: Consider items 9.68-9.69 together.

9.68. After a bupivacaine spinal anesthetic and resection of 52 g of prostate tissue by transurethral approach, a patient's bladder would *most likely* be irrigated with titrated:

a. sterile distilled water.

b. hypertonic colloid solution.

c. sterile normal saline.

d. hypotonic electrolyte solution.

9.69. The patient states he has pressure sensation to his iliac crests and cannot move his legs. Urine currently appears bright red and clot free. The urologist applies traction to the patient's triple-lumen urinary catheter. The nurse now expects the patient to experience:

a. strong abdominal pain, large urinary clots, and tissue shreds.

b. tachycardia and urge incontinence around the catheter.

c. pink-tinged urine and suprapubic pain as spinal effect ends.

d. referred flank pain and cherry red, clotless irrigation returns.

NOTE: Consider the scenario and items 9.70-9.72 together.

For the past 9 months, a female patient has undergone home dialysis even though she still produces about 500 mL of urine each day. She was admitted to the hospital 18 days ago for peritonitis treatment. One week ago, a small colon lesion was discovered, and the patient has undergone an intraoperative colonoscopy and transverse colon resection.

9.70. This patient's renal disease affects the pharmacokinetics of anesthetic medications in a way that increases:
   a. circulating unbound medication.
   b. protein-bound anesthetic.
   c. blood-brain barrier permeability.
   d. Hofmann elimination.

9.71. The patient begins to complain of post-operative pain while in the PACU. The nurse is ***most*** likely to give:
   a. meperidine 50 mg IM.
   b. fentanyl 50 mcg IV every 10 minutes.
   c. ketorolac 30 mg IV.
   d. morphine 2 mg IV every 5 minutes.

9.72. The nursing plan of care related to care of a hemodialysis patient with a synthetic graft inserted into the left arm considers all the following ***except*** that the:

   a. blood sampling occurs in the right arm.
   b. bruit is audible during left blood pressure cuff inflation.
   c. nurse's fingertips palpate a venous thrill.
   d. neurovascular status of the left arm is unaltered.

9.73. A 68-year-old man arrives in the PACU after a transurethral resection of the prostate (TURP). The perioperative nurse reports that a large amount of irrigation solution was used during the procedure while hemostasis was being achieved. The Foley catheter bag shows 200 mL of red-tinged urine; 3 L of sterile isotonic solution is hanging for continuous bladder irrigation. No clots are observed. The patient is awake and showing some signs of confusion. After attempting to reorient the patient, he remains restless and confused. He is also complaining of abdominal discomfort. The patient's confusion is ***least*** likely to be related to:
   a. anesthetic agents.
   b. TUR syndrome.
   c. anemia.
   d. orientation before procedure.

SET 1

ANSWER KEY

9.1.	b		**9.14.**	b
9.2.	c		**9.15.**	c
9.3.	d		**9.16.**	a
9.4.	c		**9.17.**	b
9.5.	b		**9.18.**	d
9.6.	c		**9.19.**	c
9.7.	a		**9.20.**	b
9.8.	b		**9.21.**	c
9.9.	d		**9.22.**	b
9.10.	a		**9.23.**	d
9.11.	b		**9.24.**	b
9.12.	a		**9.25.**	a
9.13.	c		**9.26.**	c

SET 1

9.1. Correct Answer: **b**
Oliguria defined literally means "reduced urine volume" and clinically indicates urine production of less than 400 mL/day. There is a reduction in the kidney's ability to properly filter the end products of metabolism. This may or may not result in retention of nitrogenous wastes and acidosis. Urinary catheter obstruction may be one cause of postrenal failure; patency must be determined before any intervention for suspected acute renal failure. Other causes of acute renal failure include dehydration, vascular collapse caused by sepsis, antihypertensive drug therapy, or third spacing. (Copstead LC, Banasik JL: *Pathophysiology: biological and behavioral perspectives*, ed 2, Philadelphia, 2000, Saunders; Tanagho EA, McAninch JW, editors: *Smith's general urology*, ed 15, New York, 2000, McGraw-Hill.)

9.2. Correct Answer: **c**
Aspiration is a concern for any sedated patient with a nasogastric tube. Ensuring tube patency and elevating the patient's head to semi-Fowler's position help decrease risk. A nasogastric tube snaked into the stomach enhances the likelihood of gastroesophageal reflux because it passes through (opening) the lower esophageal sphincter. Acidic stomach contents can creep up the outside of the tube, particularly if the tube is obstructed. Like fluid traveling on a wick, gastric contents can then move down the trachea into the lungs. The gastroesophageal and pharyngoesophageal sphincters normally prevent aspiration. The nasogastric tube and depression of the central nervous system by various anesthetic and adjunctive drugs interfere with these defenses and increase the aspiration risk. Gastric peristalsis slowly returns 3 to 6 days postoperatively. Thrombophlebitis *is* a potential complication though less immediate than the risk of aspiration in a sedated patient with a gastric tube in place. (Carter S: The surgical team and outcomes management: focus on postoperative ileus, *J PeriAnesth Nurs* 21[2A suppl]:S2-S6, 2006; Doherty GM: *Current surgical diagnosis & treatment*, ed 12, New York, 2006, McGraw-Hill.)

9.3. Correct Answer: **d**
A newly created stoma should be pink or red, not bluish or light gray. The nurse must inform the surgeon of this observation because interrupted blood flow to the stoma is possible. The nurse can expect no bowel sounds, a soft abdomen when palpated, and small amounts of nasogastric returns. (Drain C, editor: *Perianesthesia nursing: a critical care approach*, ed 4, Philadelphia, 2003, Saunders; Quinn D, Schick L, editors: *ASPAN's perianesthesia nursing core curriculum: preoperative, Phase I and Phase II PACU nursing*, Philadelphia, 2004, Saunders.)

9.4. Correct Answer: **c**
The patient requires a patent intravenous line. Significant cardiopulmonary compromise could immediately occur during the test dose. Malposition or migration of the epidural catheter after insertion could result in an unplanned intravascular or intraspinal injection. Emergency treatment of the resulting hypotension and respiratory suppression may include rapid

intravenous fluid volume and infusion of vasopressors and a pure opioid agonist (naloxone). The registered nurse's responsibility when delivering intraspinal medications is clear: administering a test or initial dose to determine catheter placement is the responsibility only of "licensed professionals who are educated in the specialty of anesthesia." (ASPAN: *2006-2008 Standards of perianesthesia nursing practice*, Cherry Hill, NJ, 2006, ASPAN; Morton PG et al: *Critical care nursing: a holistic approach*, ed 8, Philadelphia, 2005, Lippincott Williams & Wilkins.)

9.5. Correct Answer: **b**
The PACU nurse's scope of practice may permit the nurse to *reinject* and *alter* the infusion *rate with physician direction* when managing the analgesia of a nonobstetric patient. State law, practice codes, and facility policies must state this. Establishing dosage parameters and catheter placement are specific physician responsibilities. Up to 2 hours may be needed to achieve an effective dose of an epidural opioid. Therefore an alternative approach could be to administer supplemental doses of intravenous opioid in addition to reconsidering the dose of epidural opioid. (ASPAN: *2006-2008 Standards of perianesthesia nursing practice*, Cherry Hill, NJ, 2006, ASPAN; Morton PG et al: *Critical care nursing: a holistic approach*, ed 8, Philadelphia, 2005, Lippincott Williams & Wilkins.)

9.6. Correct Answer: **c**
This patient's bile drainage should be reported. Postoperative drainage of bile after cholecystectomy is typically less than 30 mL/hour. Obstruction, fistula, and severed common bile duct are conditions that increase volume of bile drainage. Bleeding with the bile drainage can indicate cystic artery hemorrhage, a serious consequence. (Drain C, editor: *Perianesthesia nursing: a critical care approach*, ed 4, Philadelphia, 2003, Saunders.)

9.7. Correct Answer: **a**
Glucose-insulin imbalance is expected after a pancreaticoduodenectomy (Whipple procedure) to resect a pancreatic tumor. The pancreas' insulin-producing function is disrupted by both the tumor and the surgery. Frequent measures of serum glucose determine the required insulin dose to maintain a glucose level between 80-110 mg/dL. These often poorly nourished patients also frequently receive hyperalimentation, a high-glucose fluid that contributes to serum glucose elevations. (American College of Endocrinology Task Force on Inpatient Diabetes and Metabolic Control: American College of Endocrinology position statement on inpatient diabetes and metabolic control, *Endocr Pract* 1[suppl 2]: 3-108; Drain C, editor: *Perianesthesia nursing: a critical care approach*, ed 4, Philadelphia, 2003, Saunders.)

9.8. Correct Answer: **b**
Particularly after a major resection and "reconnection" of gastrointestinal structures, the surgeon should inform the nurse of type and purpose of any abdominal tubes and of expected drainage volumes. To avoid disrupting a fragile anastomosis after gastric surgery, a nasogastric tube should *never* be irrigated, manipulated at whim, or reinserted by the nurse until approved by the surgeon. Often the nasogastric tube is precisely positioned by direct visualization during surgery. Abdominal distention after this surgery could herald a leaking anastomosis with intraabdominal

hemorrhage or leaking gastric contents. (Drain C, editor: *Perianesthesia nursing: a critical care approach*, ed 4, Philadelphia, 2003, Saunders.)

9.9.
Correct Answer: **d**
A pancreaticojejunostomy involves resection of major gastrointestinal organs and creating new connections, usually to treat pancreatic cancer. The distal (lower) stomach, part of the common bile duct, ampulla (head) of the pancreas, and adjoining duodenum are removed. Appropriate biliary, hepatic, gastric, and intestinal reconnections (anastomoses) are made to restore some integrity and function to the gastrointestinal tract. (Drain C, editor: *Perianesthesia nursing: a critical care approach*, ed 4, Philadelphia, 2003, Saunders.)

9.10.
Correct Answer: **a**
Any reduction in renal perfusion is interpreted by the kidney as reason to increase blood pressure and retain fluid. Renin released from the kidney activates angiotensinogen to produce angiotensin I. Angiotensin-converting enzyme (ACE) converts angiotensin I to angiotensin II, considered one of the most potent vasoconstrictors known. Unfortunately, this further decreases renal blood flow. Aldosterone's effect on the nephron's distal tubule promotes sodium reabsorption. Antidiuretic hormone secretion, not suppression, prompts fluid retention and decreases urine volume. (Copstead LC, Banasik JL: *Pathophysiology: biological and behavioral perspectives*, ed 2, Philadelphia, 2000, Saunders; Quinn D, Schick L, editors: *ASPAN's perianesthesia nursing core curriculum: preoperative, Phase I and Phase II PACU nursing*, Philadelphia, 2004, Saunders.)

9.11.
Correct Answer: **b**
Scopolamine, like atropine, is an anticholinergic medication that blocks the action of the neurotransmitter *acetylcholine* on the brain's vomiting center. As such, it can be a potent antiemetic. In addition, disorientation or drowsiness may develop. Risk factors including female gender and a history of postoperative nausea and vomiting have been associated with higher likelihood for postoperative nausea and vomiting. (Golembiewski J, Tokumaru S: Pharmacological prophylaxis and management of adult postoperative/postdischarge nausea and vomiting, *J PeriAnesth Nurs* 21[6]:385-397, 2006; Quinn D, Schick L, editors: *ASPAN's perianesthesia nursing core curriculum: preoperative, Phase I and Phase II PACU nursing*, Philadelphia, 2004, Saunders.)

9.12.
Correct Answer: **a**
Central nervous system (CNS) effects of anticholinergic medications include visual disturbances, sedation or disorientation, combativeness, and agitation. Hypoxia and acid-base imbalances *must* be excluded as causes of any delirium before attributing delirium solely to the scopolamine. The likelihood of emergence delirium increases when opioids are not used with the anticholinergic. Preoperative anxiety and fear, pain, and hypoxia also contribute to emergence delirium. (Drain C, editor: *Perianesthesia nursing: a critical care approach*, ed 4, Philadelphia, 2003, Saunders.)

9.13.
Correct Answer: **c**
The nurse must consider the patient's potential for deep vein thrombosis (DVT) in her legs, suggested by calf or posterior knee tenderness, erythema, or heat. Both her surgery (gynecologic) and her intraoperative position (lithotomy)

can alter circulation and damage nerves. Gynecologic procedures reportedly reduce blood flow from the legs by more than 50%, though the actual incidence of DVT is less than 10%. The nurse should assess and document that the patient's peripheral pulses are present. Back, hip, and leg pain likely are of muscular origin and therefore self-limiting. Though abdominal cramping is expected, true distention and unrelieved pain may indicate uterine perforation. Most patients have minimal postoperative drainage in PACU. (Burden N et al: *Ambulatory surgical nursing*, ed 2, Philadelphia, 2000, Saunders; Karlet MC: *Nurse anesthesia secrets*, St. Louis, 2005, Mosby; Quinn D, Schick L, editors: *ASPAN's perianesthesia nursing core curriculum: preoperative, Phase I and Phase II PACU nursing*, Philadelphia, 2004, Saunders.)

9.14. Correct Answer: **b**
Both regional and general anesthetic techniques expose the patient to changes in muscle and vascular tone, ability to move and feel pain, and altered circulation to surface areas, particularly the pressure-susceptible bony sites. More than 2 hours in a surgical position, elderly age, pre-existing (and often age-related) arthritis, diabetes, cardiovascular diseases, and nutritional status greatly affect the potential for position-related injury. (APRN: Recommended practices for positioning the patient in the perioperative practice setting, *AORN J* 73[1]:231-235, 2001.)

9.15. Correct Answer: **c**
The patient regularly takes prednisone; her steroid-induced adrenal atrophy requires timely postoperative hydrocortisone supplementation to support her stress responses. If an intraoperative

dose of hydrocortisone was not administered and no postoperative doses are ordered, the PACU nurse needs to contact the physician. Steroids cannot be abruptly interrupted without physiologic consequences; dexamethasone does not provide sufficient replacement. Cortisol is not stored in the body yet is essential to systemic function, particularly to sustain adequate serum glucose and for stress adaptation. The patient's surgical procedure and intraoperative position increase her potential for thromboembolism; she needs antiembolic stockings or pneumatic leg compression devices. (Connery LE, Coursin DB: Assessment and therapy of selected endocrine disorders, *Anesthesiol Clin North America* 22[1]:93-123, 2004; Drain C, editor: *Perianesthesia nursing: a critical care approach*, ed 4, Philadelphia, 2003, Saunders.)

9.16. Correct Answer: **a**
This elderly woman has risk for hypoxia and hypercarbia from age-related alterations in respiratory volumes. A moderate head-elevated position and encouraged deep breathing allow the greatest chest expansion. Surgically, this patient can assume a position of comfort. A high-Fowler's position is avoided to better promote blood flow to and from the legs and prevent stasis. (Drain C, editor: *Perianesthesia nursing: a critical care approach*, ed 4, Philadelphia, 2003, Saunders; Quinn D, Schick L, editors: *ASPAN's perianesthesia nursing core curriculum: preoperative, Phase I and Phase II PACU nursing*, Philadelphia, 2004, Saunders.)

9.17. Correct Answer: **b**
Unrecognized infection, impaired wound healing, thinner, more fragile skin tissue, osteoporosis, fluid

retention, and hyperglycemia are among physiologic changes produced by chronic use of synthetic corticosteroids. Any symptoms of infection can be masked by suppressed inflammatory responses. Therefore the patient requires particular attention to her nutritional status and asepsis during wound observation and dressing changes. (Burden N et al: *Ambulatory surgical nursing*, ed 2, Philadelphia, 2000, Saunders; Karlet MC: *Nurse anesthesia secrets*, St. Louis, 2005, Mosby; USPDI *Drug Information For The Health Care Professional*, (internet database). Greenwood Village, Colo, Thomson Micromedex.)

9.18. Correct Answer: **d**
The nursing process should be achieved through a series of integrated steps focusing on total patient care through team effort. The perianesthesia nurse should be able to recognize patients with increased risk for acute renal failure (ARF). This helps with a timely diagnosis and treatment to prevent any further damage. Preexisting renal dysfunction can be a predictor to postoperative ARF. Patients undergoing surgical procedures such as cardiopulmonary bypass and other vascular surgeries involving the aorta potentially have up to a 30% chance of experiencing ARF. Any condition or procedure that results in hypoperfusion of the kidneys can result in ARF. (Agodoa L: Acute renal failure in the PACU, *J PeriAnesth Nurs* 17[6]:377-383, 2002; Quinn D, Schick L, editors: *ASPAN's perianesthesia nursing core curriculum: preoperative, Phase I and Phase II PACU nursing*, Philadelphia, 2004, Saunders.)

9.19. Correct Answer: **c**
Renal function arising from prerenal failure may be improved by increasing cardiac output and sodium excretion. Furosemide (Lasix) is a potent diuretic that increases sodium excretion (followed by fluid) at the loop of Henle and distal renal tubules. Sodium and fluid are retained in prerenal failure when the kidneys "sense" low fluid volume and low cardiac output. Correcting a fluid volume deficit and supporting cardiac output also may sufficiently increase renal blood flow to improve the renal failure. Dopamine promotes renal perfusion, though the "renal dose" of dopamine is small, approximately 0.5 mg/kg; aminoglycosides are strongly nephrotoxic and should not be used in azotemic patients. Patency of any ureteral stent is essential to renal function but addresses a *post*renal cause of oliguria. (Copstead LC, Banasik JL: *Pathophysiology: biological and behavioral perspectives*, ed 2, Philadelphia, 2000, Saunders; Quinn D, Schick L, editors: *ASPAN's perianesthesia nursing core curriculum: preoperative, Phase I and Phase II PACU nursing*, Philadelphia, 2004, Saunders.)

9.20. Correct Answer: **b**
Hospital protocols and state laws govern criteria for administering medications for intravenous conscious sedation. Nursing responsibility includes continuous monitoring and assessment of airway, respiratory rate, oxygen saturation, blood pressure, and cardiac rate and rhythm. The nurse observing the patient must have no other responsibilities and must be able to both intervene in emergency situations and contact additional personnel for support. Back-up personnel should be in place who are experts in airway management, emergency intubations, and advanced cardiopulmonary resuscitation should the

need arise. (ASPAN: *2006-2008 Standards of perianesthesia nursing practice*, Cherry Hill, NJ, 2006, ASPAN; Odom-Forren J, Watson DS: *Practical guide to moderate sedation/analgesia*, ed 2, St. Louis, 2005, Mosby.)

9.21. Correct Answer: **c**
These symptoms after a transurethral resection of the prostate (TURP) are consistent with bladder perforation. Fluid pouring into the abdomen contributes to the referred pain into the shoulder. The urologist must be contacted; best outcomes require cystectomy, preferably within 1 to 2 hours after perforation. Bladder spasm is a frequent event after TURP and can cause pain (usually over the bladder area) and a strong urge to urinate. Increased bleeding and perhaps clots in the returns of the bladder irrigation solution may be noted with spasms; bladder relaxation, increased rate of irrigation, and observation are interventions for bladder spasms. (Rothrock J, editor: *Alexander's care of the patient in surgery*, ed 12, St. Louis, 2003, Mosby; Tanagho EA, McAninch JW, editors: *Smith's general urology*, ed 15, New York, 2000, McGraw-Hill.)

9.22. Correct Answer: **b**
After extracorporeal shock wave lithotripsy (ESWL), patients often are discharged home and must understand that high-volume fluid intake and straining urine are essential. ESWL directs multiple high-frequency shocks through the skin to pulverize renal calculi. The patient must excrete the stone fragments through the urine. Copious fluid intake is expected to promote an increase in urine output to flush the stones through the renal system. The patient should also be encouraged to maintain an active

ambulatory status to facilitate stone passage. Pain is usually minimal after ESWL, though flank tenderness and slight skin redness occur. (Quinn D, Schick L, editors: *ASPAN's perianesthesia nursing core curriculum: preoperative, Phase I and Phase II PACU nursing*, Philadelphia, 2004, Saunders; Tanagho EA, McAninch JW, editors: *Smith's general urology*, ed 15, New York, 2000, McGraw-Hill.)

9.23. Correct Answer: **d**
Despite adequate overall fluid volume replacement, the patient's hypotension likely results when fluid translocates from his vascular compartment into abdominal tissues and spaces that normally contain little fluid. This sequestered volume is unavailable to support cardiac output. Extensive bowel manipulation, tissue trauma or infection, decreased serum protein, and altered capillary permeability are among forces that could allow fluids to exit the vascular compartment after a major abdominal surgical procedure. (Drain C, editor: *Perianesthesia nursing: a critical care approach*, ed 4, Philadelphia, 2003, Saunders; Quinn D, Schick L, editors: *ASPAN's perianesthesia nursing core curriculum: preoperative, Phase I and Phase II PACU nursing*, Philadelphia, 2004, Saunders.)

9.24. Correct Answer: **b**
To improve cardiac output and ensure sufficient renal blood flow are appropriate responses to treat the patient's decreased circulating blood volume and fluid shifts. Supporting circulation may initially require several liters of crystalloid, or alternatively and controversially, colloid support, and then judicious monitoring to detect evidence of cardiac overload. (Drain C, editor: *Perianesthesia nursing: a critical*

care approach, ed 4, Philadelphia, 2003, Saunders; Quinn D, Schick L, editors: *ASPAN's perianesthesia nursing core curriculum: preoperative, Phase I and Phase II PACU nursing*, Philadelphia, 2004, Saunders.)

9.25. Correct Answer: **a**
The fluid volume given in the PACU to fill the patient's vascular compartment and support his cardiac output eventually is reabsorbed and excreted by the kidneys. Intestinal tissue injuries must first heal, and capillary permeability must return to normal; fluid translocation can continue for up to 72 hours. Until then, the patient still has risk of circulatory overload and requires close observation of vital signs, renal output and urine concentrating ability, and pulmonary infiltration. He still requires fluids as prescribed by the physician, as much as 200 mL/hour of hypertonic fluid. Pain can increase both preload and afterload, possibly overtaxing cardiac muscle. (Drain C, editor: *Perianesthesia nursing: a critical*

care approach, ed 4, Philadelphia, 2003, Saunders; Quinn D, Schick L, editors: *ASPAN's perianesthesia nursing core curriculum: preoperative, Phase I and Phase II PACU nursing*, Philadelphia, 2004, Saunders.)

9.26. Correct Answer: **c**
In prerenal failure, the nephron remains undamaged even though the volume of blood filtered at the glomerulus and therefore the amount of urine produced decrease. Hypovolemia from over-diuresis, shock, cardiac failure, or dehydration (outcomes produced by events unrelated to kidney anatomy) causes prerenal failure. Acute tubular necrosis results from actual damage to kidney tissue, thereby affecting the kidney's ability to concentrate fluid and excrete wastes. (Copstead LC, Banasik JL: *Pathophysiology: biological and behavioral perspectives*, ed 2, Philadelphia, 2000, Saunders; Tanagho EA, McAninch JW, editors: *Smith's general urology*, ed 15, New York, 2000, McGraw-Hill.)

SET 2

9.27.	c		**9.38.**	b
9.28.	d		**9.39.**	a
9.29.	a		**9.40.**	d
9.30.	b		**9.41.**	d
9.31.	b		**9.42.**	a
9.32.	d		**9.43.**	d
9.33.	a		**9.44.**	a
9.34.	b		**9.45.**	a
9.35.	d		**9.46.**	b
9.36.	b		**9.47.**	d
9.37.	c			

SET 2

9.27. Correct Answer: **c**
After succinylcholine-induced relaxation, muscle function returns first to the respiratory (intercostal) muscles and then to shoulders and abdomen, followed by neck and extremities. Eye, finger, and toe muscles recover last. The patient is presumed to have an atypical (congenital) pseudocholinesterase deficiency that delayed her metabolism of succinylcholine; succinylcholine is usually hydrolyzed quickly. Recovery of muscle function depends upon the amount of active circulating pseudocholinesterase. Her rash may result from a normal release of histamine. (Quinn D, Schick L, editors: *ASPAN's perianesthesia nursing core curriculum: preoperative, Phase I and Phase II PACU nursing,* Philadelphia, 2004, Saunders.)

9.28. Correct Answer: **d**
Especially after brief surgical procedures and single intubating doses of succinylcholine, nearly one half of patients state muscle aching when moving their face, neck, shoulder, rib, or abdomen. Postoperative bedrest seems to lessen the pain. Muscle tremors (fasciculations) occur during cellular depolarization; the contractions produce pain, which is noticed as the postoperative patient becomes mobile. Though nerve compression is possible from any intraoperative position, the patient's lithotomy position more likely would produce back pain. Vomiting may occur after laparoscopic and endometrial surgery, though the patient apparently tolerates fluids. (Drain C, editor: *Perianesthesia nursing: a critical care approach,* ed 4, Philadelphia, 2003, Saunders;

Quinn D, Schick L, editors: *ASPAN's perianesthesia nursing core curriculum: preoperative, Phase I and Phase II PACU nursing,* Philadelphia, 2004, Saunders.)

9.29. Correct Answer: **a**
This patient may be sensitive to latex. Eye swelling and hand dermatitis at work are important bits of preoperative information. Exposing him to the array of latex products in the anesthesia environment can result in systemic responses like bronchospasm, severe hypotension, or cardiac arrest (anaphylaxis). Health care workers such as dentists, hygienists, physicians, and nurses regularly wear latex gloves. Over time, multiple exposures to latex antigen sensitize the health care worker either by direct contact with a latex product or by inhaling airborne particles. Latex reactions range from a localized rash with redness and itching to a systemic hypersensitivity reaction with anaphylaxis. (Quinn D, Schick L, editors: *ASPAN's perianesthesia nursing core curriculum: preoperative, Phase I and Phase II PACU nursing,* Philadelphia, 2004, Saunders; Rothrock J, editor: *Alexander's care of the patient in surgery,* ed 12, St. Louis, 2003, Mosby.)

9.30. Correct Answer: **b**
Normal bladder volume ranges from about 400 to 500 mL. Urge to void generally occurs when the bladder fills with 300 to 400 mL. Deferring micturition stretches bladder walls and, over time, could alter muscle contraction and emptying. Regional anesthesia, surgical procedures, lack of privacy, and

"unnatural" positions can affect bladder emptying during the immediate postanesthesia period. (Quinn D, Schick L, editors: *ASPAN's perianesthesia nursing core curriculum: preoperative, Phase I and Phase II PACU nursing,* Philadelphia, 2004, Saunders; Tanagho EA, McAninch JW, editors: *Smith's general urology,* ed 15, New York, 2000, McGraw-Hill.)

9.31. Correct Answer: **b**
Mortality for sepsis ranges from 20% to more than 50%. Infection results from many possible sources and can initiate a progression of events that contribute to shock, disseminated intravascular coagulation (DIC), renal failure, gastrointestinal bleeding, and pulmonary failure. Vigilant effort is directed toward finding and eradicating the infectious source. The nurse will monitor the patient's currently acceptable platelets and urine output; the patient's hemoglobin level, though less than the accepted normal of 12 to 15 g/dL, may reflect hemodilution, not necessarily new bleeding, after abdominal exploration. (Drain C, editor: *Perianesthesia nursing: a critical care approach,* ed 4, Philadelphia, 2003, Saunders; Kleinpell RM et al: Incidence, pathogenesis, and management of sepsis: an overview, *AACN Adv Crit Care* 17[4]:385-393, 2006; Quinn D, Schick L, editors: *ASPAN's perianesthesia nursing core curriculum: preoperative, Phase I and Phase II PACU nursing,* Philadelphia, 2004, Saunders.)

9.32. Correct Answer: **d**
A patient with early hyperdynamic septic shock has warm, dry extremities and flushed skin. This hyperdynamic phase of septic shock is characterized by peripheral vasodilation and markedly increased cardiac output, up to 2 to 3 times

normal. Sepsis must be a primary concern for any patient with potential for multisystem organ failure, even though pain or hypothermia also occurs. This patient's shivering is not hypothermia induced; intravenous butorphanol might further increase intracardiac pressures, cardiac work, and vascular resistance; other medication options are preferable after determining respiratory adequacy. Providing analgesia should not be an "automatic" response. (Drain C, editor: *Perianesthesia nursing: a critical care approach,* ed 4, Philadelphia, 2003, Saunders; Quinn D, Schick L, editors: *ASPAN's perianesthesia nursing core curriculum: preoperative, Phase I and Phase II PACU nursing,* Philadelphia, 2004, Saunders.)

9.33. Correct Answer: **a**
Hyperventilation and $paCO_2$ of less than 32 mmHg (respiratory alkalosis) are hallmarks of septic shock. The alkalosis is the body's initial attempt to compensate for metabolic acidosis, indicated by a still elevated serum lactate. Hypoxemia heralds development of adult respiratory distress syndrome (ARDS). Sepsis stresses all body organ systems. (Drain C, editor: *Perianesthesia nursing: a critical care approach,* ed 4, Philadelphia, 2003, Saunders; Kleinpell RM et al: Incidence, pathogenesis, and management of sepsis: an overview, *AACN Adv Crit Care* 17[4]:385-393, 2006; Quinn D, Schick L, editors: *ASPAN's perianesthesia nursing core curriculum: preoperative, Phase I and Phase II PACU nursing,* Philadelphia, 2004, Saunders.)

9.34. Correct Answer: **b**
Reversing fluid volume deficits and acidemia are among interventions that can reduce renal damage (nephrotoxicity) from aminoglycoside antibiotics. Elderly

age, NSAIDs, and large doses of potent diuretics are other risk factors that can increase the incidence of renal damage during treatment with this class of antibiotics. Serum levels can adequately predict potential for renal damage and generally should be checked in all patients receiving sustained therapy. (Copstead LC, Banasik JL: *Pathophysiology: biological and behavioral perspectives*, ed 2, Philadelphia, 2000, Saunders; Tanagho EA, McAninch JW, editors: *Smith's general urology*, ed 15, New York, 2000, McGraw-Hill.)

9.35. Correct Answer: **d**
The patient's tachycardia and relatively low blood pressures may reflect absolute hypovolemia, either from hemoperitoneum and low hemoglobin or insufficient fluid volume replacement. To preserve adequate cardiac output, heart rate often reflexively increases to the tachycardic range (>100 bpm) to compensate for decreased venous blood return. The caregiver must recognize that only 2 hours after abdominal hysterectomy, the patient may be actively bleeding into her abdomen, a not-so-rare complication in the first several postoperative hours. The nurse actually may consider sepsis, hypothermia, and myocardial infarction, as well as hypovolemia, as causing the patient's hypotension but must discern the correct underlying pathophysiologic process. (Drain C, editor: *Perianesthesia nursing: a critical care approach*, ed 4, Philadelphia, 2003, Saunders; Quinn D, Schick L, editors: *ASPAN's perianesthesia nursing core curriculum: preoperative, Phase I and Phase II PACU nursing*, Philadelphia, 2004, Saunders.)

9.36. Correct Answer: **b**
The patient's current hemoglobin should be verified and her abdomen examined for increased distention (girth), rigidity, and pain. The nurse increases the infusion rate of intravenous crystalloids and perhaps adds colloids or blood cell transfusions as ordered. Persistent tachycardia should not be treated with vasodilating or beta blocking medications until fluid volume deficits are corrected. Once adequate circulating volume is restored, tachycardia often self-resolves. (Drain C, editor: *Perianesthesia nursing: a critical care approach*, ed 4, Philadelphia, 2003, Saunders.)

9.37. Correct Answer: **c**
ASPAN's *Standards of Perianesthesia Nursing Practice* recommends that "two registered nurses, one of whom is an RN competent in Phase I postanesthesia nursing, are in the same room where the patient is receiving Phase I level of care." (ASPAN: *2006-2008 Standards of perianesthesia nursing practice*, Cherry Hill, NJ, 2006, ASPAN.)

9.38. Correct Answer: **b**
The patient's fetus may have been Rh positive, having inherited this red blood cell antibody from the father. The patient has no antibodies to the Rh positive antigen. An Rh positive fetus can stimulate antibody formation in the Rh negative patient. Her future Rh positive fetuses face erythrocyte destruction when these new Rh positive maternal antibodies cross the placenta. Sensitivity to the Rh antigen can be reduced or eliminated by injecting immune globulin (RhoGAM) to Rh negative women. (Burden N et al: *Ambulatory surgical nursing*, ed 2, Philadelphia, 2000, Saunders; Karlet MC: *Nurse anesthesia secrets*, St. Louis, 2005, Mosby; Springhouse: *Handbook of*

pathophysiology, Philadelphia, 2001, Lippincott Williams & Wilkins.)

9.39. Correct Answer: **a**

During laparoscopy, patients are placed in Trendelenburg and lithotomy positions, increasing the potential for aspiration. Efforts to reduce gastric volume and acidity may be necessary preoperatively. An empty bladder is desired for laparoscopy. (Burden N et al: *Ambulatory surgical nursing*, ed 2, Philadelphia, 2000, Saunders; Karlet MC: *Nurse anesthesia secrets*, St. Louis, 2005, Mosby.)

9.40. Correct Answer: **d**

Occurrence of hypotension, tachycardia, and significant abdominal distention, perhaps with severe pain and blood oozing through bandages that cover the laparoscope puncture sites, strongly suggests intraabdominal hemorrhage. Large amounts of blood can pour into the abdomen before severe pain, an initial symptom, occurs. Hemorrhage, viscous perforation, atelectasis, air (gas) embolism, and infection are among the serious, and rare, post-laparoscopic complications. Shoulder pain, typically right-sided, some residual abdominal distention, and mild vaginal bleeding are expected events. Bradycardia may occur during the procedure because of peritoneal stretching. (Burden N et al: *Ambulatory surgical nursing*, ed 2, Philadelphia, 2000, Saunders; Karlet MC: *Nurse anesthesia secrets*, St. Louis, 2005, Mosby; Quinn D, Schick L, editors: *ASPAN's perianesthesia nursing core curriculum: preoperative, Phase I and Phase II PACU nursing*, Philadelphia, 2004, Saunders.)

9.41. Correct Answer: **d**

One assessment of peroneal nerve function is determining the ability to dorsiflex the great toe and sensation atop the foot. Ischemia, compression, or stretch from surgical position quite commonly affects the peroneal nerve during surgery and anesthesia. Recovery of function varies with extent of nerve damage and amount of regrowth necessary. (Drain C, editor: *Perianesthesia nursing: a critical care approach*, ed 4, Philadelphia, 2003, Saunders.)

9.42. Correct Answer: **a**

During laparoscopy, lithotomy and Trendelenburg positions are used. If improperly positioned or inadequately padded, the patient's leg could rest against leg supports. This lateral pressure against the leg can damage the peroneal nerve. (Drain C, editor: *Perianesthesia nursing: a critical care approach*, ed 4, Philadelphia, 2003, Saunders; Winfree CJ, Kline DG: Intraoperative positioning nerve injuries, *Surg Neurol* 63[1]:5-18, 2005.)

9.43. Correct Answer: **d**

Cisatracurium is an intermediate-acting nondepolarizing muscle relaxant. Onset of effect is longer than succinylcholine, the only depolarizing muscle relaxant currently in use. Spontaneous recovery is expected within 40 to 50 minutes and even more rapidly when reversal medications are used. Warming speeds reversal. Unlike atracurium, it is less likely to cause histamine release. (Drain C, editor: *Perianesthesia nursing: a critical care approach*, ed 4, Philadelphia, 2003, Saunders.)

9.44. Correct Answer: **a**

Neostigmine is an anticholinesterase that *reverses* muscle relaxant effects to allow acetylcholine to remain active. Medications that potentiate the effects of muscle relaxants include "mycin" antibiotics, local anesthetics, and volatile anesthetics. (Drain C, editor: *Perianesthesia nursing: a critical care approach*, ed 4, Philadelphia, 2003, Saunders; Stoelting RK, Hillier SC: *Handbook of pharmacology and physiology in anesthetic practice*, ed 2, Philadelphia, 2006, Lippincott Williams & Wilkins.)

9.45. Correct Answer: **a**
Drainage and bleeding are minimal after hemorrhoidectomy and repair of rectal fistulae. The nurse informs the surgeon when large volumes of sanguineous drainage are observed. Urinary retention is common after rectal surgery; some surgeons restrict fluids to prevent bladder distention until voiding occurs. Sharp or burning pain and rectal tenderness are likely; rectal packing often produces perineal pressure. Some surgeons infiltrate the rectal area with local anesthetic medications though, so absence of perineal pain and sensation immediately after surgery is also possible. (Drain C, editor: *Perianesthesia nursing: a critical care approach*, ed 4, Philadelphia, 2003, Saunders.)

9.46. Correct Answer: **b**
The nurse slightly supports the patient's legs so her heels do not touch the mattress. The patient's back pain and heel tenderness are probably results of her 3½-hour anesthetized, supine position. Skin circulation over bony prominences like the heels, scapulae, elbows, and sacrum is easily compromised. Ischemia with blanching, edema, or even skin breakdown develops. Muscle aches respond to analgesia, repositioning, and heat. The nurse should also anticipate postural hypotension and assess for nerve injuries, particularly to upper extremities. (APRN: Recommended practices for positioning the patient in the perioperative practice setting, *AORN J* 73[1]:231-235, 2001; Schultz A: Predicting and preventing pressure ulcers in surgical patients, *AORN J* 81[5]:986-1006, 2005.)

9.47. Correct Answer: **d**
Azotemia refers to retention of metabolic wastes in the blood because of lack of renal clearance. These by-products are nitrogen based. Urea, peptides, creatine, and creatinine result from protein or amino acid metabolism. Normal creatinine is 0.4 to 1.2 mg/dL, and BUN is 5 to 25 mg/dL. The azotemic patient who retains metabolic by-products may indeed have oliguria, with urine less than 400 mL/day. The clinical syndrome, uremia, may develop and is demonstrated with symptoms related to the effect of these toxins on other body systems. (Agodoa L: Acute renal failure in the PACU, *J PeriAnesth Nurs* 17[6]:377-383, 2002; Copstead LC, Banasik JL: *Pathophysiology: biological and behavioral perspectives*, ed 2, Philadelphia, 2000, Saunders.)

SET 3

ANSWER KEY			
9.48.	c	**9.61.**	a
9.49.	d	**9.62.**	b
9.50.	a	**9.63.**	a
9.51.	b	**9.64.**	b
9.52.	c	**9.65.**	d
9.53.	a	**9.66.**	b
9.54.	c	**9.67.**	b
9.55.	a	**9.68.**	c
9.56.	b	**9.69.**	c
9.57.	d	**9.70.**	a
9.58.	d	**9.71.**	d
9.59.	c	**9.72.**	b
9.60.	b	**9.73.**	c

Set 3

Rationales and References

9.48. Correct Answer: **c**
Blood pressure can plummet during vancomycin dosing if the drug is infused rapidly. The low blood pressure response resolves, but resolution occurs over hours. Recommended rate is 0.5 to 1 g delivered over a minimum of 60 minutes. Although ototoxicity is serious and common, the rate of infusion does not affect its development. (Stoelting RK, Hillier SC: *Handbook of pharmacology and physiology in anesthetic practice*, ed 2, Philadelphia, 2006, Lippincott Williams & Wilkins.)

9.49. Correct Answer: **d**
Hypothermia is signaled by core temperature measures of less than 36° C. Peripheral vasoconstriction, slowing blood flow, and decreasing tissue perfusion occur. Cardiac work and the potential for both dysrhythmias and hypertension increase. Shivering increases oxygen consumption, decreases ventilation, and promotes metabolic and respiratory acidosis. Hypothermia also decreases hepatic blood flow and alters rate of medication clearance, so the patient's return to alertness may be slowed. (Jeran L: Patient temperature: an introduction to the clinical guideline for the prevention of unplanned perioperative hypothermia, *J PeriAnesth Nurs* 16[5]:305-304, 2001.)

9.50. Correct Answer: **a**
The physiologic alterations associated with hypothermia increase oxygen consumption, alter oxygenation, and produce metabolic acidosis. Acidosis usually resolves as temperature increases; therefore sodium bicarbonate is not usually an *initial* therapy. Maintaining head and body skin coverage is important; nearly 50% of heat loss reportedly occurs by radiation from the head. Shivering reduction with rewarming techniques and/or medication minimizes physiologic damage and increases patient comfort. (Jeran L: Patient temperature: an introduction to the clinical guideline for the prevention of unplanned perioperative hypothermia, *J PeriAnesth Nurs* 16[5]:305-304, 2001; Noble KA: Chill can kill, *J PeriAnesth Nurs* 21[3]:204-207, 2006.)

9.51. Correct Answer: **b**
Peripheral vascular tone relaxes as the patient warms; the resulting vasodilation can produce major hypotension. Shivering consumes energy, producing carbon dioxide and consuming oxygen. Rewarming after hypothermia should be gradual. As the hypothalamus regains temperature regulating control after general anesthesia, further significant heat loss is unlikely. The mildly hypothermic patient may have "cold-induced" diuresis and altered coagulation, including fibrinolysis and clot destruction. (Jeran L: Patient temperature: an introduction to the clinical guideline for the prevention of unplanned perioperative hypothermia, *J PeriAnesth Nurs* 16[5]:305-304, 2001; Noble KA: Chill can kill, *J PeriAnesth Nurs* 21[3]:204-207, 2006; Good KK et al: Postoperative hypothermia—the chilling consequences, *AORN J* 83[5]:1055-1070, 2006.)

9.52. Correct Answer: **c**
Muscle movement involved in active shivering may produce muscle aching (myalgia) the next day. Both hypothermic and normothermic patients may

shiver postoperatively. The hypothalamus begins to function when anesthesia suppression stops; "rebound" hyperthermia is unlikely the next day. Muscle relaxant effects, or reparalysis, may recur while the patient rewarms in the PACU, but residual effects are most certainly unlikely the next day. (Quinn D, Schick L, editors: *ASPAN's perianesthesia nursing core curriculum: preoperative, Phase I and Phase II PACU nursing,* Philadelphia, 2004, Saunders.)

9.53. Correct Answer: **a**
Poor ventilation, atelectasis, and pneumonia are likely outcomes if the patient does not move, breathe deeply and often, and have adequate pain management to participate in her pulmonary care. After the high upper abdominal incision used for gastrectomy, the patient is likely to "splint" her incision and restrict her breathing to limit her pain. Her nasogastric tube is likely to drain *small* amounts of bright residual gastric blood; more than 75 mL/hr should be reported. After resection, a gastric tube for balloon tamponade should not be needed. (Quinn D, Schick L, editors: *ASPAN's perianesthesia nursing core curriculum: preoperative, Phase I and Phase II PACU nursing,* Philadelphia, 2004, Saunders.)

9.54. Correct Answer: **c**
Although rare, testicular cancer is the most common cancer in men between the ages of 15 and 35 years. Diagnosis of testicular cancer is confirmed after orchiectomy is performed. After the tumor is staged, the patient will then decide with his physician the mode of treatment. Supportive management for this patient is extremely important during this stressful time. Nurses should focus on issues surrounding the patient's concerns

related to altered sexuality, altered body image, altered role function, fertility, grief, and mortality. (Copstead LC, Banasik JL: *Pathophysiology: biological and behavioral perspectives,* ed 2, Philadelphia, 2000, Saunders; SUNA: *Urologic nursing: a study guide,* ed 2, Pitman, NJ, 2001, Society of Urologic Nurses and Associates.)

9.55. Correct Answer: **a**
The fast onset of the analgesic fentanyl makes it an ideal choice for rapid pain relief. The perianesthesia nurse should be aware that this medication does have all the usual opioid-induced adverse effects, such as nausea, constipation, pruritus, sedation, and respiratory depression. (Odom-Forren J, Watson DS: *Practical guide to moderate sedation/analgesia,* ed 2, St. Louis, 2005, Mosby; Pasero C: Fentanyl for acute pain management, *J PeriAnesth Nurs* 20[4]:279-284, 2005.)

9.56. Correct Answer: **b**
Frequent contact with blood or blood products increases risk of exposure to hepatitis B virus (HBV). Both HBV and human immunodeficiency virus (HIV) are transmitted through blood contact. Hepatitis A virus (HAV) exposure occurs through fecal, not blood, contamination to the mouth. Standard Precautions are guidelines that are to be used in all patient care situations. These guidelines are designed to block the pathogen's portal of exit route of transmission and portals of entry. (Copstead LC, Banasik JL: *Pathophysiology: biological and behavioral perspectives,* ed 2, Philadelphia, 2000, Saunders; Rothrock J, editor: *Alexander's care of the patient in surgery,* ed 12, St. Louis, 2003, Mosby.)

9.57. Correct Answer: **d**

Saturating through vaginal packing *and* a perineal pad is significant bleeding. The nurse notifies the surgeon and monitors the patient closely for hypotension, fluid deficit, and shock. Hypotension without overt bleeding may relate to surgical manipulation and pressure when vaginally removing the uterus. Abdominal cramping and pressure are expected and usually are adequately treated with opioids in moderate doses. A suprapubic catheter should *not* have tension. Intraoperative lithotomy position commonly results in low back pain. Tingling likely indicates a position-related transient nerve ischemia from peroneal nerve compression; the nurse evaluates neurovascular status, checks for edema, and then reassesses for improvement within 30 minutes. (APRN: Recommended practices for positioning the patient in the perioperative practice setting, *AORN J* 73[1]:231-235, 2001; Quinn D, Schick L, editors: *ASPAN's perianesthesia nursing core curriculum: preoperative, Phase I and Phase II PACU nursing,* Philadelphia, 2004, Saunders.)

9.58. Correct Answer: **d**

Obese patients are prone to sleep apnea and easy airway obstruction and are very sensitive to airway depression. Decreased functional reserve capacity and greater oxygen consumption increase the obese patient's work of breathing. Supine position aggravates these factors, which all contribute to hypoventilation, hypoxia, and hypercarbia. (Crum BS: Practicing safe care of the bariatric population, *Perioperative Nursing Clinics* 1[1]:67-71, 2006; Drain C, editor: *Perianesthesia nursing: a critical care approach,* ed 4, Philadelphia, 2003, Saunders.)

9.59. Correct Answer: **c**

Bladder distention can contribute to postoperative hypertension, tachycardia, and restlessness. These same symptoms also indicate hypoxia, which must be presumed as the primary cause of restlessness and disorientation until ruled out. Emergence delirium may be an additional cause of restlessness. (Quinn D, Schick L, editors: *ASPAN's perianesthesia nursing core curriculum: preoperative, Phase I and Phase II PACU nursing,* Philadelphia, 2004, Saunders.)

9.60. Correct Answer: **b**

Based on extensive research, the combination of restrictive and malabsorptive response to the Roux-en-Y gastric bypass procedure results in better long-term weight loss. The laparoscopic adjustable gastric banding is the least invasive surgery available. Vertical banded gastroplasty will not significantly decrease ingestion of sweets, junk food, milk shakes, non-diet soft drinks, or ice creams, leading to reduced weight loss or regaining lost weight. Bariatric patients frequently suffer from obstructive sleep apnea, and the surgical procedure will generally improve their sleep apnea as they lose weight. (Ackert-Burr C: Weight-loss surgery education for the health care provider and the weight-loss surgery patient, *Perioperative Nursing Clinics* 1[1]:31-45, 2006; Woodward BG: Bariatric surgery options, *Crit Care Nurs Q* 26[2]:89-100, 2003.)

9.61. Correct Answer: **a**

Surgical treatment of obesity will be successful only if the patient understands the need to modify diet and lifestyle. Early ambulation and mobility are important to prevent thrombophlebitis and deep vein thromboembolism. Clear liquids will be started on postoperative day 1. Small portions and avoidance of calorie-dense foods will minimize discomfort and enhance weight loss. (O' Brien D, Palazzolo WC: Patient preparation and education: bariatric surgery, *Perioperative Nursing Clinics* 1[1]:47-53, 2006.)

9.62. Correct Answer: **b**
Oxygen saturation is measured by pulse oximetry, a noninvasive monitoring technique used to estimate arterial oxygen saturation. Ventilation is measured by auscultation to assess air movement and more definitively through end-tidal carbon dioxide monitoring devices or direct measurement of $PaCO_2$ in an arterial blood sample. Reduced oxygen levels may assist the nurse in identifying the patient at risk for respiratory depression or oversedation by opioids, but it is not the only reason for measuring oxygen saturation. (AACN: *AACN procedure manual for critical care*, ed 5, Philadelphia, 2005, Saunders; O' Brien D, Palazzolo WC: Patient preparation and education: bariatric surgery, *Perioperative Nursing Clinics* 1[1]:47-53, 2006.)

9.63. Correct Answer: **a**
Isoflurane is a useful anesthetic for maintenance of general anesthesia with rare toxic effects. It is eliminated primarily by exhalation as an intact molecule with 0.2% metabolism occurring in the liver. The kidneys excrete the metabolites. Enflurane has a slow elimination and is the most likely of all volatile anesthetics to produce a lingering CNS depressant effect in the PACU. Sevoflurane can be nephrotoxic if levels of metabolites are allowed to rise high enough. (Quinn D, Schick L, editors: *ASPAN's perianesthesia nursing core curriculum: preoperative,*

Phase I and Phase II PACU nursing, Philadelphia, 2004, Saunders.)

9.64. Correct Answer: **b**
A moderate fluid challenge can increase urine volume. Decreased urine output from prerenal causes arises from non-kidney origins. Examples include hypovolemia from hemorrhage, surgical blood losses, ascites removal, decreased myocardial performance, and "third space" fluid shifts or gastrointestinal losses. Diuretics do increase renal perfusion, but consider that a diuretic might further accentuate volume depletion. Catheter function addresses a postrenal cause. Myoglobin and aminoglycoside antibiotics like gentamicin are associated with acute renal failure and nephron damage, which are not prerenal conditions. (Agodoa L: Acute renal failure in the PACU, *J PeriAnesth Nurs* 17[6]:377-383, 2002; Copstead LC, Banasik JL: *Pathophysiology: biological and behavioral perspectives*, ed 2, Philadelphia, 2000, Saunders.)

9.65. Correct Answer: **d**
Creatinine, a product of muscle metabolism, is filtered by the renal glomerulus and not reabsorbed. It is excreted exclusively by the kidneys. Blood urea nitrogen (BUN) varies with the rate of protein metabolism; osmolality and potassium also vary with nonrenal influences. Normal fasting serum creatinine (0.7-1.5 mg/dL) measures usually indicate adequate glomerular filtration, as the rate of muscle metabolism is constant. The only two factors that affect serum creatinine are: (1) the rate of creatinine produced from muscle, which is relatively constant in the absence of muscle breakdown, and (2) the rate of creatinine excreted by the kidney, which is determined primarily by the glomerular filtration rate.

(Copstead LC, Banasik JL: *Pathophysiology: biological and behavioral perspectives*, ed 2, Philadelphia, 2000, Saunders.)

9.66. Correct Answer: **b**
One of the objectives when caring for a patient with ARF is the avoidance and treatment of infection because of the immuno-suppressive state of the patient. Awareness of the patient's heightened risk and attention to aseptic technique are crucial to positive outcomes for this patient. (Copstead LC, Banasik JL: *Pathophysiology: biological and behavioral perspectives*, ed 2, Philadelphia, 2000, Saunders; Tanagho EA, McAninch JW, editors: *Smith's general urology*, ed 15, New York, 2000, McGraw-Hill.)

9.67. Correct Answer: **b**
Stress, surgical lysis of tissues, and acidosis promote release of intracellular potassium to extracellular fluid. The failing kidney, whether the result of acute or chronic disease, cannot adjust electrolyte imbalances; serum potassium increases to cardiotoxic, life-threatening levels. Hyperkalemia causes muscle dysfunction with hypopolarization to the extent that the resting membrane potentials lie above their threshold potentials. Hyperkalemia also decreases the duration and rate of rise of cardiac action potentials and decreases the conduction velocity in the heart. Severe hyperkalemia can cause cardiac arrest. (Copstead LC, Banasik JL: *Pathophysiology: biological and behavioral perspectives*, ed 2, Philadelphia, 2000, Saunders.)

9.68. Correct Answer: **c**
Postoperatively, isotonic solutions (physiologic fluids that are neither hypertonic nor hypotonic) should be used to irrigate the bladder. Movement of solutions into the circulation by osmosis or vascular absorption can cause significant dilutional hyponatremia and produce symptoms of water intoxication. Water can cause hemolysis of red blood cells after absorption into the blood stream through highly vascular prostate tissue. Isotonic and nonhemolytic solutions are used during surgery to avoid electrical conduction through ionic solutions and ensure clear visualization. (Quinn D, Schick L, editors: *ASPAN's perianesthesia nursing core curriculum: preoperative, Phase I and Phase II PACU nursing*, Philadelphia, 2004, Saunders; Rothrock J, editor: *Alexander's care of the patient in surgery*, ed 12, St. Louis, 2003, Mosby.)

9.69. Correct Answer: **c**
Traction on a urethral bladder catheter after transurethral resection of the prostate (TURP) applies pressure to the bladder outlet and is intended to decrease bleeding. The urine should clear to a light red or pale pink color. The nurse observes the urinary returns while the sensory and smooth muscle effects of the spinal anesthetic abate. Irrigation returns that again become either intermittently or continuously bright red suggest a bladder spasm. Clots may obstruct the catheter. The patient may feel strong bladder pain over his pubis. The nurse increases the irrigation's titrated rate to clear blood and clots from the bladder and administers a belladonna and opium suppository to relax irritable bladder muscle. (Quinn D, Schick L, editors: *ASPAN's perianesthesia nursing core curriculum: preoperative, Phase I and Phase II PACU nursing*, Philadelphia, 2004, Saunders;

Rothrock J, editor: *Alexander's care of the patient in surgery*, ed 12, St. Louis, 2003, Mosby.)

9.70. Correct Answer: **a**
All patients with renal failure, whether acute or chronic, must have their medications carefully scrutinized. Because most medications are excreted by the kidneys, dosages and frequencies must be modified. Some medications are eliminated during dialysis, whereas others have their effects potentiated. Unbound drug circulates freely in the blood and has prolonged effect in a patient whose failing kidneys cannot eliminate the drug. (Copstead LC, Banasik JL: *Pathophysiology: biological and behavioral perspectives*, ed 2, Philadelphia, 2000, Saunders.)

9.71. Correct Answer: **d**
Fentanyl is becoming a common drug given in the PACU for pain control; however, for the patient with renal insufficiency, caution is recommended. Reduced clearance of the drug can result in accumulation that may cause increased sedation or respiratory depression. The use of ketorolac is discouraged in patients with renal disease because of its possible renal damage as a result of decreased prostaglandin levels in kidney cells. The pain scale should be used with the administration of any analgesic to ensure that the nurse is meeting the objective of pain control and comfort. The level of acceptable pain should be defined by the patient. (Anthony D, Jasinski DM: Postoperative pain management: morphine versus ketorolac, *J PeriAnesth Nurs* 17[1]:30-42, 2002; ASPAN: *2006-2008 Standards of perianesthesia nursing practice*, Cherry Hill, NJ, 2006, ASPAN; Pasero C: Fentanyl for acute pain

management, *J PeriAnesth Nurs* 20[4]:279-284, 2005.)

9.72. Correct Answer: **b**
This type of vascular access has no external components. The graft is made from a synthetic material, bovine carotid artery, human umbilical vein graft, or the patient's own vessels. One end is grafted to the artery and tunneled under the skin. The other end is anastomosed to a large vein. Nursing care includes avoiding situations that could compress blood flow through this graft or promote thrombosis obstruction. Therefore *no* blood pressure inflation or venipuncture tourniquets can be placed on the affected arm. Hypotension can also compromise vascular flow. Patency of the access is detected by palpating above the venous anastomosis to feel a rush of blood flowing through the tubing. Bruit can also be audibly detected by stethoscope. (Rothrock J, editor: *Alexander's care of the patient in surgery*, ed 12, St. Louis, 2003, Mosby.)

9.73. Correct Answer: **c**
Although the effects of anesthesia can commonly cause transient confusion, it is important to assess the patient after transurethral resection of a prostate (TURP) for signs of TUR syndrome. This is characterized by dilution hyponatremia that results from large amounts of fluid absorption into the venous sinusoids during the procedure. Other observations would include abdominal rigidity and swelling. Part of the report should have included the patient's mental status before the procedure along with duration and extent of the TUR procedure. The nurse's priority in the care of this patient should be providing a safe environment for the confused patient.

(Eaton J: Detecting hyponatremia in the PACU, *J PeriAnesth Nurs* 18[6]: 392-397, 2003; Rothrock J, editor: *Alexander's care of the patient in surgery*, ed 12, St. Louis, 2003, Mosby; Tanagho EA, McAninch JW, editors: *Smith's general urology*, ed 15, New York, 2000, McGraw-Hill.)

Chapter 10

Maxillofacial, Nasopharyngeal, Ophthalmic, Otologic, and Reconstructive Concepts

The content of this section focuses on perianesthesia considerations related to *ophthalmic* (eye), *otologic* (ear), *rhinologic* (nasal), *maxillofacial* (oral), *laryngologic* (neck or throat), and *reconstructive* (plastic) surgical procedures. These issues are considered together because:

- Surgery on the eye, ear, mouth, nose, or throat involves facial and neck structures that may require additional surgical reconstruction

- Special care is needed to promote positive outcomes for eye, facial, and reconstructive procedures that all share common postanesthesia priorities: hemostasis to promote healing, management of airway and positioning, and limiting pressure-increasing activities like coughing, stretching, straining, or vomiting

ESSENTIAL CORE CONCEPTS	AFFILIATED CORE CURRICULUM CHAPTERS
Nursing Process	**Chapter 2**
Assessment	
Planning and Implementation	
Evaluation	
Ophthalmic Concerns	**Chapter 47**
Nursing Process	
Optic Structures and Physiology	
Pathology	
Abrasions, Ptosis, and Detachments	
Cataracts and Glaucoma	
Pharmacology	
Miotics and Mydriatics	
Cycloplegics and Osmotics	
Perianesthesia Priorities	
Nausea-Free, Coughless, Bloodless, Painless	
Surgical Procedures and Reconstruction	
Tumors, Ulcerations, and –plasty's	

Otologic Concerns

Chapter 50

Nursing Process
Otic Structures and Physiology
Function and Innervation
Pathology
Otitis, Trauma, and Tumors
Perianesthesia Priorities
Bleeding and Spinal Fluid Leaks
Instructions and Dressings
Neurologic Weaknesses and Hearing Deficit
Pain and Position
Vertigo and Vomiting
Surgical Procedures and Reconstruction
-ectomy's, -otomy's, and –plasty's

Nasopharyngeal Concerns

Chapter 50

Nasal Structures and Physiology
Nursing Process
Pathology
Mucus, Polyps, Septum, and Sinuses
Perianesthesia Priorities
Airway, Bleeding, and Emesis
Packing, Pain, and Position
Surgical Procedures and Reconstruction
-ectomy's, -otomy's, and –plasty's
Fractures, Reconstructions, and Windows

Maxillofacial and Laryngeal Concerns

Chapters 48, 50

Nursing Process
Oral and Pharyngeal Structures and Physiology
Pathology
Adenoids, Tonsils, and Nodules
Fractures and Tumors
Perianesthesia Priorities
Airway Patency and Oxygenation
Emesis, Hemorrhage, and Mucus
Endocrine Balance and Nerve Function
Extubation, Tracheal Tubes, and Jaw Wires
Position and Communication
Sepsis, Suction, and Drains
Surgical Procedures and Reconstruction
-ectomy's, -otomy's, and –plasty's
-oscopy's and Laser Excisions

Issues of Reconstructive Surgery

Chapter 52

Coagulation, Healing, and Infection Potential
Nursing Process
Perianesthesia Priorities
Airway Patency and Oxygenation
Bleeding, Ecchymosis, and Edema
Coughing, Straining, and Vomiting
Fluid Volume, Position, and Pain
Surgical Procedures
Augmentations and Reductions
Congenital Clefts and Cosmetic Images
Expanders, Flaps, Grafts, and Implants
Lipectomies, Lifts, and -plasty's
Repairs and Reconstructions
Repositions and Reshapings

SET 1

10.1. After surgery to correct strabismus, the anesthesia provider reports that the patient had one intraoperative episode of severe bradycardia requiring treatment with atropine. The ***most likely*** reason for the drop in heart rate during eye surgery is:
   a. surgical manipulation of the rectus muscle.
   b. overdilation of the pupil.
   c. temporary loss of vitreous pressures.
   d. pain response to ineffective eye block.

10.2. A 68-year-old woman is undergoing a resection of an acoustic neuroma. When she arrives in Phase I PACU after surgery, her vital signs, including blood pressure, heart rate, respiratory rate, temperature, and oxygen saturation, are assessed. Upon the initial assessment she is found to be tachypneic and tachycardic. Her blood pressure is 84/45, and oxygen saturations is 83%. The patient is extremely agitated and disoriented. The most serious complication to explain this assessment is:
   a. acute hearing loss.
   b. dizziness and tinnitus.
   c. air embolism.
   d. denervation of the acoustic nerve.

NOTE: Consider items 10.3-10.5 together.

10.3. A 4-year-old male is admitted through same-day surgery for a tonsillectomy and adenoidectomy. All the following are appropriate indications for this surgery *except:*
   a. recurrent otitis media.
   b. obstructive sleep apnea.
   c. tonsillar enlargement.
   d. frequent episodes of tonsillitis.

10.4. As a preschooler, this boy will best be prepared for his surgical experience by:
   a. allowing him to handle any equipment or supplies that are nearby.
   b. hiding any equipment or supplies so that he is not frightened.
   c. focusing on abstract aspects of his procedure.
   d. providing two 30-minute teaching sessions.

10.5. Preoperatively this child was diagnosed with obstructive sleep apnea. Diagnostic symptoms include but are not limited to all the following *except:*
   a. excessive mouth breathing.
   b. frequent nighttime awakening.
   c. encopresis.
   d. snoring.

NOTE: Consider items 10.6-10.7 together.

10.6. A male patient was involved in a motor vehicle accident in the past 24 hours and sustained a Le Forte I fracture of the left mandible. He has arch bars to provide jaw stability and is temporarily nasally intubated and therefore unable to speak. This patient is demonstrating symptoms of discomfort including clenching of his fists and grimacing. The plan to provide comfort to him should include:
   a. administering benzodiazepines to provide amnesia.
   b. offering nonpharmacologic therapies, such as distraction techniques.
   c. providing only limited opioids to avoid oversedation.
   d. determining a pain-rating goal.

10.7. The patient was maintained under hypotensive anesthesia. The ***primary*** reason that hypotensive anesthesia is selected as a technique is to:
   a. avert a hypertensive crisis.
   b. minimize damage to delicate blood vessels in the mandible.
   c. reduce the volume of surgical blood loss.
   d. protect the patient from premature cardiac disease.

10.8. After ocular surgery, the optic nerve is protected by:
a. prophylactic antiemetics.
b. supine bedrest for 3 hours.
c. osmotic diuretics.
d. intravenous corticosteroids.

NOTE: Consider items 10.9-10.10 together.

10.9. A male diabetic patient begins complaining of abdominal pain, nausea, and vomiting after a wide excision of a mid-thigh melanoma. It is noted that the patient has a sweet odor to his breath. His serum glucose is 400 mg/dL. The perianesthesia nurse suspects that he has ketoacidosis and is concerned that he may also develop:
a. potassium depletion.
b. Biot respirations.
c. profound and transient bradycardia.
d. diabetic fibrosis.

10.10. Once the patient has met discharge criteria from the Phase I PACU, he is transferred to the surgical intensive care unit for additional monitoring and treatment of his diabetes. He is now at risk for delayed healing and infection of his surgical wound. Which of the following statements below is *true?*
a. Elevated blood sugars decrease the risk for peripheral vascular disease.
b. Poor glycemic control impairs the body's ability to eliminate bacteria.
c. Elevated blood glucose increases the diffusion rate of glucose into the cells.
d. Hyperglycemia increases oxygen demand and blood flow to the tissues.

10.11. The optimal candidate for an endoscopic facelift:
a. has very delicate and thin skin.
b. has multiple expressions of wrinkles.
c. demonstrates moderate skin laxity and a strong desire to avoid facial incisions.
d. possesses "classic" skin changes associated with cigarette smoking.

10.12. According to recommended staffing guidelines, the last and only patient in an ambulatory facility who is still receiving Phase I level of care can expect:
a. two registered nurses, one who is competent in Phase I postanesthesia nursing, to be present in the room with him or her.
b. one registered nurse competent in Phase I postanesthesia nursing and a family member at the bedside.
c. one registered nurse competent in Phase I postanesthesia nursing and a certified respiratory therapist to help with airway management.
d. one registered nurse competent in Phase I postanesthesia nursing and a second registered nurse available in the building by beeper.

10.13. Within 5 minutes of admission to PACU after a uvulopalatopharyngoplasty (UPPP), a previously healthy but drowsy patient is observed to have rocking respirations and abdominal movement. Prompt intervention includes:
a. an antiemetic per protocol.
b. suction of bloody secretions.
c. a semi-Fowler's position.
d. repositioning the head.

10.14. The immediate discomfort from an augmentation mammoplasty can be reduced or alleviated by:
a. initiating gentle arm circling exercises and passive arm raises to improve circulation.
b. pre-medicating and then applying deep tissue massage to treat pectoralis spasms.
c. withholding medication combinations such as muscle relaxants and oral narcotics to minimize drowsiness.
d. applying 2- or 3-inch ACE wrap bandages around the chest and applying ice packs.

10.15. After radical neck dissection in an attempt to control the spread of squamous cell carcinoma of the larynx, the patient may experience:
a. inability to raise both shoulders against resistance.
b. partial paralysis of uvula with deviation to surgical side.

c. asymmetric mouth opening.

d. inability to close both eyes tightly.

10.16. Perioperative hypothermia has been associated with:

a. stabilized cardiovascular status because of decreased vascular resistance.

b. more rapid metabolism of anesthetic agents.

c. increased risk of infection and impaired wound healing.

d. decreased pain experienced because of decreased peripheral sensation.

10.17. Risk factors for developing methicillin-resistant *Staphylococcus aureus* (MRSA) include:

a. frequent urinary catheterizations.

b. no prior contact with the healthcare system.

c. history of recent upper respiratory infection.

d. no prior exposure to antibiotics.

10.18. Signs of the oculocardiac reflex include:

a. decreased blood pressure, pulse, and consciousness.

b. miosis and widened pulse pressure with anxiety.

c. hypertension and tachycardia with hyperthermia.

d. vomiting, pulsus paradoxus and mydriasis.

10.19. The most critical nursing assessments of the post-thymectomy patient focus on preventing:

a. autonomic hyperreflexia.

b. malignant hyperthermia.

c. hypothyroid crisis.

d. respiratory muscle failure.

10.20. To minimize damage to a 3-year-old patient's tracheal tissue while ensuring adequate airway protection, the optimal endotracheal cuff pressure is:

a. uninflated.

b. near 20 mmHg.

c. fully inflated.

d. near 30 mmHg.

10.21. Agents commonly used for moderate sedation include:

a. benzodiazepines and central nervous system (CNS) stimulants.

b. opioids and barbiturates.

c. benzodiazepines and opioids.

d. opioids and CNS stimulants.

10.22. According to The Joint Commission, which of these statements is *true?*

a. Moderate or deep sedation can be provided by any licensed individuals.

b. Only patients with a cardiac history are required to be monitored.

c. Pre-sedation assessments must be done on each patient.

d. Post-sedation assessments are required only on patients younger than 18 years or older than 60 years.

10.23. In preparation for an ethmoidectomy and nasal polypectomy, cocaine may be used to promote:

a. dissociative sedation.

b. localized hemostasis.

c. long-term analgesia.

d. craniofacial relaxation.

10.24. After an ethmoidectomy and nasal polypectomy, the nurse would contact the surgeon if the patient develops which of the following?

a. Reoccurring nausea

b. Serous rhinorrhea

c. Unabated dizziness

d. Inability to inhale nasally

10.25. Potential for postoperative nausea and vomiting (PONV) is *least* likely to occur after:

a. strabismus repair.

b. tympanomastoidectomy.

c. laparoscopic ovum retrieval.

d. transurethral resection of the prostate.

10.26. Which of the following patients is *most* likely to experience postoperative nausea and vomiting (PONV)?

a. Female, nonsmoker, and history of PONV

b. Male, nonsmoker, and general anesthesia
c. Female, smoker, and general anesthesia
d. Male, smoker, and history of motion sickness

10.27. After general anesthesia for removal of a preauricular cyst, a 24-year-old female patient arrives with a laryngeal mask airway (LMA) in place. It is best to extubate this patient when:
a. the cuff has been deflated by 50%.
b. the patient is deeply anesthetized or awake to avoid laryngospasm.
c. frequent stimulation restores protective reflexes.
d. the patient maintains adequate oxygen saturation on room air.

NOTE: Consider items 10.28-10.29 together.

10.28. After tympanoplasty and excision of a cholesteatoma, an 8-year-old child must learn:
a. ear irrigation with antibiotic solution.
b. atraumatic sneezing techniques.
c. to cope with an altered self-image.
d. how to insert a hearing device.

10.29. As the child becomes more responsive, he is asked to grimace, grin, and purse his lips. This is to assess the function of the:
a. cochlea.
b. facial nerve.

c. temporal lobe.
d. cranial nerve VIII.

10.30. Intraocular pressure is decreased during surgery by:
a. coughing and hyperventilation.
b. hypocarbia and hypovolemia.
c. respiratory acidosis and elevated central venous pressure.
d. hypoventilation and Valsalva effect.

10.31. After a right carotid endarterectomy, the most appropriate positioning for a patient is:
a. semiprone off of the operative side with head of bed flat.
b. supine with head of bed elevated 25 to 30 degrees.
c. supine with head of bed elevated 90 degrees.
d. Trendelenburg with head of bed slightly elevated.

10.32. After a right carotid endarterectomy, the nurse would carefully monitor for changes in which of the following cranial nerves?
a. VII (facial), IX (glossopharyngeal), X (vagus), and XII (hypoglossopharyngeal)
b. VII (facial), VIII (acoustic), and XI (spinal accessory)
c. X (vagus) and XI (spinal accessory)
d. V (trigeminal), VII (facial), and X (vagus)

SET 1

ANSWER KEY

10.1.	a		**10.17.**	a
10.2.	c		**10.18.**	a
10.3.	c		**10.19.**	d
10.4.	a		**10.20.**	a
10.5.	c		**10.21.**	c
10.6.	d		**10.22.**	c
10.7.	c		**10.23.**	b
10.8.	d		**10.24.**	b
10.9.	a		**10.25.**	d
10.10.	b		**10.26.**	a
10.11.	c		**10.27.**	b
10.12.	a		**10.28.**	b
10.13.	d		**10.29.**	b
10.14.	d		**10.30.**	b
10.15.	a		**10.31.**	b
10.16.	c		**10.32.**	a

SET 1

RATIONALES AND REFERENCES

10.1. Correct Answer: **a**
Surgery to correct strabismus improves the strength of weakened, dystrophic, or paralyzed extraocular muscles. To achieve this outcome, a surgeon must resect a portion of the muscles, recess the muscle posteriorly, or transplant a muscle to improve eye coordination. During this process, incidental manipulation of the rectus muscle will cause transient and sometimes profound bradycardia. (Quinn D, Schick L, editors: *ASPAN's perianesthesia nursing core curriculum: preoperative, Phase I and Phase II PACU nursing*, Philadelphia, 2004, Saunders.)

10.2. Correct Answer: **c**
Air embolisms are a potential perioperative complication for any surgery requiring the patient to be in a sitting position. (Quinn D, Schick L, editors: *ASPAN's perianesthesia nursing core curriculum: preoperative, Phase I and Phase II PACU nursing*, Philadelphia, 2004, Saunders; Barash PG, Cullen BF, Stoelting RK, editors: *Clinical anesthesia*, ed 4, Philadelphia, 2001, Lippincott Williams & Wilkins.)

10.3. Correct Answer: **c**
Enlargement of the tonsils is rarely an indication for surgical removal. Most children have normally large tonsils that atrophy as the child ages. Tonsillectomies are usually done to treat recurrent tonsillitis, hypertrophy that causes pharyngeal occlusion and apnea, and recurrent purulent otitis media. (Smeltzer SC, Bare BG: *Brunner & Suddarth's textbook of medical-surgical nursing*, ed 10, Philadelphia, 2004, Lippincott Williams & Wilkins.)

10.4. Correct Answer: **a**
The best educational strategies for a preschooler are based on developmental characteristics that include magical thinking, immature coping, fear of body mutilation, and understanding of concrete explanations. (Quinn D, Schick L, editors: *ASPAN's perianesthesia nursing core curriculum: preoperative, Phase I and Phase II PACU nursing*, Philadelphia, 2004, Saunders.)

10.5. Correct Answer: **c**
The presenting diagnostic symptoms in children with obstructive sleep apnea depend on the child's age. In children younger than 5 years, snoring is the most common complaint. Other symptoms frequently reported by parents include mouth breathing, diaphoresis, paradoxical rib cage movement, restlessness, frequent awakenings, and witnessed episodes of apnea. Children ages 5 years and older commonly exhibit bedwetting, behavioral problems, attention deficits, and failure to thrive, in addition to snoring. (Chan J, Edman JC, Koltai PJ: Obstructive sleep apnea in children, *Am Fam Physician* 69[5]:1147-1154, 2004.)

10.6. Correct Answer: **d**
Whenever possible, the patient's plan of care for pain management should begin during the preoperative interview. Because 24 hours had passed since the patient's accident, critical opportunities for

preoperative teaching regarding pain management options were available. Pain relief/comfort goals should be established with the patient. The patient's self-report of pain is the best measurement tool to use when assessing pain. Although distraction is a valuable tool, it is best used before pain actually begins. (ASPAN pain and comfort clinical guideline, *J PeriAnesth Nurs* 18[4]:232-236, 2003.)

10.7. Correct Answer: **c**
Correction of dentofacial deformities by orthognathic surgery may cause significant bleeding. The blood loss during orthognathic surgery under hypotensive anesthesia can be significantly reduced. (Zellin G et al: Evaluation of hemorrhage depressors on blood loss during orthognathic surgery: a retrospective study, *J Oral Maxillofac Surg* 62[6]:662-666, 2004.)

10.8. Correct Answer: **d**
Intravenous antibiotics are common for the prevention of infection, particularly after fracture repairs and removal of foreign bodies. Topical instillation of antibiotics and external application of ointments to external sutures are typical postoperative interventions. However, concern about optic nerve swelling is usually treated prophylactically with intravenous corticosteroids. (Smeltzer SC, Bare BG: *Brunner & Suddarth's textbook of medical-surgical nursing*, ed 10, Philadelphia, 2004, Lippincott Williams & Wilkins.)

10.9. Correct Answer: **a**
This hyperglycemic patient is metabolizing fat, causing diabetic ketoacidosis (DKA). Potassium replacement is a primary

intervention for patients with DKA. Total body potassium stores are depleted by the process of diuresis. Acidosis releases intracellular potassium to extracellular fluid, initially producing hyperkalemia. As insulin treatment gradually decreases serum glucose, potassium replacement and close monitoring are necessary. Deep and regular Kussmaul respirations, not Biot respirations, correct metabolic acidosis. (Barash PG, Cullen BF, Stoelting RK, editors: *Clinical anesthesia*, ed 4, Philadelphia, 2001, Lippincott Williams & Wilkins.)

10.10. Correct Answer: **b**
When the blood glucose level is elevated, glucose does not diffuse easily through the pores of the cell membrane, which creates a dehydrating effect. Both extracellular and intracellular dehydration can occur, which affects the healing time of the skin. Poor glycemic control impairs the body's ability to eliminate bacteria and can lead to an increase in infections. In addition, hyperglycemia decreases oxygen to the tissues. Delivery of leukocytes and antibiotic agents to the wound is impaired because of lack of blood flow. Oxygen is necessary for macrophage mobility and growth of granulation tissue during wound healing. (Posthauer ME: Diet, diabetes, and wound management, *Holist Nurs Pract* 18[6]: 318-320, 2004.)

10.11. Correct Answer: **c**
The optimal candidate for endoscopic facial surgery has good skin quality that is not too thin and has minimal facial wrinkles and sagging skin. This candidate should also have no dermal changes associated with exposure to sun or cigarette damage. (McCain LA: Endoscopic

facial surgery, *Plast Surg Nurs* 21[3]:129-133, 2001.)

10.12. Correct Answer: **a**
Phase I level of care staffing guidelines as described by the ASPAN Standards indicate that two registered nurses, one of whom is an RN competent in Phase I postanesthesia nursing, are present (being in the particular place where the patient is receiving the care) whenever a patient is receiving Phase I level of care. (ASPAN: *2006-2008 Standards of perianesthesia nursing practice,* Cherry Hill, NJ, 2006, ASPAN.)

10.13. Correct Answer: **d**
Chest and abdominal "rocking" in a sedated patient indicate an acute airway obstruction. Indications for the UPPP include obstructive sleep apnea and profound snoring. Repositioning the head; extending the neck; head jaw support; or lateral positioning likely will relieve the obstruction. The relaxed tongue and intraoral swelling are frequently the sources of an obstruction that limits air passage through the mouth. (Quinn D, Schick L, editors: *ASPAN's perianesthesia nursing core curriculum: preoperative, Phase I and Phase II PACU nursing,* Philadelphia, 2004, Saunders.)

10.14. Correct Answer: **d**
Perianesthesia care of the patient after aesthetic breast surgery includes providing multimodal drug therapy, restricting arm activity, teaching the patient massage of the prosthesis only within the first 2 weeks, and applying ACE wrap bandages with ice for comfort and support. (Quinn D, Schick L, editors: *ASPAN's perianesthesia*

nursing core curriculum: preoperative, Phase I and Phase II PACU nursing, Philadelphia, 2004, Saunders.)

10.15. Correct Answer: **a**
Generally, radical neck surgery involves the removal of the sternocleidomastoid muscle, omohyoid muscle, internal and external jugular veins, and all lymphatic tissue on one side of the neck, as well as the resection of the XIth cranial nerve. The XIth cranial nerve is also known as the *spinal accessory nerve,* which relays motor information to the sternocleidomastoid and trapezius muscles. (Drain C, editor: *Perianesthesia nursing: a critical care approach,* ed 4, Philadelphia, 2003, Saunders.)

10.16. Correct Answer: **c**
Negative consequences of surgical hypothermia include shivering discomfort, untoward cardiac events, increased circulating catecholamines, impaired platelet function, altered drug metabolism, and impaired wound healing with increased susceptibility to infection. (ASPAN: *2006-2008 Standards of perianesthesia nursing practice,* Cherry Hill, NJ, 2006, ASPAN.)

10.17. Correct Answer: **a**
Certain conditions increase the risk of colonization and infection with drug-resistant organisms. These include severity of illness, frequent use of antibiotics, and co-morbid medical conditions including chronic renal disease and diabetes. In addition, repeated and invasive procedures, such as dialysis and urinary catheterizations, and repeated contact with the health care system predispose patients to risk. (CDC: *Multidrug-resistant organisms in non-hospital healthcare settings.* In

Issues in Healthcare Settings, Centers for Disease Control and Prevention, December 2000.)

10.18. Correct Answer: **a**
The oculocardiac reflex is a response to manipulation of eye muscles and tissue. Heart rate, blood pressure, and level of consciousness decrease. An oculocardiac reflex can be elicited preoperatively during placement of a retrobulbar block with a local anesthetic. During surgery, direct pressure on the eyeball, traction on eye muscles, a child's strabismus repair, or retinal surgery can also evoke this reflex response. Hypotension and varied intracardiac conduction blocks can continue into the postoperative period. (Barash PG, Cullen BF, Stoelting RK, editors: *Clinical anesthesia*, ed 4, Philadelphia, 2001, Lippincott Williams & Wilkins.)

10.19. Correct Answer: **d**
Myasthenia gravis may be treated with surgical removal of the thymus gland (thymectomy). A patent airway, preventing respiratory muscle fatigue, maintaining careful cardiac monitoring, and observing overall muscle strength are important considerations. Anticholinesterase medications continue after thymectomy, perhaps at reduced doses. (Drain C, editor: *Perianesthesia nursing: a critical care approach,* ed 4, Philadelphia, 2003, Saunders.)

10.20. Correct Answer: **a**
The pediatric airway differs from the adult airway in that the narrowest part of an adult airway is by the trachea but is at the cricoid cartilage in the child. The endotracheal tube predisposes the trachea to edema from mechanical irritation and pressure. As a result, uncuffed endotracheal tubes are used until the child is 8 to 10 years old. (Drain C, editor: *Perianesthesia nursing: a critical care approach,* ed 4, Philadelphia, 2003, Saunders.)

10.21. Correct Answer: **c**
Pharmacologic agents used during moderate sedation include midazolam, diazepam, fentanyl, meperidine, and morphine. Sedatives, hypnotics, and dissociative medications can be added to deepen the level of sedation. (Quinn D, Schick L, editors: *ASPAN's perianesthesia nursing core curriculum: preoperative, Phase I and Phase II PACU nursing,* Philadelphia, 2004, Saunders.)

10.22. Correct Answer: **c**
The Joint Commission (TJC) has taken on an active role concerning moderate sedation practices. TJC recommends that every patient's physiologic status is monitored continuously. The physiologic parameters to be monitored include but are not limited to respiratory rate, oxygen saturation, blood pressure, cardiac rate and rhythm, and level of consciousness. (Quinn D, Schick L, editors: *ASPAN's perianesthesia nursing core curriculum: preoperative, Phase I and Phase II PACU nursing,* Philadelphia, 2004, Saunders.)

10.23. Correct Answer: **b**
Cocaine is a local anesthetic used (legally) in surgery for its strong vasoconstrictive properties. This action contrasts with the dilating actions of other local anesthetics. Cocaine shrinks mucous membranes, reduces bleeding, and

provides brief, topical anesthesia during intranasal surgery. (Dixson RK: The why, what, and how of endoscopic sinus surgery, *Semin Perioper Nurs* 9[4]:163-167, 2000.)

10.24. Correct Answer: **b**
Clear fluid draining from the patient's nose after any sinus procedure may be indicative of a cerebrospinal fluid leak. The surgeon must be notified. Severe pain should also be reported. Sensations of nausea and dizziness, though troublesome to manage, occur regularly; persistent vomiting, despite nursing and pharmacologic intervention, should be reported. (Quinn D, Schick L, editors: *ASPAN's perianesthesia nursing core curriculum: preoperative, Phase I and Phase II PACU nursing*, Philadelphia, 2004, Saunders.)

10.25. Correct Answer: **d**
Controversy surrounds establishing any relationship between specific surgical procedures and the undesired outcome of postoperative nausea and vomiting (PONV). PONV is not specifically linked with uncomplicated transurethral prostate resection. However, ophthalmic surgery may produce significant PONV. In general, laparoscopic procedures are associated with increased nausea. PONV is also often reported after ear procedures. (Golembiewski J, Chernin E, Chopra T: Prevention and treatment of postoperative nausea and vomiting, *Am J Health Syst Pharm* 62[12]:1247, 2005.)

10.26. Correct Answer: **a**
Studies have shown that adult patients undergoing general anesthesia with inhalational anesthetic agents who are more at risk for PONV include female, history of PONV or motion sickness, nonsmoker, surgical duration of more than 60 minutes, and use of postoperative opioids. In these studies, the frequency of PONV was 10% to 20% for patients with no or one risk factor and 40% to 80% for patients with two or more risk factors. Other factors included the use of perioperative opioids, gynecologic laparoscopy, laparoscopic cholecystectomy, and middle-ear surgery. (Golembiewski J, Chernin E, Chopra T: Prevention and treatment of postoperative nausea and vomiting, *Am J Health Syst Pharm* 62[12]:1247, 2005.)

10.27. Correct Answer: **b**
The laryngeal mask airway is often indicated as an adequate substitute for masks or endotracheal tubes for the delivery of anesthesia. The LMA should be removed with the patient deeply anesthetized or awake because premature extubation predisposes the patient to laryngospasm, aspiration, coughing, retching, and obstruction. (Quinn D, Schick L, editors: *ASPAN's perianesthesia nursing core curriculum: preoperative, Phase I and Phase II PACU nursing*, Philadelphia, 2004, Saunders.)

10.28. Correct Answer: **b**
Immediately postoperatively, this child must learn to sneeze with the mouth and both nostrils open to prevent pressure increases within the ear. In addition, the child must be instructed not to blow the nose or to cough to maintain integrity of the grafts. (Drain C, editor: *Perianesthesia nursing: a critical care approach*, ed 4, Philadelphia, 2003, Saunders.)

10.29. Correct Answer: **b**
The facial nerve lies behind the ear and is very near the surgical incision used for tympanoplasty, which is performed to improve hearing. Mouth drooping, drooling, and facial asymmetry when grinning, grimacing, wrinkling the forehead, or closing the eyes are reportable outcomes related to facial nerve injury. Surgical edema, infiltration of local anesthetic, inflammation, or trauma to a specific nerve may compromise muscular function. (Quinn D, Schick L, editors: *ASPAN's perianesthesia nursing core curriculum: preoperative, Phase I and Phase II PACU nursing*, Philadelphia, 2004, Saunders.)

10.30. Correct Answer: **b**
Normal intraocular pressure (IOP) is 10 to 20 mmHg. During surgery, a rise in IOP can lead to permanent visual loss. Hypocarbia (decreased pCO_2 through hyperventilation and respiratory alkalosis) vasoconstricts and reduces aqueous humor production, which decreases IOP. Anesthesia-related events like coughing, Valsalva maneuvers, straining, or vomiting strongly increase intrathoracic pressure and therefore central venous pressure. These activities increase IOP by as much as 40 mmHg. (Barash PG, Cullen BF, Stoelting RK, editors: *Clinical anesthesia*, ed 4, Philadelphia, 2001, Lippincott Williams & Wilkins.)

10.31. Correct Answer: **b**
Sudden changes in position for the patient after carotid endarterectomy could result in hypotension or hypertension because of the temporary inability of the vascular structures to compensate for changes in head position. Patients are optimally placed in a supine position with the head of the bed elevated 25° to 30°. (Drain C, editor: *Perianesthesia nursing: a critical care approach,* ed 4, Philadelphia, 2003, Saunders.)

10.32. Correct answer: **a**
In addition to assessing the patient's vital signs and condition of the dressings and observing for any indications of neurologic insults, the nurse will assess the post–carotid endarterectomy patient for the function of cranial nerves VII, IX, X, and XII. This is conducted by instructing the patient to smile, frown, swallow, speak, and stick out the tongue. Any deficits in this examination need to be reported to the surgeon. (Drain C, editor: *Perianesthesia nursing: a critical care approach,* ed 4, Philadelphia, 2003, Saunders.)

Index

In this index entries are located by page number for Chapter 1, and by item (question) number for Chapters 2-10. For example, item 4.61 is found in Chapter 4, and is question #61 within the chapter. Also, refer to Core Concepts at the beginning of each chapter, master these concepts, and refer to information contained in the affiliated chapter of *ASPAN's perianesthesia nursing core curriculum: preoperative, Phase I and Phase II PACU nursing.*

Epinephrine
  added to local anesthetics, 4.25; 8.23
  interaction with inhaled anesthetics, 5.35
  racemic for post-extubation laryngeal edema, 6.54
  tetracaine with, 8.22
Equipment
  bedside, 2.74
  malignant hyperthermia, 2.74
  medical
    available during sedation, 2.37
    reporting malfunctions of, 2.32
ERC. *See* Examination Review Committees
EREM. *See* Extended-release epidural morphine
Erythrocyte. *See* Red blood cells
Erythropoietin, 7.23
Estimated blood loss
  ectopic pregnancy, 3.48
  postdelivery, 3.36; 3.37
ESWL. *See* Extracorporeal shock wave lithotripsy
ET. *See* Endotracheal tube
Ethics, 2.54
  accountability and responsibility, 2.62
  data collection for research, 5.38
  decision making, 2.66; 2.69; 2.70
  deontology, 2.69
  duties to self, 2.64
  justice in, 2.58
  nurse's personal convictions and, 2.56
  pain management, 2.73
  reporting of questionable behavior in, 2.57
  transport of patients, 5.27
  veracity in, 2.55
Ethmoidectomy, 10.23; 10.24
Ethrane. *See* Enflurane
Etomidate, 4.12; 6.114
Eutectic mixture of local anesthetic, 5.54
Euthanasia, 2.72
Examination Review Committees, 2
Extended-release epidural morphine, 5.37
Extracellular fluid, percentage of total body weight in child's, 7.10
Extracorporeal shock wave lithotripsy, 9.22
Extubation
  criteria for, 5.60; 6.46
  delayed tracheal tube, 6.65
  difficult airway and, 6.55
  inadequate reversal of muscle relaxants and, 6.62
  laryngeal edema following, 6.53; 6.54
  laryngeal mask airway, 10.27
  readiness for, 6.64
  timing of, 6.46
Eye abrasion due to intraoperative positioning, 8.50

F
Facelift, endoscopic, 10.11
Facemask for oxygen delivery, 6.28

Facial nerve function, 10.29
Facial trauma, airway difficulties and, 6.45
False imprisonment, 2.25
Family visitation, 5.5
Fat embolus, 6.123; 6.124; 8.2
FDA. *See* Food and Drug Administration
Feminist ethics, 2.66; 2.69
Femoral neck fracture, 8.62
Femoral sheath, 6.99; 6.100
Fentanyl
  epidural, 8.47
    aspiration of catheter, 8.52
    blood pressure and, 8.53
    catheter placement, 5.22
    onset of action, 5.21
  properties of, 5.67
  renal insufficiency and, 9.71
  side effects, 8.41; 9.55
  supplemental IV narcotics and, 8.51
  for symptomatic bradycardia, 6.50
  transdermal patch placement, 8.30
Fever. *See* Body temperature
FFP. *See* Fresh frozen plasma
Fiberoptic bronchoscope, 6.77
Fibrillation
  atrial, 6.57; 6.58; 6.59
    cardiac valvular dysfunction and, 6.117; 6.118; 6.119; 6.120
  ventricular, 6.149
Fistula
  arteriovenous, 6.96
  rectal, 9.45
5-HT$_3$ receptor antagonists, 4.14; 5.20
Flexion, abnormal, 8.34
Fluid overload, 6.103; 8.18; 8.19
Fluid therapy
  colloids *versus* crystalloids, 6.142
  in elderly, 3.30
  following abdominal surgery, 9.25
  hypotension in pediatric patient and, 3.57
  in preterm labor, 3.53
  for prevention of dehydration in sickle cell disease, 7.31
Flumazenil, 4.39; 6.19
Food and Drug Administration, reporting of medical device malfunctions to, 2.32
Forane. *See* Isoflurane
Fracture
  fat embolus and, 6.123; 6.124; 8.1
  femoral neck, 8.62
Free-flap reconstruction, 6.106; 6.107; 6.108
Fresh frozen plasma
  for coagulation deficiencies, 7.20
  for postpartum hemorrhage, 3.51
Frontal lobe
  Broca's area lesion in, 8.64
  function of, 8.61

Magnesium, increased concentration of, 7.63

Magnesium sulfate, 3.18; 3.34

Malicious prosecution, 2.22

Malignant hyperthermia
  in capnography diagnosis, 6.24
  patients at risk for, 8.13
  renal failure due to, 6.56
  signs of, 6.51
  treatment, 2.30, 2.74; 7.37; 8.1

Malpractice
  civil law associated with, 2.1
  four key elements, 2.2; 2.3
  informed consent, 2.17; 2.18; 2.19

Mammoplasty, augmentation, 10.14

Mannitol, 8.39; 8.46

MAP. *See* Mean arterial pressure

Massage
  uterine, 5.30

Massive transfusion therapy
  following cesarean section, 5.31

Mean arterial pressure, 6.22
  in cerebral perfusion pressure, 8.78
  in renal assessment following cardiac ischemic
    event, 6.121

Mechanical ventilation, 6.36; 6.82; 6.83

Mediastinal chest tube, 6.109

Mediastinoscopy, 6.131

Medical devices
  reporting of malfunctions of, 2.32

Medical malpractice
  civil law associated with, 2.1
  four key elements, 2.2; 2.3
  informed consent, 2.17; 2.18; 2.19

Medical record. *See* Documentation

Meningioma, 8.79; 8.80; 8.81; 8.82; 8.83

Meperidine, 2.34; 2.35; 4.29; 4.49

Mepivicaine, 5.3

Metabolic acidosis, 6.89; 7.68; 7.69

Metabolic alkalosis, 6.10

Metabolism
  drug
    elderly, 3.31
  increased in hypothermic infant, 7.53
  muscle relaxants, 4.27

Methamphetamine, 4.28

Methicillin-resistant *Staphylococcus
  Aureus,* 10.17

Methohexital, 2.38, 4.5

Metoclopramide, 4.45

Metoprolol, 4.28

MH. *See* Malignant hyperthermia

MI. *See* Myocardial infarction

Midazolam, 2.34; 5.36
  diazepam dosing *versus,* 4.9
  dosing, 8.14
    pediatric, 3.4
  for symptomatic bradycardia, 6.50

Minimal sedation
  effects of on cardiovascular and respiratory
    systems, 6.14

Minimum alveolar concentration, 4.6; 4.7; 5.49

Mitral valve regurgitation
  atrial fibrillation and, 6.117; 6.118; 6.119; 6.120

Mivacurium, 4.27

MOAIs. *See* Monoamine oxidase inhibitors

Moderate sedation/analgesia
  agents used for, 10.21
  clinical parameters, 5.12
  effects of on cardiovascular and respiratory
    systems, 6.14
  The Joint Commission recommendations, 10.22
  patient assessment, 5.13

MONA acronym, 6.72

Monitoring of patient
  during sedation, 2.34; 2.36

Monoamine oxidase inhibitors, 2.35

Monro-Kellie hypothesis, 8.77

Moral framework for ethical decision
    making, 2.70

Morals, 2.54; 2.59

Morphine
  cautionary use of, 8.99
  conscious sedation, 4.51
  epidural, 8.47
    intramuscular *versus,* 4.23
  extended-release epidural, 5.37
  for myocardial infarction, 6.72
  opiate abstinence, 5.58
  for renal patients, 9.71
  respiratory assessment, 4.46
  supplemental intravenous, 8.51
  toxicity, 4.42

Motor block, 8.26; 8.27

MRSA. *See* Methicillin-resistant *Staphylococcus
    Aureus*

Multidisciplinary approach, 2.61

Muscle necrosis in compartment syndrome,
    6.42; 6.43

Muscle relaxants
  cisatracurium as, 9.43; 9.44
  depolarizing, 4.40
  effect of magnesium on, 4.33
  hypocalcemia and, 7.41
  inadequate reversal of, 6.62
  metabolism, 4.27
  nondepolarizing, 4.47
  potentiation of, 9.44
  return of muscle function following, 9.27

Muscle strength assessment, 8.85

Myalgia due to postoperative shivering, 9.52

Myasthenia gravis, 8.16; 10.19

Myasthenic crisis, 8.17

Myelocytic leukemia, *7.42*

Myocardial infarction, 6.70; 6.71; 6.72